W9-CGW-625

Biopharmaceutics and Pharmacokinetics

Biopharmaceutics and Pharmacokinetics

AN INTRODUCTION

Second Edition, Revised and Expanded

ROBERT E. NOTARI

College of Pharmacy
The Ohio State University
Columbus, Ohio

With the Assistance of

JOYCE L. DeYOUNG

Pharmaceutical Research and Development
Merrell—National Laboratories
Cincinnati, Ohio

and

RAYMOND C. ANDERSON

College of Pharmacy
The Ohio State University
Columbus, Ohio

MARCEL DEKKER INC. NEW YORK

MARCEL DEKKER, INC.

270 Madison Avenue, New York, New York 10016

LIBRARY OF CONGRESS CATALOG CARD NUMBER: 75-4039

ISBN: 0-8247-6248-7

Current printing (last digit):

10 9 8 7 6 5 4 3 2 1

Printed in the United States of America

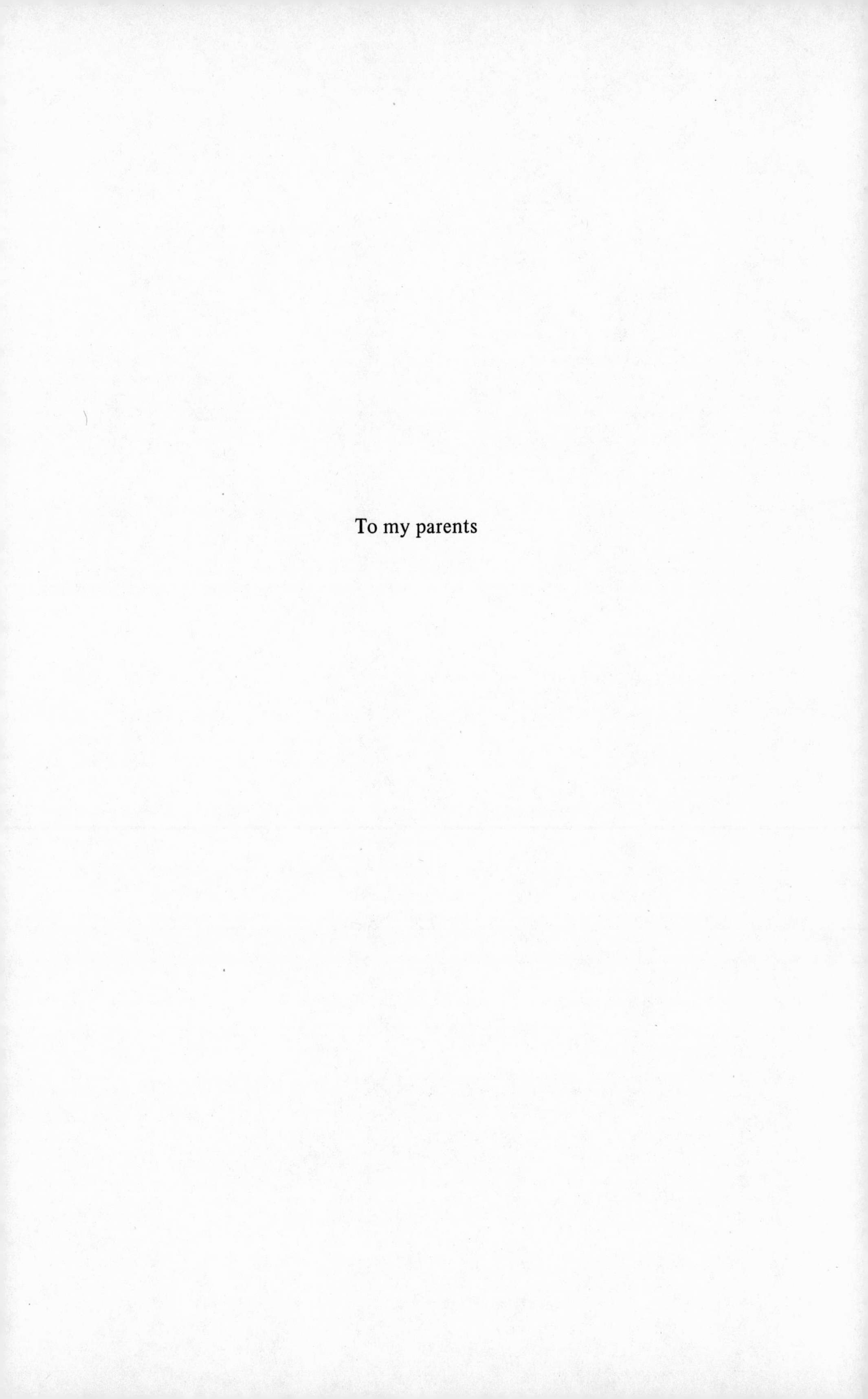

To my parents

Preface To The First Edition

This book is designed as an introductory text for use in formal courses or for self-study. It is aimed at both biomedical researchers and practitioners. The book assumes no prior knowledge of either kinetics or calculus on the part of the reader. Derivations are provided for those who are mathematically inclined. Those who are not may simply make use of the final or "working" equations. None of the subjects is beyond the level of comprehension of an advanced undergraduate with no calculus background. However, one must approach this book "actively," with graph paper and pencil in hand and with desire to learn well in mind. The material is presented in "building-block" fashion, and it is imperative that the user solve the examples and practice problems to have all of the pieces necessary to build a solid foundation. Topics are covered in a cumulative manner, and skipping a principle will almost certainly result in an inability to understand a subsequent topic fully. Although it is not a programmed text, it must be approached in the same fashion—as a work book. Casual reading will not suffice.

One problem that faces those who develop an interest in learning biopharmaceutics and pharmacokinetics for the first time is how to get started. Byron once wrote, "Nothing is more difficult than a beginning." This is certainly true for the present subject. Most current references are not written at the basic introductory level. They assume that the reader has some level of sophistication in either calculus or kinetics or both. In addition they do not provide for active participation in the form of problem solving. A teacher wishing to develop a course would have to do so from the literature. Yet it is difficult to read the literature without a fundamental knowledge of the field. This book is meant to provide that knowledge for teachers, students, biomedical practitioners, and research scientists in medicinal chemistry, pharmacology, pharmacy, and other biomedical disciplines. Chapters 2 and 3 comprise the basic introductory materials, and Chapter 4 illustrates some of the applications. An understanding of this text should provide sufficient introduction to the field to allow further reading of more complex applications in the literature.

During the past six years I have been teaching biopharmaceutics to senior students in the College of Pharmacy of The Ohio State University. The absence of a textbook for the course has presented a number of difficulties. Although assigned readings of review articles and selected chapters have proven helpful, they fail to provide the structural foundation that a textbook achieves. Students repeatedly failed to visualize the total structure of the subject material until the course was nearly complete in spite of the fact that detailed syllabi and other outlines were distributed each quarter. Students were generally accustomed to working with a required text which serves to define the course goals in much more detail and provides a means for reading ahead. Furthermore, when a student experienced difficulties in solving homework problems, there was no reference book to provide additional information over and above that found in the lecture notes. Problem sets had to be created, printed, and distributed in lieu of an available source such as a required text. There was no provision for additional practice problems for the student who felt the need for such experience.

As a result, the outlines, problem sets, graphic demonstrations, classroom handouts, short presentations of principles, etc., grew in both number and in size until some of the materials distributed to the class approached the size of a chapter or even a small book. Most of the contents of this text have evolved from the development of these undergraduate teaching aids. Some of the subject matter was added later to accommodate an intermediate level graduate course. All of the examples and practice problems have been worked many times over by undergraduate and graduate students alike. Over the past two years (and prior to its publication) the book has been successfully used as a required text in both undergraduate and graduate courses here at Ohio State.

It would be impossible to list the names of all those students whose comments and general interest served to stimulate the writing of this book as well as to influence its contents and mode of presentation. Certainly I must acknowledge the graduating classes of the College of Pharmacy of The Ohio State University from 1965 through 1971, who had the dubious honor of serving as "guinea pigs" for the development of this course. Sincere thanks for their patience and enthusiasm. It is with pleasure that I thank the graduate students and faculty who read the text and in some cases helped develop the problems and examples. Among them I wish especially to acknowledge the efforts of Miss Marilyn Lue Chin, Mrs. Joyce DeYoung, Imtiaz Chaudry, Raymond Anderson, and Dr. Richard H. Reuning. The physical appearance of the text is a testimonial to the fine art work of Mrs. Yvonne Holsinger and the excellent typing of Miss Carol J. Lusk.

Finally, any comments, criticisms, suggestions, errors or improvements would be most gratefully received by the author.

Robert E. Notari

Preface to the Second Edition

The objectives of this book are identical to those of the first edition. It is a place to begin your studies—an introduction. Hopefully, it is both simple and accurate. And the agreement between reader and author has also remained constant. This is a workbook. If you are willing to work the problems, the principles should become meaningful to you by the process of discovery.

To that end the second edition has been modified to make it more self-sufficient. As each new principle is introduced, two types of problems are presented. Sample problems are completely solved so that you can diagnose your error when your answer is not correct (and assuming that mine is!). Practice problems are designed to test your ability to apply what you have learned. They are generally slightly more difficult.

The constancy of objectives is not a reflection of a lack of progress in the field or a lack of change between the editions. Indeed, the second edition is largely a new book. In accomplishing the updating and improving of the book, the author gratefully acknowledges the indispensable contributions of co-authors Joyce L. DeYoung (Chapters 2 and 3) and Raymond C. Anderson (Chapter 5).

Those who are familiar with the first edition will find it helpful to know what changes have been made. Chapters 2 and 3 have been completely rewritten and restyled. While they cover the same subject matter, the order of presentation is different. Chapter 2 now contains pharmacokinetic models and the basic kinetics required to understand them. For example, a beaker is still used to teach two-compartment model kinetics, but it is immediately followed by the analogous situation in pharmacokinetics. The basic kinetics are therefore kept minimal and limited to models with pharmacokinetic counterparts. Chapter 3 contains methods and discussions for calculating pharmacokinetic parameters. Among the notable changes is the expansion of the section dealing with the apparent volume of distribution. This has been completely updated to include both discussion and equations regarding variation in calculated values obtained by different methods for multicompartmental drugs.

Chapter 4 has been expanded. It begins with a revised section on the interpretation of blood level curves and ends with a new addition covering dosage regimen calculations in patients with normal renal function or with renal failure. This latter area is one of the most widely recognized contributions of pharmacokinetic sciences to improved clinical therapy.

Chapter 5 is a new addition to the book. It is aimed at fostering both an understanding and an interest in the effects of molecular manipulation on pharmacokinetic parameters and the resultant pharmacologic impact. This is a field which is relatively undeveloped (as compared with studies on dosage-form effects) but which will be a key to future evaluation and development of new drugs.

The second edition is amply referenced. Each chapter provides sufficient citations for the interested reader to check on the validity or limitations of the subject matter presented or to become more familiar with a particular field.

Again, I would greatly appreciate receiving comments, criticisms, suggestions, opinions, or notifications of errors regarding any section of the book. A similar invitation in the preface to the first edition was accepted by several people, whose comments had a direct influence on the production of the second edition. While I cannot cite them all, I would particularly like to thank Dr. Adam Danek, Dr. Gerald E. Schumacher, Dr. Donald A. Zuck, and Dr. James W. Ayres for their helpful suggestions, encouraging comments, and poignant questions.

Robert E. Notari

Contents

Biopharmaceutics and Pharmacokinetics

Chapter 1

BIOAVAILABILITY

It is both an enlightening and astonishing experience to read the labels on so-called cure-alls and tonics on display in museums and occasionally found collecting dust in remote corners of storerooms in old established pharmacies. Since we are no longer obliged to take these medicines when we become ill, we may even see a great deal of humor in their claims. Therapeutic effectiveness was generally certified on the basis of testimonials or anecdotal evidence. Modesty was not a characteristic of promotional statements. *Hamlin's Wizard Oil*, "The Great Medical Wonder," recognized no limitations in stating "There is no sore it will not heal. No pain it will not subdue." *Dr. King's New Discovery* was favorably compared with other recent inventions such as the steamship, steam engine, automobile, telephone, telegraph, and radio. According to the advertisement it rated well as "The Greatest of All." "*No-To-Bac* made a man of me," another advertisement read, and picturing a young man embracing a young woman it noted that by use of this product he had "thrown away his pipe and tobacco and thereby won the love of this stunning girl." A delightful review of that era can be found in the book, *One for a Man, Two for a Horse* [1]. That title in itself shows that individualization of dosage regimens (discussed in Chap. 4 of this text) is not as innovative as one might think. As a final example of immodest claims and an unbelievable dosage regimen, consider the statement regarding *Pond's Extract* and made by the popular fictional character, Buster Brown: "From my own personal experiences, *Pond's Extract* is the best remedy for all inflammations, hemorrhages, sprains, cuts, bruises, chill blains, burns, scalds, frostbite." So much for the indications. Now for the clinical results: "It has made a better and healthier boy of me and is my best friend." And finally the dosage regimen: "Used externally, internally, and *eternally*."

How well did the products and claims of yesteryear measure up to the standards of today? One might use the following criteria:

1. Contents
2. Percent strength

3. Purity
4. Safety
*5. Clinical effectiveness
*6. Bioavailability

Not only did the contents of such products not appear on the label, but it is unlikely that the manufacturer himself knew the ingredients. If the contents are not known, the question of percent strength becomes meaningless. Plant sources sold for the production of drug products were often adulterated. Even if the plants used were pure, the active ingredients, if there were any, were not known. Chemical analyses were neither possible nor of great concern to a naive society. Some awareness of the danger in such a system probably evolved as a direct result of unfortunate experiences with products that not only failed to cure but also caused toxic effects that may have been worse than the malady. Initially, society responded with legislation aimed at ensuring that medicines were safe and free from adulterants. No doubt these seemingly simple goals presented tremendous problems, without adding concern for therapeutic effectiveness which was generally certified on the basis of testimonials or anecdotal evidence.

The development of analytical chemistry brought about an acute awareness of the importance of controlling the contents of a product. That each drug should have an adequate purity rubric became the concern of those given the responsibility for setting standards for the protection of society. Tests for physical characteristics were introduced, and as analytical technology advanced the sophistication of product tests increased. Trace analysis made limitations on allowable contamination practical. Chemical content and product purity advanced to a scientific level commensurate with the analytical technology of the day.

And so we can observe that since the turn of the century, product development has evolved from cure-all herb teas to stable, pure formulations containing known amounts of chemicals that have been defined as drugs. It was quite natural that the scientific community and society at large had confidence in a product which adhered to its purity rubric. This philosophy dominated from 1938 (when the final drug safety amendments to the Federal Food, Drug, and Cosmetic Act were made) until relatively recent years. During that time it was widely assumed that all products containing equal doses of the same drug were equipotent when put to use by the clinician. The first four criteria in our list were regarded as sufficient. More recently, we have come to the sometimes surprising realization that percentage chemical strength is not the sole criterion for clinical effectiveness. In fact, formulations were produced and marketed which satisfied all of the required legal standards but were not therapeutically active. It became obvious that a dosage form must not only contain the correct amount of the labeled drug but must also release that drug upon administration to the patient. *Clinical effectiveness* and *bioavailability* were thus added to the criteria for effective drug product development. A drug should be not only safe, but beneficial as well, and its therapeutic claims must be based upon sound clinical evidence. Furthermore, a drug which has been proven effective can be rendered ineffective due to lack of bioavailability.

What is bioavailability? The simplest concept to consider is that of a *bioavailable dose*. This is the dose available to the patient, in contrast to the dose stated on the label. Only a drug that is completely absorbed into the bloodstream will have a bioavailable dose equal to that stated on the label. In the case of tablets or capsules administered orally, the bioavailable dose will generally be less than the administered dose. Bioavailability therefore deals with the transfer of drug from the site of administration into the body itself as evidenced by its appearance in the general circulation. Since a transfer process is involved, it may be characterized by both the rate of transfer and the total amount transferred. The bioavailable dose refers only to the total amount transferred. A complete description of the bioavailability of a drug from a dosage form must include both the rate and the amount. Methods for such characterizations are discussed in this book. Bioavailability has been defined in various ways [2-5]. Those which ignore the rate of transfer [2,3] are inadequate to explain cases where products show differences in blood levels and/or clinical response due in total or in part to rate of release of drug. A more acceptable definition for *bioavailability* is therefore [5]: "A term used to indicate the rate and relative amount of the administered drug which reaches the general circulation intact."

The measure of success in the use of any drug is the degree to which the results obtained agree with those expected. Therefore, the degree of success achieved by the use of a drug product may be altered by factors which affect bioavailability, such as certain foods, other drugs, the dosage regimen, the route of administration, a less than optimum formulation, or the inappropriate use of a suitable formulation. Biopharmaceutics deals with such problems. It is concerned with obtaining the expected therapeutic effect from a drug product when it is in use by the patient. One such definition has been offered as follows [5]: "*Biopharmaceutics* is the study of the factors influencing the bioavailability of a drug in man and animals and the use of this information to optimize pharmacologic or therapeutic activity of drug products in clinical application."

Since studies involving the rates of drug transfer employ kinetic methods, biopharmaceutics is closely linked to pharmacokinetics. Indeed, the terms have been interchanged often in the literature. In this book the following definition [5] will be used: "*Pharmacokinetics* is the study of the kinetics of absorption, distribution, metabolism, and excretion of drugs and their pharmacologic, therapeutic, or toxic response in animals and man."

Finally, consider the term *bioequivalency*. Like the others, it has been defined in various ways. We shall use the simplest interpretation. Two drug products containing equal doses of a drug will be said to be bioequivalent if they do not differ significantly in either their bioavailable dose or its rate of supply.

Thus, the time course for drug in the blood following administration of either product would be identical. Bioequivalency therefore includes not only the amount of active ingredient available but also the rate at which it is available.

A corollary to the more recent concerns for product quality and effectiveness is the challenge to physicians and pharmacists to consider the impact of these sciences on clinical practice. For example, the clinician must be informed when the co-administration of other drugs or foods may influence the bioavailability of an active ingredient. As research defines the critical factors influencing the absorption of drugs, the information must be put to clinical use so that practitioners are aware of those situations that should be avoided.

This concept can be further extended into all areas of biomedical drug research. Let us consider pharmacology as a case in point. In a broader sense the concept of bioavailability cannot be circumvented by choice of route of administration. Regardless of where the experiment begins, the final observations are a function of the bioavailability of the drug to the site of action, and the factors influencing its arrival there are many. Since the movement of drug from the site of administration to the site of action requires time, the overall process may best be analyzed by pharmacokinetics. Thus, the bioavailability time profile is again critical in the comparison of drugs or drug analogs. A pharmacological study is greatly enhanced by a knowledge of how much of the drug has reached the receptor as a function of time.

The concept of bioavailability in biomedical drug research, pharmaceutical product development, and rational clinical use of formulations is the subject of this book.

REFERENCES

1. G. Carson, *One for a Man, Two for a Horse*, Bramhall House, New York, 1961.
2. *National Formulary XVIII*, American Pharmaceutical Association, Washington, D.C., 1970.
3. Food and Drug Administration, *Federal Register*, *38* No. 3, 885-887 (Jan. 5, 1973).
4. *Guidelines for Biopharmaceutical Studies in Man*, A.Ph.A. Academy of Pharmaceutical Science, Washington, D.C., Feb. 1972.
5. Pharmacokinetics and Biopharmaceutics: A Definition of Terms, *J. Pharmacokin. and Biopharm.*, *1*, 3 (1973).

Chapter 2

RATE PROCESSES IN BIOLOGICAL SYSTEMS

I. INTRODUCTION

After a drug is introduced into a biological system it is subject to a number of processes whose rates control the concentration of drug in that elusive region known as the "site of action," thus affecting its onset, its duration of action, and the intensity of the biological response. Some knowledge of these rate processes governing the fate of a drug is therefore necessary for a full understanding of the observed pharmacological activity of the drug.

While presupposing no formal background in kinetics, pharmacokinetics, or calculus, this chapter is designed to teach the basic principles of compartmental modeling. A limited number of simple derivations are included in the text, but it is possible to make use of the results without having the mathematical skill to carry out the derivations. For those who have some proficiency in calculus there are a few more advanced derivations and brief discussions regarding their significance in the Appendix.

In assuming minimal experience on the part of the reader, the chapter presents the subject using a "self-study" approach. Each topic is followed by a sample problem for which a method of solution is provided. A practice problem covering the same principles but including only the final answers follows each sample. Solutions to the samples and practice problems may appear obvious, but the experience acquired by working them through is prerequisite to a complete comprehension of the subject matter. You will need semilog paper (2 cycles × 10 to the inch and 1 cycle × 60 divisions) and coordinate paper (20 squares to the inch). A natural log table is included at the end of this book.

II. TRANSPORT OF DRUGS

A. Passive Diffusion

1. Two-compartment Closed Model

Consider the case where both compartments in Fig. 1 contain equal volumes of water. Both compartments are therefore equivalent in all respects. Let us dissolve some drug in the water contained in compartment A. Since the barrier is

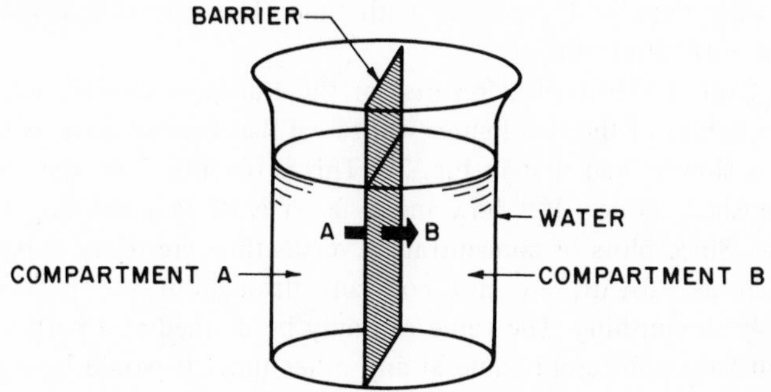

Fig. 1. Model illustrating passive transfer of a drug from compartment A to B through a permeable membrane.

permeable to drug, we would expect drug molecules to pass freely from compartment A to compartment B and vice versa. However, there will be a net transfer of drug from compartment A to B during the process. This transport of drug from the solution of higher concentration to that of lower concentration is indicated by the arrow in Fig. 1. The arrow is not meant to imply that the passage of molecules through the membrane is a one-way process, but rather that the net transfer of drug is from the high-concentration solution to the low-concentration solution. We shall refer to this as a *passive transport process*, meaning that a net transfer of drug will occur from compartment A to B until the concentrations in both compartments become equal. At that time the system will be in equilibrium, which is to say that although there is movement across the barrier in both directions there is no net transfer in either direction. The concentrations in each compartment then remain equal.

In pharmacokinetics we will be concerned with the amount of drug transferred across a membrane and the rate of transfer. That is, we are interested in both the equilibrium state and the rate of achieving equilibrium. We shall consider both of these aspects and their analysis in the following sections. (For a discussion of the relationship of Fick's law rate constants to the observed first-order constants discussed in this chapter, see the Appendix.)

a. Time Course for Concentration in A and B. Let us define the concentration of drug in compartment A as A and that in compartment B as B. The transport of drug may then be illustrated as

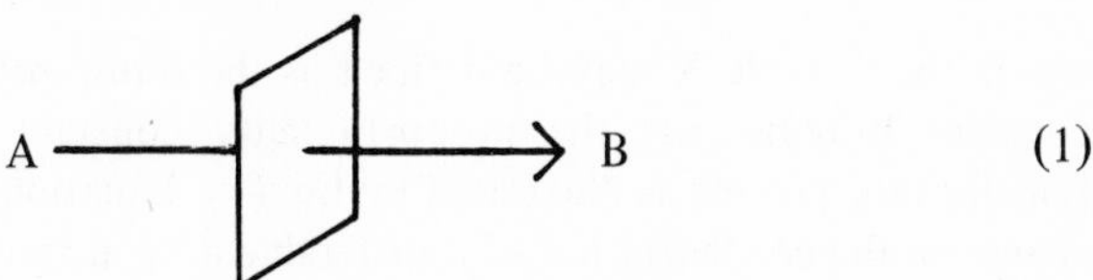

The rate of transfer of drug may be examined by observing the way in which A

decreases with time or B *increases* with time. This rate of transport may be expressed as $-dA/dt$ or $+dB/dt$.

Figure 2 illustrates typical results for the transport process defined in Eq. (1). A comparison of the two figures will reveal that the *rate process* represented in Fig. 2a is slower than that in Fig. 2b. This is obvious from the fact that the latter is finished sooner. But how much faster is it? It is not easy to compare rates per se. Since plots of concentration versus time are really curves, the rate values, such as $-dA/dt$, are not constant throughout the process but are continuously diminishing. The value can only be defined at a particular time t, since it will have a different value at any other time. It would be convenient if one could compare some parameter which is constant for a given rate process.

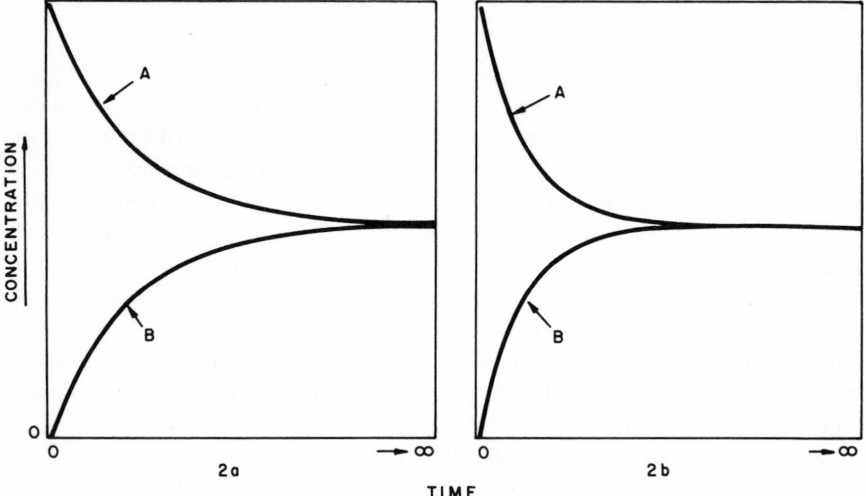

Fig. 2. Concentration time course for drug in compartments A and B following introduction of drug into compartment A in Fig. 1. The barrier employed in Fig. 2a is thicker than that in Fig. 2b.

b. The Rate Constant: A Time-independent Parameter. Often a rate process may be found experimentally to behave according to the general expression

$$\frac{dX}{dt} = -kX^n \tag{2}$$

where the variable X may be defined as the *transferable concentration* and the constant k represents the proportionality constant associated with the net transfer rate process as illustrated by Eq. (1). Equation (2) states that the rate of change in the concentration of transferable drug at time t is equal to the product of a proportionality constant k times the transferable concentration raised to the n-th power. The constant k is referred to as the *rate constant* and the power, n, defines the *order* of the process. These parameters are usually determined graphically and will be the subject of subsequent sections.

It is imperative that the reader clearly understand the physical meaning of the variable X. Equation (2) illustrates that X is a variable that changes with time. It is defined as the transferable concentration remaining at any given time. At equilibrium or t_∞, X will always be equal to zero. In terms of Eq. (1) and Figs. 1 and 2, we can calculate X at any given time from the expression $(A_t - A_\infty)$. Since A_∞ represents the final concentration left in compartment A, the concentration yet to be transferred at any time t is the difference between the concentrations at times t and ∞ or $(A_t - A_\infty)$. By employing the material balance equation $A_t + B_t = A_0$, one can calculate the variable X from data representing the B compartment. Since $(A_0 - A_\infty) = B_\infty$, we can substitute first for A_t and then for $(A_0 - A_\infty)$ to obtain $(B_\infty - B_t)$. Thus the variable X is *transferable concentration* and may be calculated according to the equation

$$X = (A_t - A_\infty) = (B_\infty - B_t) \tag{3}$$

It is apparent from Eq. (2) that a rate process may have a convenient parameter associated with it in the form of the rate constant, k. Since this is a numerical constant, it will not be time-dependent. Thus we will have only one rate constant associated with the overall rate process. Two rate processes, of the same order, may conveniently be compared by comparison of their rate constants. The calculation of first-order rate constants is discussed in the following section.

c. *The Determination of First-order Rate Constants.* For a first-order process the value of n in Eq. (2) will be one. Equation (4) represents the differential equation for a first-order process,

$$\frac{dX}{dt} = -k_1 X \tag{4}$$

where k_1 is the first-order rate constant. Separating the variables yields

$$\frac{dX}{X} = -k_1\, dt \tag{5}$$

which integrates to

$$\ln X \Big|_{X_0}^{X_t} = -k_1 t \Big|_0^t \tag{6}$$

yielding

$$\ln X_t = \ln X_0 - k_1 t \tag{7}$$

Equation (7) is the *working equation* which we will use to calculate the value of the first-order rate constant, k_1. If we are using data for decrease in A with time, we can simply substitute for X in terms of A according to Eq. (3) to yield

$$\ln(A_t - A_\infty) = \ln(A_0 - A_\infty) - k_1 t \tag{8}$$

For the case presented in Fig. 1, $B_0 = 0$. Therefore, $B_t = A_0 - A_t$ and $B_\infty = A_0 - A_\infty$. Substituting in Eq. (8) yields

$$\ln (B_\infty - B_t) = \ln B_\infty - k_1 t \tag{9}$$

Equation (9) can be used to solve for k_1 from data representing the increase in drug concentration in the B compartment as a function of time.

According to Eq. (7), a plot of the natural logarithm of the variable X, where X is $(A_t - A_\infty)$ or $(B_\infty - B_t)$, versus time will be linear with slope $-k_1$ and intercept $\ln X_0$. The intercept is thus the natural logarithm of the total concentration change which can occur. Thus we can apply Eq. (7) to data to determine whether or not the rate process is described by Eq. (4). If a good first-order plot results, we may conclude that the process is first-order and calculate the first-order rate constant from the slope of the plot. This is illustrated in the following example.

Sample Problem 1

A drug is dissolved in the water contained in compartment A in the beaker illustrated in Fig. 1. Calculate the first-order rate constant for transfer using the concentration in compartment A, measured as a function of time, as given in Table 1.

Table 1

Decrease in Drug Concentration (mg%) in Compartment A as a Function of Time

t (min)	Conc (mg%)	t (min)	Conc (mg%)
0	10.00	100	5.20
10	8.56	110	5.17
20	7.58	120	5.14
30	6.88	130	5.11
40	6.35	140	5.09
50	5.98	150	5.06
60	5.70	160	5.04
70	5.51	170	5.02
80	5.39	180	5.01
90	5.29	190	5.00

Solution: The first-order rate constant for transfer from A to B may be calculated from a plot based on Eq. 7. In this problem the variable $X_t = (A_t - A_\infty)$, where A_∞ is equal to 5.00 since the compartments are equivalent. The values for X_t, calculated in this way, may be plotted on semilog paper as shown in Fig. 3a. The rate constant is calculated from this plot as follows:

$$k_1 = \frac{\ln 5.00 - \ln 0.50}{70 \text{ min}}$$

$$k_1 = 3.26 \times 10^{-2} \text{ min}^{-1}$$

There are some important guidelines to observe in estimating rate constants by this graphical method. Generally it is best to limit the plot to values of X that are greater than $0.2X_0$ to avoid using data representing small differences in relatively large numbers. Figure 3a exceeds this limit, since it includes the value $0.1X_0$ at 70 min. The graph paper should be chosen and labeled in such a way that the plot is expanded over the maximum distance. The slope should be calculated from the line which best fits the data and not from experimental points. The reason for this approach is illustrated in Fig. 3b, where the data points do not fall on the line of best fit.

Practice Problem 1

A drug-transfer experiment was conducted in a beaker arranged as in Fig. 1. A solution containing 100 mg of drug in 100 ml of buffer was put into compartment A, with 100 ml of the same buffer in compartment B. The concentration of drug in B was assayed as a function of time (Table 2).

Table 2

Drug in Compartment B as a Function of Time

t(min)	Conc (mg%)
0	0
10	9.2
20	18.5
35	27.0
60	35.3
80	41.0
115	45.5
240	50.4
360	49.7

(a) What is the rate constant for the transfer of drug from A to B?
Answer: $k_1 = 2.12 \times 10^{-2} \text{ min}^{-1}$

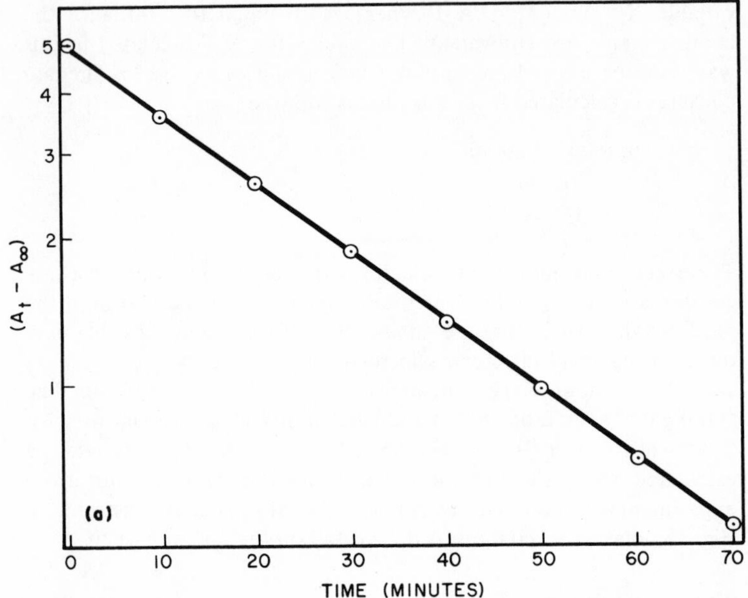

Fig. 3a. First-order plot for data in Sample Problem 1. The variable X_t = $(A_t - 5.00)$ is plotted on semilog paper as a function of time.

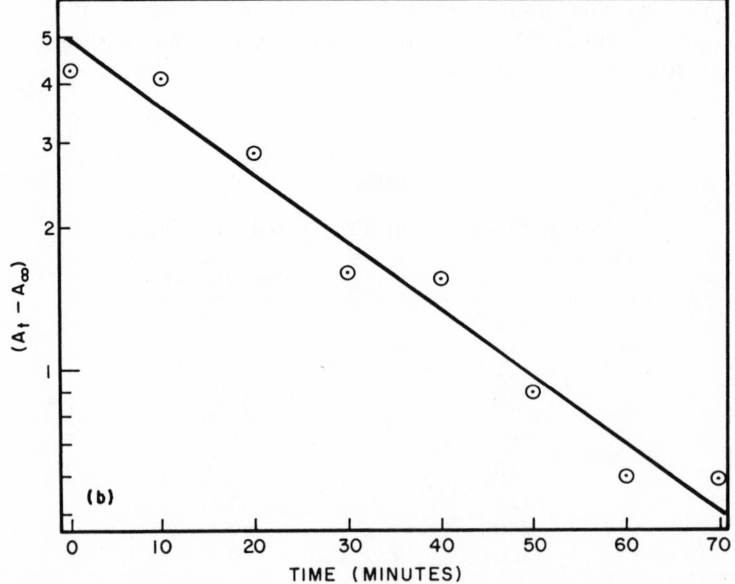

Fig. 3b. First-order plot for data which illustrate experimental error. The rate constant for the line of best fit is identical to that in Fig. 3a. Any pair of experimental points, chosen from this data, will not provide the value for $-k_1$.

(b) What value would be obtained for k_1 using a plot based on data for the A compartment?
Answer: $k_1 = 2.12 \times 10^{-2}\ \text{min}^{-1}$

d. Nonequivalent Compartments. Since a system such as that described by Fig. 1 is reversible, it is more accurate to write Eq. (1) as

$$A \underset{k_r}{\overset{k_f}{\rightleftharpoons}} B \tag{10}$$

where k_f is the first-order rate constant for the forward rate process and k_r is the first-order rate constant for the reverse process. The rate expression may be written

$$\frac{-dA}{dt} = k_f A - k_r B \tag{11}$$

It is evident, then, that the apparent first-order rate constant k_1 is actually a combination of the microconstants k_f and k_r. The exact nature of this relationship will be defined later. First, we will examine the system at equilibrium.

At equilibrium, the concentrations in compartments A and B remain constant. That is,

$$\frac{-dA}{dt} = 0 = k_f A_\infty - k_r B_\infty$$

or

$$k_f A_\infty = k_r B_\infty \tag{12}$$

Upon rearrangement, we obtain

$$\frac{k_f}{k_r} = \frac{B_\infty}{A_\infty} = K \tag{13}$$

where K is the apparent equilibrium constant. Note that in the previous cases of equivalent compartments, $A_\infty = B_\infty$, and necessarily, $k_f = k_r$. Now however, we are considering nonequivalent compartments, so that the concentrations of *total* drug in A and B are not necessarily equal when equilibrium is attained. On the other hand, the concentrations of *transferable* species *are* always equal at equilibrium, since that species determines the concentration gradient for diffusion. (See Appendix A.)

Since $B_t = A_0 - A_t$, this may be combined with Eqs. (11) and (12) to derive

$$\ln(A_t - A_\infty) = -(k_f + k_r)t + \ln(A_0 - A_\infty) \tag{14}$$

which becomes

$$\ln(A_t - A_\infty) = -(k_f + k_r)t + \ln A_\infty \tag{15}$$

for the case of equivalent compartments where $B_\infty = A_\infty$. A comparison of Eqs. (14) and (8) shows that the observed first-order rate constant, k_1, calculated from the slope of plots such as that shown in Fig. 3 is defined by

$$k_1 = k_f + k_r \tag{16}$$

This relationship is derived in several kinetics texts [1-4]. The values for the individual constants may be calculated from Eqs. (13) and (16), since both k_1 and K may be determined experimentally. Thus the apparent first-order rate constant for the reverse rate process may be determined from

$$k_r = \frac{k_1}{K + 1} \tag{17}$$

and for the forward rate process from

$$k_f = \frac{k_1 K}{K + 1} \tag{18}$$

or from Eq. (16).

Sample Problem 2

A weakly acidic drug is dissolved in compartment A of a beaker arranged as in Fig. 4. The results are given in Table 3. Compartment B has a pH of 4, and the pK_a of the drug is 3. Only unionized drug may pass through the membrane.

Table 3

Decrease in Drug Concentration in Compartment A as a Function of Time

t (min)	Total Conc (mg%)	t (min)	Total Conc (mg%)
0	6.60	40	0.68
5	4.15	50	0.63
10	2.69	60	0.61
15	1.89	70	0.60
20	1.32	80	0.60
30	0.85	90	0.60

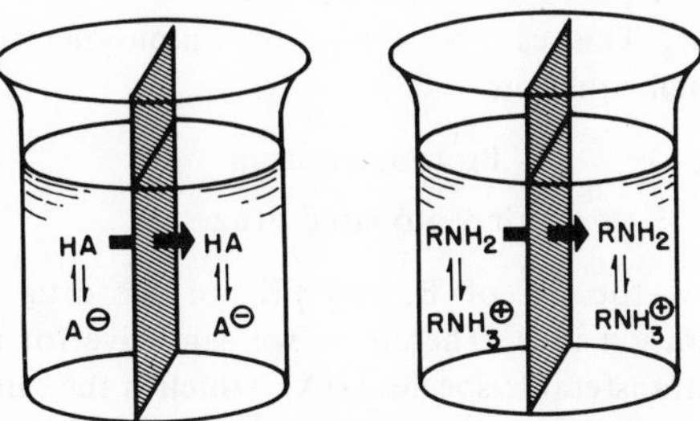

Fig. 4. Passive transport is limited to uncharged species in this model. Transfer of a weak acid, HA, or an amine base, RNH_2, will be influenced by the pH of compartments A and B since the concentration of uncharged species must be equal when the two compartments achieve equilibrium.

(a) Calculate the value of the apparent first-order rate constant, k_1. *Solution:* A semilog plot of $(A_t - A_\infty)$ vs t, similar to that shown in Fig. 3, is linear with slope equal to -1.06×10^{-1} min^{-1}. It follows that $k_1 = 1.06 \times 10^{-1}$ min^{-1}. Note that a plot of data for the B compartment would yield an identical line.

(b) What is the value of the apparent equilibrium constant, K? What is the value of the equilibrium constant if the concentration of unionized drug only is considered?
Solution: In the first instance,

$$K = \frac{B_\infty}{A_\infty} \quad \text{(Eq. 13)}$$

$$K = \frac{6.00}{0.60} = 10$$

In the second case, however, we know that at equilibrium the concentration of transferable species in each compartment must be equal, so

$$K' = 1$$

(c) Solve for k_f and k_r.
Solution: We know that K = 10 and $k_1 = 1.06 \times 10^{-1}$ min^{-1}. Using Eq. (17), which states

$$k_r = \frac{k_1}{K + 1}$$

$$k_r = 0.964 \times 10^{-2} \text{ min}^{-1}$$

and from Eq. (16),

$$k_f = 9.64 \times 10^{-2} \text{ min}^{-1}$$

(d) What is the pH of the A compartment?

Solution: This can be solved by employing the Henderson-Hasselbach equation:

$$pH = pK_a - \log \frac{\text{Protonated drug}}{\text{Unprotonated drug}}$$

We know the pH of B, and pK_a of the drug, and the total concentration in B. Therefore, we can solve for the concentration of transferable species (HA), which is the same in B as in A at equilibrium.

$$HA = \frac{6.00 \text{ mg\%}}{11} = 0.545 \text{ mg\%}$$

This value may be substituted into the equation

$$\text{pH of A} = 3 - \log \frac{HA}{A^-}$$

to yield

$$\text{pH of A} = 3 - \log 9.9 \cong 2$$

Practice Problem 2

Sulfadimethoxine is placed into compartment A, which contains human blood serum. A membrane separates it from compartment B, which contains only water. The experiment is illustrated in Fig. 5. Free sulfadimethoxine, S_f, passes through the membrane, while the protein-bound sulfa, S-P, does not. The initial total concentration of sulfonamide in compartment A is 62 mg%. The data for the transfer process are found in Table 4.

Table 4

The Concentration of Sulfadimethoxine Transferred from the Blood Plasma Compartment as a Function of Time

t (min)	mg% Total Sulfa in B	t (min)	mg% Total Sulfa in B
0	0.00	180	6.52
15	1.02	240	7.16
30	1.92	300	7.53
45	2.73	360	7.73
60	3.42	400	7.85
90	4.55	640	8.00
120	5.40	880	8.00
150	6.04		

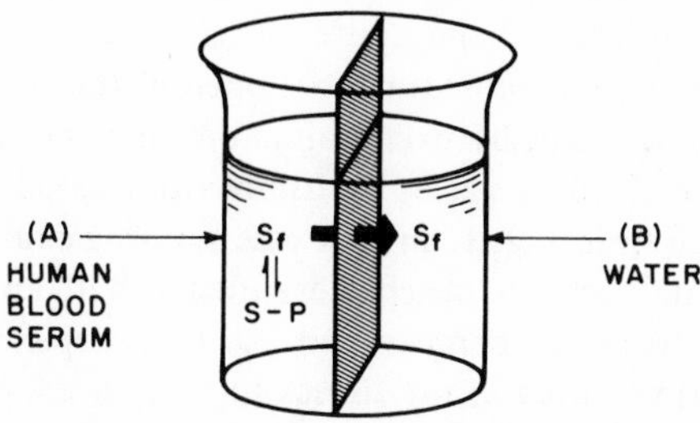

Fig. 5. In this model, passive transport is limited to unbound (free) sulfadimethoxine. The concentration of free (S_f) is assumed to be in equilibrium with that bound to plasma protein (S-P).

(a) What is the first-order rate constant?
Answer: $k_1 = 9.36 \times 10^{-3}\ \text{min}^{-1}$

(b) What is the apparent K?
Answer: 1.48×10^{-1}

(c) What are the values for k_f and k_r?
Answer: $k_f = 1.21 \times 10^{-3}\ \text{min}^{-1}$, $k_r = 8.15 \times 10^{-3}\ \text{min}^{-1}$

(d) What is the mg% bound in A at t_∞?
Answer: 46 mg%

2. *Two-compartment Open System*

a. Time Course for Concentration in B, T, and C. The two compartment open model may be illustrated as in Fig. 6. The central compartment (which will be referred to as blood), composed of blood and well-perfused tissues, is

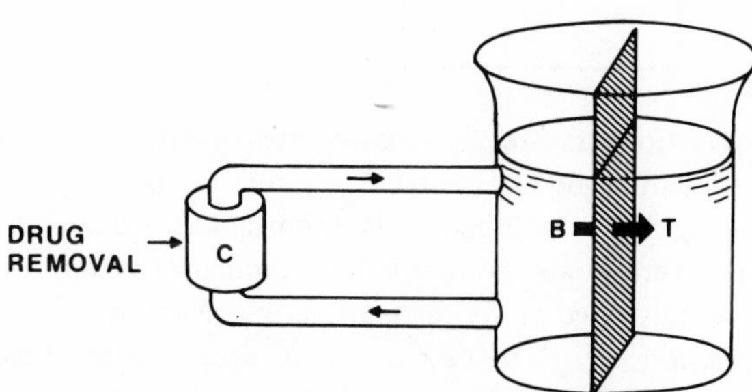

Fig. 6. A model for the two-compartment open model. Drug placed in compartment B undergoes passive transport to T and is simultaneously removed as the solution circulates through C at a constant rate. The beaker has two compartments which contain drug remaining in the system. The model is open compared with Fig. 1, since drug removed by C is considered lost from the system (the beaker).

designated by B, and the tissues or the rest of the body by T. All drug removed from the body, regardless of the route of elimination, is represented by compartment C. The central compartment is open in the sense that elimination occurs from this compartment by excretion and/or metabolism. Thus the entire system is open, since the drug passes reversibly from blood to tissue. Contrast this system to that given in Fig. 1. In that case no drug could leave the system, so an equilibrium state had to be reached eventually. With an open system, drug is always being lost from one compartment, so that, depending on the rate of equilibration, the ratio of drug in the tissues to drug in the plasma may or may not reach its equilibrium value.

The time course of the drug in each of these compartments is shown in Fig. 7, where, contrary to the case of the closed system shown in Fig. 2, the amounts of drug in B and T do not reach constant levels.

b. Rate Constants. Another way of depicting the two-compartment open model is by means of Eq. (19).

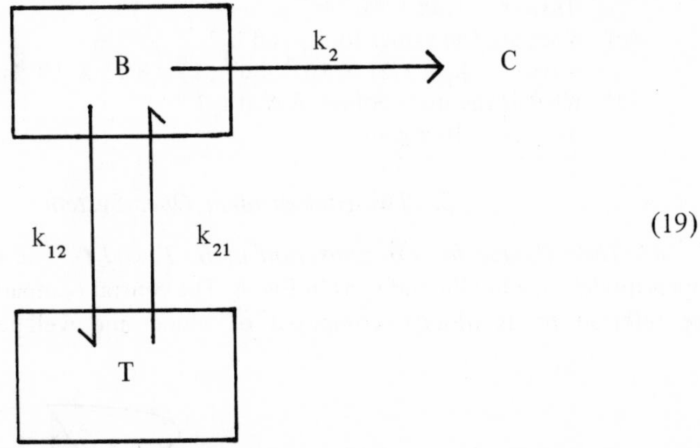

(19)

Rate constants for drug transfer between compartments 1 and 2, the blood and tissues, are represented by k_{12} and k_{21}, and k_2 is the rate constant for elimination of drug from the blood. It is important to realize that k_2 is not the same as β, the overall rate constant for elimination from the body. The difference will be illustrated in the calculations which follow.

c. Determination of Rate Constants. A drug placed directly into the bloodstream will undergo simultaneous elimination and distribution processes. The resulting decrease in drug concentration in the blood will be described by the kinetics for transport to parallel compartments. A general treatment for the kinetic analysis of competing first-order rate processes will be presented later under the discussion of elimination. Diffusion into the tissues is a reversible process with two microconstants, as discussed previously in Sec. II.A.1.d.

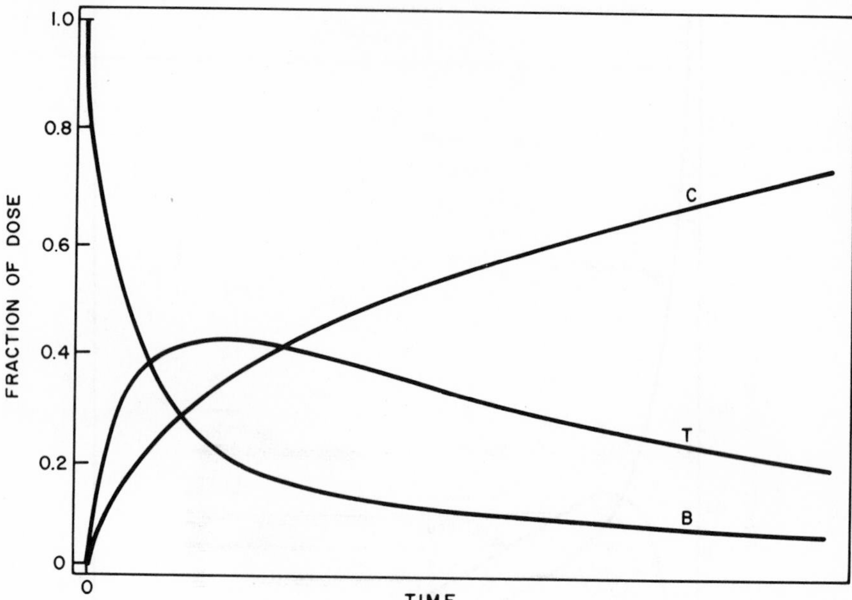

Fig. 7. Time course for drug in each compartment following introduction of a dose in B of Fig. 6. Drug is initially lost from B to both T and C and eventually from both B and T to C so that $B_\infty = T_\infty = 0$ and $C_\infty = 1$. In a closed system $B_\infty = KT_\infty$. (See Fig. 2, where $K = 1$ and $B_\infty = T_\infty = 0.5$.)

If the concentration of drug in the blood is measured as a function of time following a rapid intravenous injection, it may be possible to observe a biphasic curve. Although in truth all rate processes are occurring simultaneously throughout the curve, appropriate values for the constants in Eq. (19) make it possible to observe both a "distribution phase" and an "elimination phase." During the distribution phase the fraction of drug in the tissue compartment is seen to increase to a maximum value as shown in Fig. 8. The fraction of drug in the blood decreases due to simultaneous loss to both tissue (T) and elimination (C). During the elimination phase, drug content decreases in both the tissue and blood compartments as a function of time. If these same data are plotted on semilog paper, the elimination phase will become linear. Figure 9 illustrates such a plot. Note that these data for blood and tissue result in parallel lines, indicating that their common value for the slope represents the negative value of the rate constant for loss from the entire body, which is composed of compartments B and T in this model. A reference line, representing the sum of B plus T, is also included in the figure. This line also becomes parallel to the others during the elimination phase. It is important to note (and to remember) that the ratio of tissue content to blood content (T'/P') has approached a constant value during

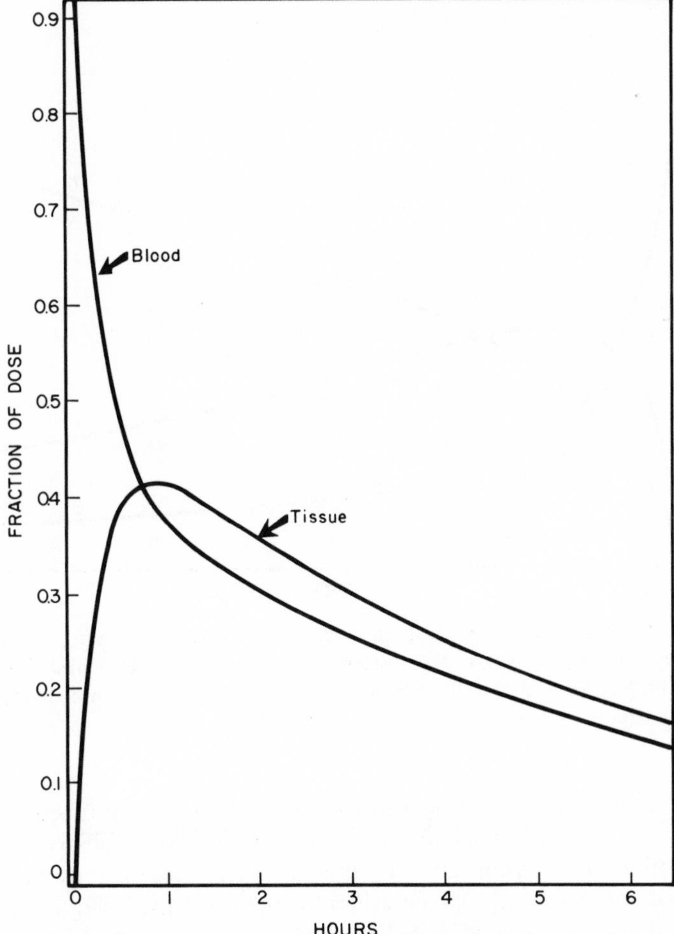

Fig. 8. Time course for drug in blood and tissue compartments of Eq. (19) following a rapid intravenous injection. The distribution phase occurs during the first 1.5 hr and is followed by an elimination phase characterized by parallel loss from both blood and tissue.

the elimination phase. (We shall not consider exceptions to this case in this text.) The elimination phase is also referred to as the β phase, and the negative value of the slope of its log plot is β. The reason for this nomenclature should become clear from the following mathematics.

A system such as this may be described by the equation

$$P = Ae^{-\alpha t} + Be^{-\beta t} \tag{20}$$

where P is the concentration of drug in plasma. Equation (20) has been derived

previoulsy by several authors [5–8]. This biexponential equation illustrates why the decrease in plasma drug concentration as a function of time is a biphasic curve. The constants, α and β, however, are complex functions of all three rate constants, k_{12} k_{21}, and k_2. The solutions to α and β are given here simply to illustrate their complexity:

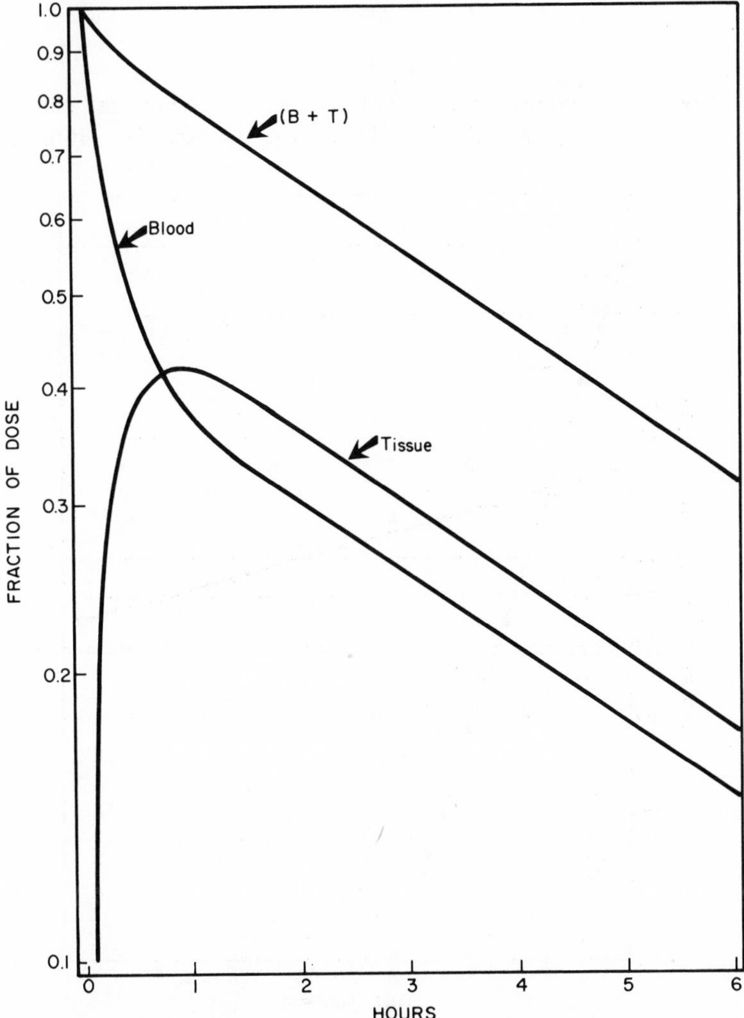

Fig. 9. A semilog plot for the data shown in Fig. 8. Loss of drug from the blood and tissue compartments is represented by parallel lines during the elimination phase. This represents loss from the entire body since the sum, B + T, is also parallel. Blood data representing the elimination phase can therefore be used to describe loss from the entire body.

$$\alpha = \frac{c_1 + \sqrt{c_1^2 - 4c_2}}{2} \tag{21}$$

and

$$\beta = \frac{c_1 - \sqrt{c_1^2 - 4c_2}}{2} \tag{22}$$

where $c_1 = k_{12} + k_{21} + k_2$ and $c_2 = k_{21}k_2$.

In spite of the imposing appearance of these terms, it is not a difficult matter to solve for k_{12}, k_{21}, and k_2 from blood level vs time data. It is simply

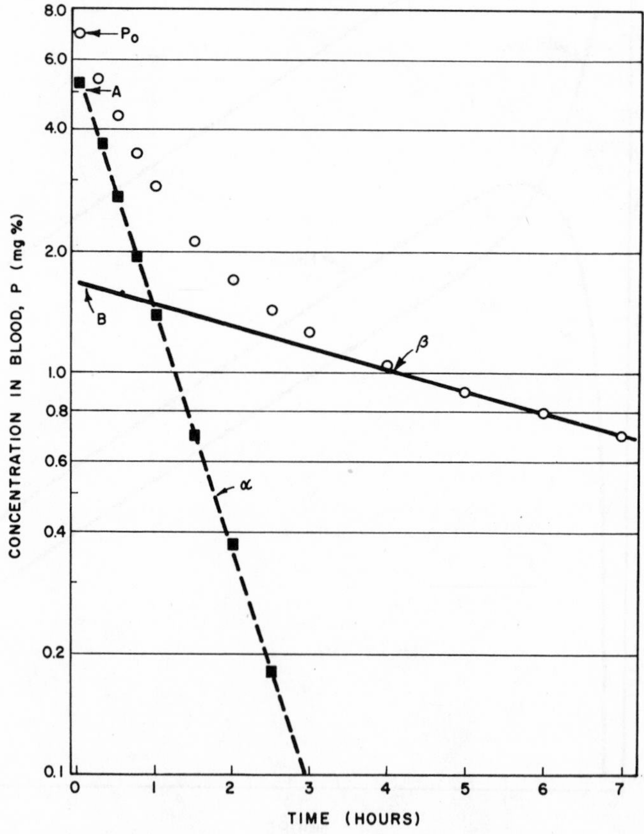

Fig. 10. "Feathering" blood level data. The best-fit line for the β phase is drawn first to obtain the slope, $-\beta$, and intercept, B. The second line represents the difference between the β line and the experimental points. The slope, $-\alpha$, and intercept, A, are obtained from this difference plot. The values A, α, B, β are used in Eqs. (23) through (28) to calculate the values for k_{12}, k_{21}, and k_2.

necessary to obtain values for α, β, A, and B from a plot of ln P vs time such as the one illustrated in Fig. 10. The following equations can then be employed to calculate the values of the individual rate constants from the blood concentration data.

$$A + B = P_0 \tag{23}$$

$$A' = \frac{A}{P_0} \tag{24}$$

$$B' = \frac{B}{P_0} \tag{25}$$

$$k_{21} = A'\beta + B'\alpha \tag{26}$$

$$k_2 = \frac{1}{A'/\alpha + B'/\beta} = \frac{\alpha\beta}{k_{21}} \tag{27}$$

$$k_{12} = \frac{A'B'(\beta - \alpha)^2}{k_{21}} = \alpha + \beta - k_2 - k_{21} \tag{28}$$

The use of these equations in pharmacokinetic analysis of plasma drug concentration data is illustrated in the following problems.

Sample Problem 3

A drug was administered by rapid intravenous injection into an adult male. An indwelling venous catheter was used to withdraw blood samples over a 7-hr. period. Samples were assayed for intact drug and results are given in Table 5. Calculate the values for k_2, k_{21}, and k_{12}.

Table 5.

Concentration of Drug in Blood
Following Intravenous Administration

t (hr)	Conc (mg%)	t (hr)	Conc (mg%)
0.00	7.00	2.50	1.43
0.25	5.38	3.00	1.26
0.50	4.33	4.00	1.05
0.75	3.50	5.00	0.90
1.00	2.91	6.00	0.80
1.50	2.12	7.00	0.70
2.00	1.70		

Solution: Construct a first-order plot representing drug concentration in the blood as shown in Fig. 10. The negative slope of the second phase, β, is derived from the best line drawn through the terminal portion of the plot. The intercept of this line with the y axis is B. (Note that semilog paper is used.) The α line, marked by solid squares in Fig. 10, is obtained as follows. From each data point (open circles) in the initial phase of the curve is subtracted the value at the corresponding time on the extrapolated portion of the β line. A plot of these values yields a line of slope equal to minus α and intercept equal to A.

The following values were obtained from Fig. 10:

$A = 5.25$ mg% $\quad B = 1.75$ mg% $\quad P_0 = 7.00$ mg%

$\alpha = 1.34\ \text{hr}^{-1} \quad \beta = 0.13\ \text{hr}^{-1}$

Application of Eqs. (24) through (28) leads to:

$k_2 = 0.40\ \text{hr}^{-1} \quad k_{21} = 0.43\ \text{hr}^{-1} \quad k_{12} = 0.64\ \text{hr}^{-1}$

Practice Problem 3

A drug was administered by intravenous injection into a patient, and the blood level data given in Table 6 were obtained. Calculate the values for k_2, k_{21}, and k_{12}.

Answer: $k_2 = 0.39\ \text{hr}^{-1}$, $k_{12} = 0.84\ \text{hr}^{-1}$, $k_{21} = 0.61\ \text{hr}^{-1}$

Table 6

Concentration of Drug in Blood as a Function of Time

t (hr)	μg/ml	t (hr)	μg/ml
0.2	5.65	2.0	1.78
0.4	4.58	3.0	1.43
0.6	3.80	4.0	1.22
0.8	3.23	5.0	1.06
1.0	2.78		

3. *Pre-equilibrium or One-compartment Open Model*

a. Equilibrium and Its Implications. Equation (20) describes the time course of a drug that is introduced into compartment B in Eq. (19). Analysis of this data as illustrated in Fig. 10 indicates that the initial slope, α, is due primarily to the distribution of drug throughout the body. If the distribution of drug throughout the body is very rapid relative to the rate of elimination, then $\alpha \gg \beta$, and Eq. (20) will approach the limit

$$P = Be^{-\beta t} \tag{29}$$

which is a monoexponential expression. This does not imply that the drug is distributed in a manner that is any different from that shown in Eq. (19). It simply means that if a single plot is made using a given time axis which will accommodate the β slope, the α slope will be too fast to be displayed on the same plot. In fact, if samples were removed at sufficiently early time periods following injection and an expanded plot of the initial time were made, the α slope could be evaluated. This one-compartment open model is therefore actually an approximation or simplification used to describe the two-compartment open model when $\alpha \gg \beta$. Since the α phase is completed very early in the process, the approximation based on Eq. (29) is valid over nearly all of the time course of the drug in the body. Indeed, it might be preferable to portray a one-compartment system as

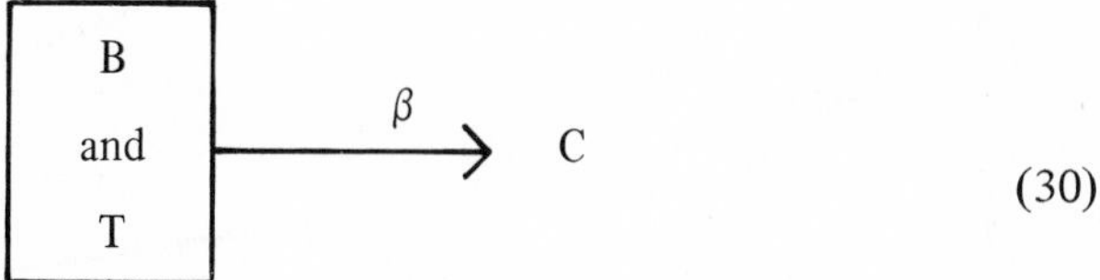

(30)

since the partitioning between blood and tissue is not observed unless very early samples are taken.

This very rapid α phase has some important consequences. The magnitude of α is, as was mentioned, largely dependent on the rate of the distribution of drug between B and T relative to the rate of elimination to C. The rate of distribution, in turn, depends on the sum of the forward and reverse rate constants, $k_{12} + k_{21}$. When the sum of these microconstants becomes large enough relative to k_2, distribution takes place so rapidly that even though elimination is occurring at the same time, the blood and tissue compartments will approach an equilibrium ratio. That is,

$$\frac{k_{12}}{k_{21}} \simeq \frac{T'}{P'} \simeq K \tag{31}$$

where T' is the amount of drug in the tissues, P' is the amount of drug in the central compartment, and K is the equilibrium constant as discussed under Eq. (13). This is illustrated in Fig. 11, where $\alpha \gg \beta$ and the ratio of k_{12}/k_{21} is 3/1. If equilibrium is achieved, the ratio of drug in tissues to that in plasma should also be 3/1. This relationship is seen to be true in Fig. 11, since the dashed line representing $3 \times P$ is identical to the time course for T. This figure also illustrates the approximate nature of Eq. (29), since the α phase is indeed present but it is too fast to display on the same time scale as the β phase.

Under what condition does Eq. (29), or equilibrium, apply? As a *first approximation* it may be assumed that Eq. (29) will apply when

$$k_{12} + k_{21} \geqslant 20k_2 \tag{32}$$

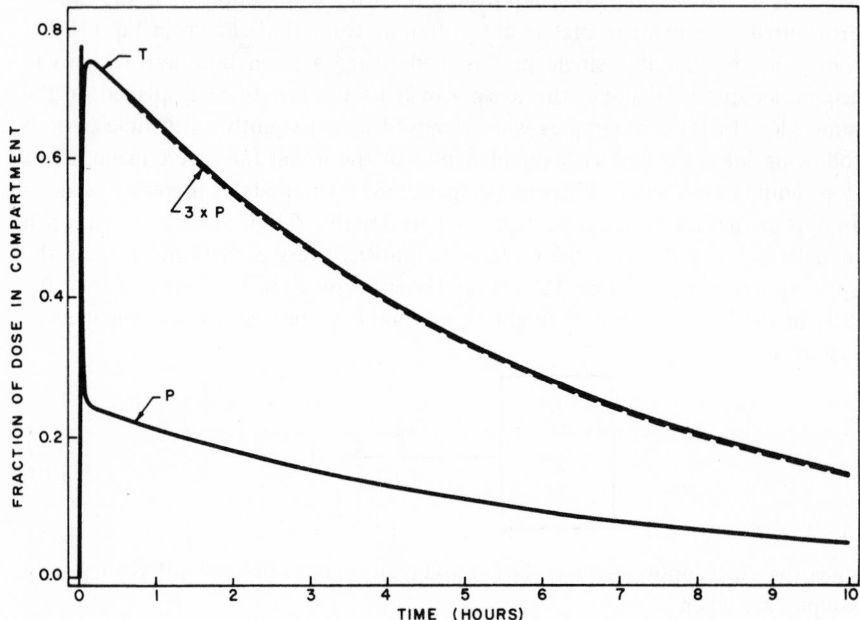

Fig. 11. A two-compartment model resembles a one-compartment model when distribution is rapid relative to elimination. The ratio $k_{12}/k_{21}/k_2$ is 90/30/1 in this example. The rate constant for distribution is therefore 120 (Eq. 16) and the equilibrium constant, K, is 3 (Eq. 13). The dashed line, 3 X P, demonstrates the agreement between the equilibrium prediction and the observed data.

In such cases the distribution is sufficiently fast to compete favorably with elimination and establish what has been referred to here as a pre-equilibrium state. In Fig. 11 the ratio $(k_{12} + k_{21})/k_2$ is 120. The ratio of T′/P′ is thus equal to the equilibrium constant, k_{12}/k_{21}. The ratio of T′/P′ is also constant during the β phase of a two-compartment open model, but it is not equal to the value k_{12}/k_{21}.

The relationship between β, the rate constant for elimination from the whole body, and k_2 is a simple one for a drug distributed by a one-compartment model. The rate of loss of drug from the body may be written as

$$-\frac{dD}{dt} = \beta D = k_2 P' \tag{33}$$

where D represents the total amount of drug remaining in the body. Since

$$D = T' + P' \tag{34}$$

substitution for T′ from Eq. (31) and then for D in Eq. (33) yields

$$\beta P'(1 + K) = k_2 P' \tag{35}$$

which reduces to

$$\beta = \frac{k_2}{1 + K} \tag{36}$$

b. Arbitrary Test for a One-compartment Model. A simple test commonly employed to determine the number of required compartments consists of examining a first-order plot of plasma level data for the existence or nonexistence of an α phase. Of course, if the time between the injection and the first blood sample is long enough, any drug will appear to be described by a one-compartment model. Thus it may be appropriate to sample shortly after injection to determine the relative rate of distribution as compared to elimination. If early sampling fails to detect an α phase, a one-compartment model will describe the data. If analysis of the α and β portion indicates that Eq. (31) is in effect, it may still be appropriate to acknowledge that pre-equilibrium exists and use a one-compartment model to describe the biphasic data. A cardinal rule in modeling or compartmental analysis is to use the fewest number of compartments necessary to describe the data adequately [9].

Depending on the purpose of the study, this number may differ. For example, Baggot [10] has compared the elimination of amphetamines from numerous animal species using a one-compartment analysis wherein the first plasma assay, taken at 30 min., lies on the β line in all cases although the $t_{1/2}$ values varied from 0.6 to 6 hr. Conversely, Kaplan [11] has determined all of the constants in Eq. (19) by determing five points during the first 20 min in a study which required 12 hr to describe the β phase.

c. Determination of β and k_2 in the One-compartment Open Model. Equation (29) may be rewritten as

$$\ln P = \ln B - \beta t \tag{37}$$

indicating that the slope of a semilogarithmic plot of blood concentration vs time will be $-\beta$. The intercept of a semilog plot is B.

Substitution of Eq. (31) into Eq. (36) yields

$$\beta = \frac{k_2 k_{21}}{k_{12} + k_{21}} \tag{38}$$

Therefore, if we knew the values of k_{12} and k_{21} we could easily calculate k_2 from β. However, in the case of a one-compartment model, there are many instances when k_{12} and k_{21} cannot be determined because the α phase either was not or could not be determined. It would be possible to calculate k_2 if the volume of B were known. Equation (26) may be rewritten as

$$k_2 = \frac{1}{A/\alpha P_0 + B/\beta P_0} \tag{39}$$

which simplifies to

$$k_2 = \frac{\beta P_0}{B} \tag{40}$$

for the one-compartment model, since $A/\alpha \ll B/\beta$. We know B from the first-order plot of the blood level data. P_0 is a hypothetical value equal to the concentration in the central compartment at time zero if all the drug remained in the central compartment. This may be easily calculated from the dose and the volume of the central compartment if this value is known. If the central compartment is assumed to be the plasma, as is often done, the volume will be approximately 5% of the body weight.

The value of the equilibrium constant, K, may also be determined from P_0 and B. Combining Eqs. (38) and (40) and rearranging yields

$$\frac{P_0}{B} - 1 = \frac{k_{12}}{k_{21}} \tag{41}$$

which of course is equal to K.

Sample Problem 4

A drug is administered to a 70-kg man and the fraction of the dose in each of three compartments is determined as a function of time with the results shown in Table 7.

Table 7

Fraction of Dose, f, in Blood, Urine, and as Metabolites Following Intravenous Injection

	f		
Time (hr)	Blood	Urine	Metabolites
1.0	0.28	0.11	0.05
2.0	0.24	0.18	0.09
3.0	0.21	0.24	0.12
4.0	0.18	0.30	0.15
5.0	0.16	0.35	0.17
6.0	0.14	0.39	0.20
8,0	0.10	0.46	0.23
10.0	0.08	0.50	0.25
48.0	0.00	0.67	0.33

(a) Is this drug described by a one- or a two-compartment model?
Solution: A first-order plot of the data does not show an α phase. From the data at hand the most reasonable choice is therefore the one-compartment open model.

(b) What is the value of β, the overall rate constant for elimination from the body? Calculate this value using urine and metabolite as well as blood data.
Solution: First-order plots of blood, urine, and metabolite data yield three parallel lines. Thus, any of these sets of data may be used to calculate β. (See the discussion concerning rate constants for elimination.)

$$\text{slope} = -\beta$$

$$\beta = 1.41 \times 10^{-1}\ \text{hr}^{-1}$$

(c) What is the value of k_2, the specific elimination constant for loss of drug from the central compartment?
Solution: We know from Eq. (40) that

$$k_2 = \frac{\beta P_0}{B} = \frac{0.141}{0.32}$$

since P_0 must equal 1, and the intercept of the semilog plot of blood data gives a value for B of 0.32. Therefore,

$$k_2 = 4.41 \times 10^{-1}\ \text{hr}^{-1}$$

(d) What is the ratio k_{12}/k_{21}?
Solution: For a one-compartment model

$$\frac{k_{12}}{k_{21}} = \frac{\text{tissue content}}{\text{blood content}} = \frac{T'}{P'}$$

Values for P' are given in the data, and T' may be calculated easily since

$$\text{total drug} = 1 = T' + P' + \text{urine} + \text{metabolites}$$

For example, at 4 hr,

$$P' = 0.18$$

$$T' = 1 - 0.18 - 0.30 - 0.15 = 0.37$$

$$\frac{k_{12}}{k_{21}} = \frac{2}{1}$$

The same value will be obtained at any other time.

Practice Problem 4

A drug was given by intravenous injection. Blood samples were taken and analyzed as a function of time with the results shown in Table 8.

Table 8

Concentration of Drug in Blood Following Intravenous Injection

t (hr)	Conc (mg%)	t (hr)	Conc (mg%)
0.05	26.4	1.00	7.2
0.10	17.4	1.50	6.4
0.15	13.6	2.00	5.8
0.20	11.3	3.00	4.6
0.30	9.2	4.00	3.7
0.40	8.5	5.00	3.0
0.50	8.1	6.00	2.3
0.75	7.6	7.00	1.9

(a) Is the time course for this drug best described by a one- or a two-compartment model?
Answer: A two-compartment model is suggested by a first-order plot of this data as shown in Fig. 12. However, most of the time profile is in the β phase, since the α phase is complete within 0.5 hr while the β phase is not finished in 7 hr. Therefore, a one-compartment model might be sufficient if equilibrium is achieved. The values for the microconstants can be used to make this appraisal as shown in part (b).

(b) What are the values for the microconstants?
Answer: Since $\alpha \gg \beta$, it is difficult to feather this data. The results are roughly A = 35 mg%, α = 12.8, B = 9 mg%, and β = 0.22, which yield the following values: k_{12} = 9.22; k_{21} = 2.79; and k_2 = 1.01. Thus the ratio, $(k_{12} + k_{21})/k_2 = 12$, indicates pre-equilibrium conditions where a one-compartment model with K = 4.3 might adequately describe the system.

4. *Multicompartment Open Models*

As has been noted [9,12], the preferred compartmental model is the one containing the fewest compartments which adequately describe the data. While one-compartment and two-compartment models accommodate a great many drugs, there are a number of cases where these are not sufficient. Significant distribution of drug in deep tissues such as bone or fat, or strong binding to any tissue, may result in the appearance of a triexponential blood level curve, indicating the presence of a third compartment.

More than three compartments are also possible, but there are practical limits on the detection of new compartments. The addition of each new compartment requires an additional phase in the first-order plots employed in the classical pharmacokinetic approach. Deciding how many phases actually

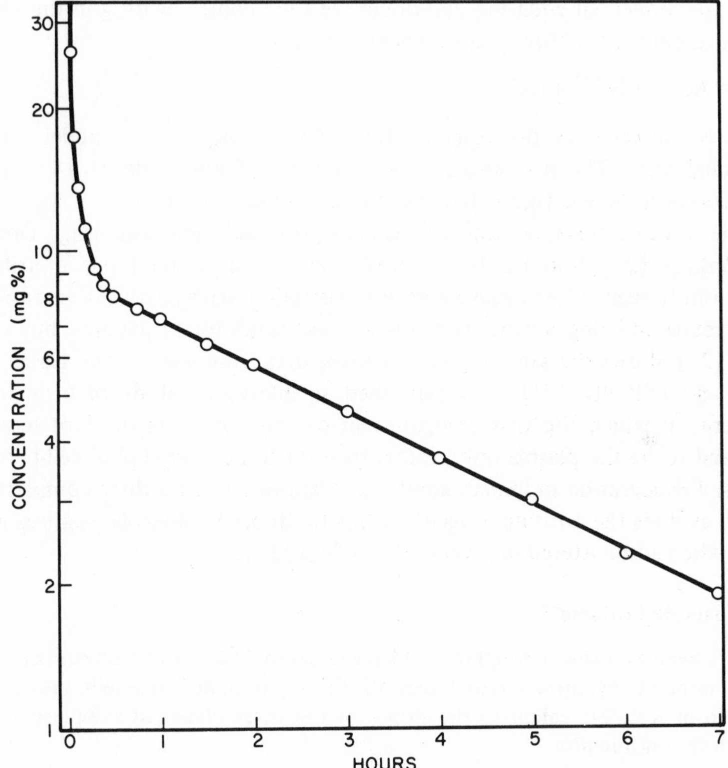

Fig. 12. A first-order plot of the data in Practice Problem 4. The system may be described by a one- or two-compartment model as discussed in the answer to this problem. If the first sample were drawn at 30 min, the α phase would not be observed and the remaining data would be treated as a one-compartment model. Analysis of the early data provides estimates for k_{12}, k_{21}, and k_2 values.

exist can be a problem. At this stage in the development of pharmacokinetics, the data seldom warrant proposing anything more complex than a three-compartment open model for intact drug. One alternative approach is based upon the rate at which the plasma flow perfuses various organs. Methotrexate, thiopental, and arabinosylcytosine are drugs which have been analyzed using this approach [13-16]. While this method may have certain advantages [17], it has the disadvantage of requiring sacrifice of the animal to determine actual organ levels of drug in order to test the validity of the proposed model. Our discussion will be limited to the classical approach for compartmental analysis using the intact animal as its own control.

A triexponential equation describing the time course of drug in the central compartment for the three-compartment model is

$$P = Ae^{-\alpha t} + Be^{-\beta t} + Ge^{-\gamma t} \tag{42}$$

which is the same as the equation for the two-compartment model with an additional term. The mathematics and treatment of this model [6,18–21] and more complex models [6,20] have been discussed in some detail.

The three-compartment model has been proposed for several drugs. Doherty and Perkins [22] found a triexponential curve for serum levels of tritiated digoxin in humans after intravenous administration. This curve suffers from the disadvantage of being constructed from average values for 11 patients, but a later paper [23] shows the same type curve using data from one patient. Nagashima, Levy, and O'Reilly [21] have published an interesting study of bishydroxy-coumarin in which the first compartment of the three-compartment model is proposed to be the plasma only, rather than the usual plasma plus well-perfused tissues. Tubocurarine in human adults [24] appears to fit a three-compartment model, as does the antitumor agent 5-(dimethyltriazo)-imidazole-4-carboxamide (DIC) when administered intravenously to dogs [19].

Sample Problem 5

A healthy subject weighing 70 kg was given 150 mg of bishydroxy-coumarin, by intravenous injection. From the data in Table 9, taken from Ref. 21, calculate the slopes of the three phases of the plasma level vs time plot.

Table 9

Concentration of Bishydroxycoumarin (BHC) in the Plasma after Intravenous Injection

t (hr)	BHC (mg/liter)	t (hr)	BHC (mg/liter)
0.17	36.2	3.0	13.9
0.33	34.0	4.0	12.0
0.50	27.0	6.0	8.7
0.67	23.0	7.7	7.7
1.0	20.8	18.0	3.2
1.5	17.8	23.0	2.4
2.0	16.5		

Solution: Three different phases of the curve can be resolved in a manner analogous to that used for the two-compartment open model. A semilogarithmic plot of the data shows a terminal linear portion with slope equal to $-\gamma$. The extrapolated portion of this line is subtracted from the corresponding experimental points to yield a biphasic curve with a final slope of $-\beta$. Finally, the extrapolated portion of the β line is subtracted from the nonlinear portion of this second plot to give the α line. The slopes and y intercepts for the lines obtained by this process are:

Slopes	Intercepts
$\alpha = 3.1\ \text{hr}^{-1}$	A = 23.5 mg/liter
$\beta = 0.44\ \text{hr}^{-1}$	B = 10.5 mg/liter
$\gamma = 0.078\ \text{hr}^{-1}$	G = 14.0 mg/liter

The microconstants for this system may be determined as outlined in Ref. 21.

Practice Problem 5

A drug is administered by intravenous injection. The plot of blood concentration vs time is found to have three phases with negative slopes of 0.75, 0.30, and 0.085 hr^{-1}.

(a) Draw a compartmental scheme which describes the data.
Answer:

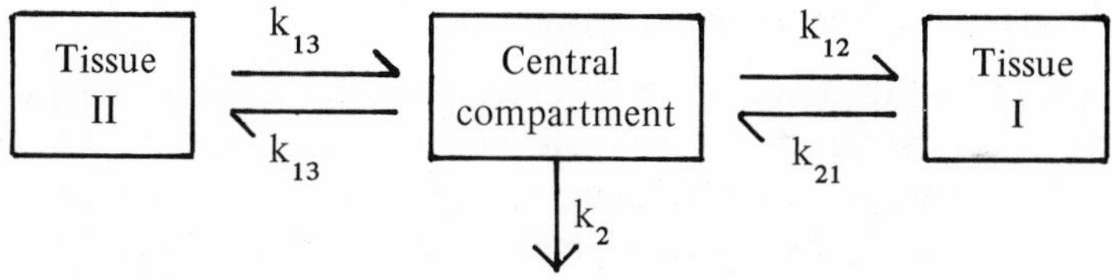

(b) What processes might be responsible for each slope?
Answer: The first slope results primarily from distribution to the tissue compartments. The second slope reflects elimination following establishment of steady-state conditions. When the less tightly held drug has been eliminated, the drug remaining in the deep tissues is not released rapidly enough to maintain a plasma-to-tissue ratio as high as in the second phase. This results in a second and slower elimination phase. You may suggest alternative descriptions which are kinetically equivalent. Try it.

B. Active Transport

1. Description

Up to this point, all the rate processes discussed have been examples of passive transport. That is, the membrane itself did not actively participate in the transfer process, but instead it simply provided a physical barrier which permitted the formation of a concentration gradient when the drug was introduced into one of the compartments. However, there are many cases where the membrane plays an active role, transporting solute molecules against an electrochemical or concentration gradient. Molecules transported in this manner include naturally occuring substances, with sodium and potassium ions representing the best-known examples. Others are amino acids [25], sugars [26], uracil [27], and thymine [28]. Some foreign molecules, such as 5-fluoro- and 5-bromouracil [29] are also actively transported.

A number of dicussions of transport mechanisms have been published [18,25,30–33]. The distinctions between passive and active transport can be briefly summarized by comparing their major properties.

Passive transport may be characterized by the following:

1. Drug molecules move from a region of relatively high concentration to one of relatively low concentration.
2. The rate of transfer is proportional to the concentration gradient between the compartments involved in the transfer.
3. The transfer process achieves equilibrium when the concentration of the transferable species is equal on both sides of the membrane.
4. Drugs which are capable of existing in both a charged and a noncharged form approach an equilibrium state primarily by transfer of the noncharged species across the membrane.

In contrast to the above, an active process involves active participation by the membrane in the transfer of molecules between compartments. A "carrier," which may be an enzyme or other component of the membrane, is responsible for effecting the transfer by a process which may be represented as follows:

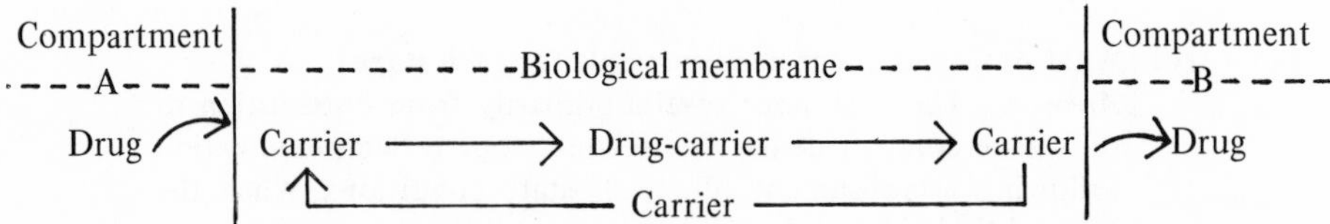

Here the drug in compartment A is picked up by the carrier at the surface of the membrane. The drug carrier complex then moves across the membrane and the drug is discharged to compartment B at the membrane surface open to B. The carrier then returns to the A compartment surface for another drug molecule.

A transfer system like this quite naturally has characteristics decidedly different from those listed for the passive system:

1. This process consumes *energy*. There is energy involved in the work done by the carrier.
2. Since the transport involves consumption of energy, it may be subject to *poisoning* by such metabolic poisons as fluorides, dinitrophenol, lack of oxygen, and so on.

3. Unlike the passive transfer process, which is dependent upon a concentration gradient, an active transfer process can work *against the concentration gradient*. That is, the carrier may transport all of the drug from one compartment to the other without any regard for an "equilibrium state" which was the endpoint in the case of a passive transport process. Indeed, the carrier transfer system will generally be a "one-way" transport process.
4. The system will be relatively *structure-specific*. The carrier will be designed to transport a specific chemical structure. Thus, it will not be completely indiscreet in its activity.
5. However, the carrier system may transport a chemical structure which is sufficiently similar to the one for which it is allegedly "specific." The transfer system is thus subject to *competition* between similar chemical structures.
6. Since there are a finite number of carriers available, the system is capacity-limited. If the total number of transferable molecules exceeds the number of carrier sites available for transfer, the system will become *saturated*. The system will then be working at full capacity and the transfer of drug may thus occur at a constant rate until the concentration of drug falls below that of the capacity limit of the system.

2. *Mixed Kinetics*

a. Zero-order Kinetics. A system in which transfer occurs at a constant rate is described by zero-order kinetics. An example of such a system is the saturated active transport system just described.

When n, the order of the rate process, becomes zero, Eq. (2) becomes

$$\frac{dX}{dt} = -k_0 \tag{43}$$

where k_0 is the zero-order rate constant. Separating variables and integrating between the limits of $t = 0$ and t, and X_0 and X_t yields

$$X_t = X_0 - k_0 t \tag{44}$$

Equation (44) is the working equation which we will use to calculate the value of the zero-order rate constant, k_0. Before we consider typical data for the calculation of a zero-order rate constant, let us briefly review some properties of a zero-order rate process.

The properties of first-order rate processes, which have previously been discussed, do not apply to zero-order processes. This will be quite evident upon examination of the zero-order rate expression. According to Eq. (43), the rate of a zero-order transfer process will be equal to a constant, k_0. On the other hand, we have previously seen how the rate of a first-order process decreases with time, being at a maximum at time zero and decreasing to a zero rate asymptotically.

Notice that equal initial rates for a zero-order and a first-order process very quickly result in a faster zero-order rate, since the first-order rate process decreases as the material is transferred and the zero-order process continues at a rate equal to the initial rate (Fig. 13a).

b. Determination of Zero-order Rate Constants. A comparison of Eqs. (44) and (7) reveals a method for distinguishing between zero- and first-order data. Equation (44) indicates that if the data are zero-order, a plot of X vs t will be a straight line of slope equal to $-k_0$ and intercept equal to X_0. First-order data plotted in this way will not yield a straight line. This situation is illustrated in Fig. 13b. The type of deviation from linearity which is observed is worth noting. First-order data on a zero-order plot show a *positive* deviation from linearity. Conversely, zero-order data on a first-order plot show a definite *negative* deviation (see also Sample Problem 6).

The zero-order rate constant is easily calculated from the slope of a graph such as that shown in Fig. 13b.

c. First-order Conditions in Active Transport. The active transport system considered in the previous example may also behave according to a first-order rate process. Consider the same transfer system under conditions where the number of sites greatly exceeds the amount of drug available for transport. The transfer process will not operate at its maximum capacity under these conditions since it is dependent upon the availability of drug. When a fruitful collision occurs between drug and carrier, then the transport of drug across the membrane

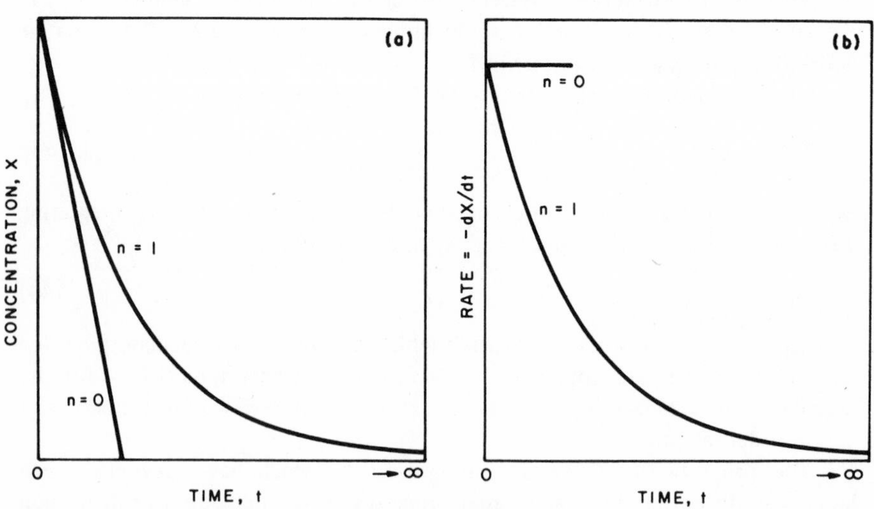

Fig. 13. (a) Rate of loss, $-dX/dt$, from compartment A as a function of time for a zero-order process, n = 0, and a first-order process, n = 1. (b) Decrease in drug concentration in compartment A as a function of time for a first-order process, n = 1, and a zero-order process, n = 0.

as a drug-carrier complex occurs in the same manner as previously outlined. However, at any given moment there is a large number of available sites not in operation. The rate is thus far below the rate at saturation.

Now let us imagine that the concentration of drug is doubled but that the available sites remain in large excess of transferable drug. We would expect the rate to increase, since on a statistical basis there are now twice as many collisions and thus twice as many chances for a fruitful carrier-drug collision. An increase in concentration will result in an equal increase in rate as long as the carrier system does not become saturated and the solutions remain sufficiently dilute so that an increase in concentration is paralleled by an increase in thermodynamic activity. In Eq. (4) we have seen that a process is first-order when the transfer rate is proportional to the concentration of transferable drug. Thus an active transport system can behave by a first-order rate process when the concentration of drug is sufficiently dilute to be the limiting factor rather than the capacity of the transfer system itself. Figure 14 illustrates the change in kinetic order when drug concentration is increased from dilute conditions to those of capacity-limited transfer.

The above discussions of zero- and first-order kinetics as indicative of saturated and nonsaturated active transport systems are analogous to the Michaelis-Menten approach to enzyme-catalyzed reactions. Wagner [34] has stated that truly zero-order urinary excretion data are not obtained regardless of dose size if Michaelis-Menten kinetics are followed. In some cases, however, apparent zero-order kinetics adequately describe a capacity-limited elimination rate process. This will be considered further in the discussion of elimination, including an example where the saturation of the metabolic process forming salicyluric acid from sodium salicylate approaches zero-order.

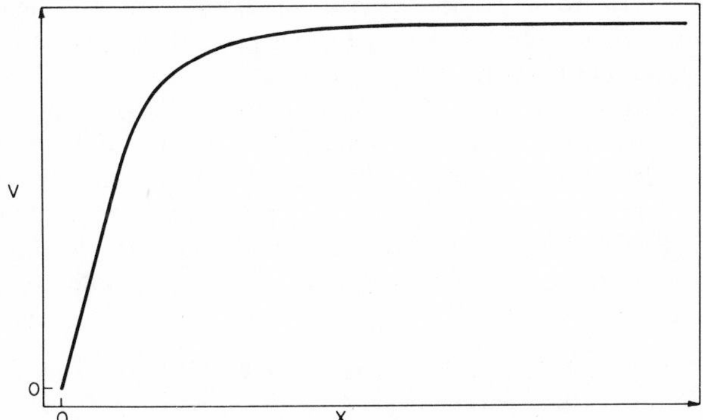

Fig. 14. Rate of transport, V, as a function of transferable concentration, X, for an active transport system at first-order conditions (low X) and pseudo zero-order conditions (high X) where the carrier system is saturated.

Sample Problem 6

A drug is being transferred from compartment A to compartment B during two experiments which are conducted under different sets of experimental conditions. In both cases the appearance of drug in the B compartment is measured as a function of time. The volume of the B compartment is identical to that of A, and the results are given in terms of the amount of drug transferred rather than the concentration of drug in the B compartment. Results are given in Table 10.

Table 10

Appearance of Drug in Compartment B During the Transfer Process from Compartment A

	Total Amount Transferred (μg) Experiment			Total Amount Transferred (μg) Experiment	
t (min)	No. 1	No. 2	t (min)	No. 1	No. 2
0	0	0	25	97	42
3	34	5	30	98	50
5	51	8	35	99	58
10	76	17	40	99	67
15	88	25	50	100	83
20	94	33	60	100	100

(a) What is the order of the transfer process in experiments 1 and 2?
Solution: A plot of $B_\infty - B_t$ on coordinate graph paper results in a straight line for data from experiment 2, while data from experiment 1 are nonlinear. The same data on semilog paper, however, are linear in the case of experiment 1. Therefore, experiment 1 illustrates a first-order process, and experiment 2 a zero-order process.

A first-order plot of data covering the first 15 min of each experiment (this includes almost 90% of the total process in experiment 1, but only 25% of the total in experiment 2) is linear for experiment 1, and is very nearly linear for experiment 2 as well. This emphasizes the importance of plotting data covering at least 50% of a process when trying to determine its order.

(b) What are the rate constants associated with both experiments?
Solution: In experiment 1,

$$k_1 = -\text{slope} = \frac{\ln 100 - \ln 24.2}{10 \text{ min}}$$

$$k_1 = 1.42 \times 10^{-1} \text{ min}^{-1}$$

In experiment 2,

$$k_0 = -\text{slope} = \frac{100\,\mu g - 0\,\mu g}{60\text{ min}}$$

$$k_0 = 1.67\,\mu g/\text{min}$$

Practice Problem 6

Two separate experiments are carried out involving the active transport of a drug through a biological membrane. In each case the drug remaining in compartment A is assayed as a function of time. Results are given in Table 11.

Table 11

Loss of Drug from Initial Compartment at Two Dosage Levels

t (min)	mg%	mg%	t (min)	mg%	mg%
0	10.0	100.0	60	0.02	32.6
5	6.0	94.5	70	0.00	21.4
10	3.5	89.0	80	0.00	10.0
15	2.1	83.5	85	–	6.0
20	1.2	77.8	90	0.00	3.5
25	0.70	72.0	95		2.1
30	0.41	66.5	100		1.2
35	0.24	60.8	105		0.7
40	0.14	55.0	110		0.4
50	0.05	43.8	115		0.0

(a) What is the order of the transport process at the 10 mg% dose level?
Answer: First order

(b) What is the value of the rate constant?
Answer: $1.04 \times 10^{-1}\text{ min}^{-1}$

(c) What is the order of the transport process at the 100 mg% dose level?
Answer: Zero order

(d) What is the value of the rate constant?
Answer: 1.1 mg%/min

(e) What is occurring between 80 and 115 min following the 100 mg% dose? (You might find it helpful to construct a plot of mg% vs. t in answering this question.)
Answer: At 80 min, when the concentration in A drops to 10 mg%, the active transport system is no longer saturated, so the process becomes first order.

REFERENCES

1. W. P. Jencks, *Catalysis in Chemistry and Enzymology*, McGraw-Hill Book Company, New York, 1969, pp. 586–589.
2. K. J. Laidler, *Chemical Kinetics*, McGraw-Hill Book Company, New York, 1950, pp. 19–21.
3. S. W. Benson, *The Foundations of Chemical Kinetics*, McGraw-Hill Book Company, New York, 1960, pp. 27–29.
4. A. A. Frost and R. G. Pearson, *Kinetics and Mechanism*, 2nd Ed., John Wiley and Sons, New York, 1961, pp. 160–162, 166–172, 186.
5. M. Mayersohn and M. Gibaldi, Mathematical Methods in Pharmacokinetics. II. Solution of the Two-compartment Open Model, *Am. J. Pharm. Educ.*, *35*, 19 (1971).
6. A. Rescigno and G. Segre, *Drug and Tracer Kinetics*, Blaisdelll Publishing Co., Waltham, Mass., 1966, pp. 24 ff., 91 ff.
7. J. G. Wagner, *A Manuscript on Pharmacokinetics*, J. M. Richards Laboratory, Grosse Pointe Park, Mich., 1969, pp. 114–122, 128.
8. S. Riegelman, J. C. K. Loo, and M. Rowland, Shortcomings in Pharmacokinetic Analysis by Conceiving the Body to Exhibit Properties of a Single Compartment, *J. Pharm. Sci.*, *57*, 117 (1968).
9. E. R. Garrett, Basic Concepts and Experimental Methods of Pharmacokinetics, in *Advances in the Biosciences 5: Schering Workshop on Pharmacokinetics* (G. Raspe, ed.), Pergamon Press-Vieweg, New York, 1970, p. 7.
10. J. D. Baggot, A Comparative Study of the Pharmacokinetics and Biotransformation of Amphetamine, Thesis, The Ohio State University, Columbus, Ohio, 1971.
11. S. A. Kaplan, R. E. Weinfeld, S. Cotter, C. W. Abruzzo, and K. Alexander, Pharmacokinetic Profile of Trimethoprim in Dog and Man, *J. Pharm. Sci.*, *59*, 358 (1970).
12. J. G. Wagner, *Biopharmaceutics and Relevant Pharmacokinetics*, Drug Intelligence Publications, Hamilton, Ill., 1971, pp. 237–238.
13. K. B. Bischoff, R. L. Dedrick, and D. S. Zaharko, Preliminary Model for Methotrexate Pharmacokinetics, *J. Pharm. Sci.*, *59*, 149 (1970).
14. K. B. Bischoff, R. L. Dedrick, D. S. Zaharko, and J. A. Longstreth, Methotrexate Pharmacokinetics, *J. Pharm. Sci.*, *60*, 1128 (1971).
15. K. B. Bischoff and R. L. Dedrick, Thiopental Pharmacokinetics, *J. Pharm. Sci.*, *57*, 1346 (1968).
16. R. L. Dedrick, D. D. Forrester, and D. H. W. Ho, In Vitro-in Vivo Correlation of Drug Metabolism—Deamination of 1-β-D-Arabinofuranosylcytosine, *Biochem. Pharmacol.*, *21*, 1 (1972).
17. D. S. Zaharko, Pharmacokinetics, *Cancer Chemother. Rep.*, Part 3, *3*, 21 (1972).
18. G. A. Portman, Pharmacokinetics, in *Current Concepts in the Pharmaceutical Sciences: Biopharmaceutics* (J. Swarbrick, ed.), Lea and Febiger, Philadelphia, 1970, pp. 11–12, 67–70.
19. T. L. Loo, B. B. Tanner, G. E. Housholder, and B. J. Shepard, Some

Pharmacokinetic Aspects of 5-(Dimethyltriazeno)-imidazole-4-carboxamide in the Dog, *J. Pharm. Sci., 57*, 2126 (1968).

20. L. Z. Benet, General Treatment of Linear Mammillary Models with Elimination from Any Compartment as Used in Pharmacokinetics, *J. Pharm. Sci., 61*, 536 (1972).
21. R. Nagashima, G. Levy, and R. A. O'Reilly, Comparative Pharmacokinetics of Coumarin Anticoagulants, IV. Application of a Three-compartmental Model to the Analysis of the Dose-dependent Kinetics of Bishydroxycoumarin Elimination, *J. Pharm. Sci., 57*, 1888 (1968).
22. J. E. Doherty and W. H. Perkins, Studies with Tritiated Digoxin in Human Subjects After Intravenous Administration, *Am. Heart J., 63*, 528 (1962).
23. J. E. Doherty, W. H. Perkins, and W. J. Flanigan, The Distribution and Concentration of Tritiated Digoxin in Human Tissues, *Ann. Int. Med., 66*, 116 (1967).
24. M. Gibaldi and G. Levy, Dose-dependent Decline of Pharmacologic Effects of Drugs with Linear Pharmacokinetic Characteristics, *J. Pharm. Sci., 61*, 567 (1972).
25. W. Wilbrandt and T. Rosenberg, The Concept of Carrier Transport and Its Corollaries in Pharmacology, *Pharmacol. Rev., 13*, 109 (1961).
26. T. H. Wilson and B. R. Landau, Specificity of Sugar Transport by the Intestine of the Hamster, *Am. J. Physiol., 198*, 99 (1960).
27. L. S. Schanker and D. J. Tocco, Characteristics of the Pyrimidine Transport Process of the Small Intestine, *Biochem. Biophys. Acta, 56*, 469 (1962).
28. L. S. Schanker and D. J. Tocco, Active Transport of Some Pyrimidines Across the Rat Intestinal Epithelium, *J. Pharmacol. Exp. Therap., 128*, 115 (1960).
29. L. S. Schanker and J. J. Jeffrey, Structural Specificity of the Pyrimidine Transport Process of the Small Intestine, *Biochem. Pharmacol., 11*, 961 (1962).
30. W. Wilbrandt, Possible Mechanisms of Active Transport, in *Enzymes and Drug Action* (J. L. Mongar and A. V. S. DeReuck, eds.), J. and A. Churchill, London, 1962, pp. 43-59.
31. W. D. Stein, *The Movement of Molecules Across Cell Membranes*, Academic Press, New York, 1967.
32. W. A. Ritschel, *Applied Biopharmaceutics I*, University of Cincinnati, Cincinnati, Ohio, 1969, pp. 138-143.
33. T. Teorell, General Physico-chemical Aspects of Drug Distribution, in *Advances in the Biosciences 5: Schering Workshop on Pharmacokinetics* (G. Raspé, ed.), Pergamon Press-Vieweg, New York, 1970, pp. 21-37.
34. J. G. Wagner, Properties of the Michaelis-Menten Equation and Its Integrated Form Which Are Useful in Pharmacokinetics, Abstracts, APhA 119th Annual Meeting, Houston, Texas, *2*, 61 (1972).

Chapter 3

Principles of Pharmacokinetics

I. INTRODUCTION

One of the problems in arriving at a more accurate dosage regimen or a more meaningful interpretation of a biological response to a dose is inaccessibility of the drug concentration at the active site. In order to approximate a solution to this problem the technique of *compartmental analysis* has come into use. This is an attempt to define quantitatively what has become of the drug as a function of time from the moment it is administered until the time it is no longer in the body. Although widespread practice of compartmental analysis is relatively recent, the principle has been with us since at least 1937, when Teorell offered a compartmental scheme. His model was virtually ignored for years because of the complexity of the kinetic equations necessary for its solution. With the advent of computers and the increased interest in understanding drug action, models such as his have been successfully employed in the pharmacokinetic analysis of many drugs. The essential components of a typical compartmental scheme are shown here.

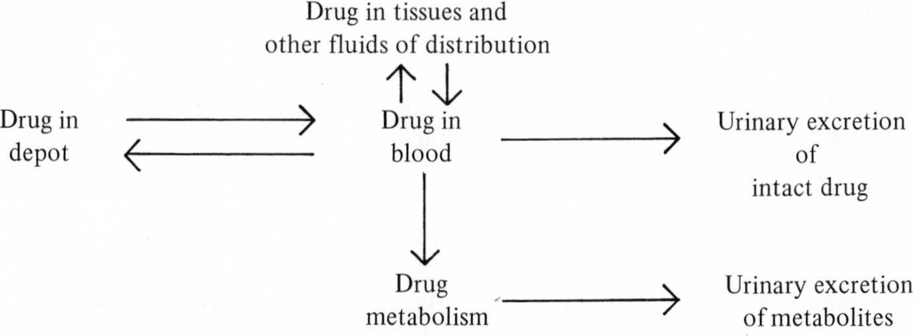

Many modifications of this scheme have been used and certainly no single scheme will apply to all drugs. For example, if protein binding occurs in the plasma, one must consider the equilibrium between bound and unbound drug and its effect on distribution which occurs by diffusion of free drug into tissues. Although many different models may be required to describe a large variety of drugs, there are some generalizations which can be made relative to this approach.

All schemes describe the distribution of drug within "compartments." Compartments generally include the blood and urine. However, while a compartment may be an anatomical entity, this is not a requirement. A compartment is defined as a kinetically distinguishable "pool" in terms of the drug concentration-time profile. If the data indicate the loss of a certain fraction of drug to some site, as a function of time, this site would constitute a compartment in the scheme regardless of whether or not the anatomical or physiological significance were known. In other words, it is possible to know the amount of drug in a compartment as a function of time without really knowing where that compartment is physically located.

In humans, the studies are generally limited to *blood* and *urine concentration* studies. This is coupled with a knowledge of the dose and other information which can be assessed separately, such as binding phenomena.

When a drug or metabolite moves from one compartment to another, there are one or more *rate constants* associated with the transfer process. In general, these rate processes will be *first-order*. Exceptions will occur in cases where a capacity-limited transport system or metabolic route becomes saturated and thus behaves as a zero-order rate process. Schemes are drawn by employing the *fewest possible number of compartments* that are compatible with the experimental results. Generally, data are tested for "best fit."

In brief, pharmacokinetics is concerned with quantitatively accounting for the whereabouts of a drug after it has been introduced into the body. The analysis is carried out throughout the entire time course for the drug in the body. By analyzing the content of accessible fluids, one uses kinetics to make deductions regarding the amount of drug in nonaccessible regions—perhaps even the site of action. The most widely sampled fluids are blood and urine, which are often analyzed for both drug and drug metabolic products. This data is used to produce a compartmental analysis. The relative volumes of distribution and rate constants derived from the analysis are significant parameters in the comparison of analogs of a given drug or a variety of dosage forms. This chapter will be devoted to the methods for determining these parameters using the technique of compartmental analysis.

Pharmacokinetic parameters may be vital to ensure a successful protocol in the clinic as well as in research on laboratory animals. Often the clinical evaluation of drugs or drug products is carried out on the basis of some secondary response because of the nonexistence of a directly measurable parameter which is related to the treatment of the disease by the drug. Many times no response is measured at all, and the clinician attempts to make objective and subjective assessments of the patient's general welfare. A dosage regimen for a new drug may in fact be based on such an evaluation and may or may not include a comparison with a standard drug or analog. Even with proper experimental design, a dosage regimen based upon such studies can be only a rough approximation at best. This point is well illustrated if one compares sulfonamide dosage regimens calculated from pharmacokinetic data to those commonly used in the clinic [1].

II. PHARMACOKINETIC PARAMETERS

A. Biological Half-life

1. Half-life

a. First-order. The half-life of a first-order process is a constant for a given rate process. It can be defined by considering the previously defined variable, X. The half-life is the time required for X_t to become equal to one-half of X_0. Thus, it is the time required for the variable X to decrease to one-half of its initial value. Equation (7) in Chap. 2 can be rearranged to give

$$\ln \frac{X_t}{X_0} = -k_1 t \tag{1}$$

By the definition of half-life, X_t/X_0 equals 0.5 at $t_{1/2}$, so

$$t_{1/2} = \frac{0.693}{k_1} \tag{2}$$

since ln(0.5) equals −0.693.

From Eq. (2) it is obvious that one way to calculate a first-order half-life is by using the rate constant determined from a first-order graph of the data. This method is most accurate, but half-lives may also be estimated directly from plots of raw data.

Figure 1 is a plot of the data from Sample Problem 1 in Chap. 2 on coordinate paper. According to the definition, the half-life is the time it takes for half of the observed change to occur. In this problem the total change is 5 mg%. Starting at zero time, the $t_{1/2}$ is therefore the time required to decrease from 10 to 7.5 mg%, or 21 min. This is the same value as that obtained using Eq. (2). What result is obtained when a different point on the curve is used as the initial value? If the time corresponding to 8 mg% drug in the A compartment, and 2 mg% in B is chosen as the starting point, the half-life is the time for a change of 1.5 mg%, or 21 min again. Try it.

This example illustrates some important points. The $t_{1/2}$ is independent of initial concentration. This can easily be understood by examining Eq. (1). Regardless of what value you choose for X_0, the value for X_t will be $0.5X_0$. Substituting into Eq. (1) yields

$$\ln \frac{0.5X_0}{X_0} = -k_1 t_{1/2} \tag{3}$$

which reduces simply to the ln of 0.5. Thus Eq. (2) will always describe the $t_{1/2}$ independent of the initial value of X chosen to make the calculation. Although the $t_{1/2}$ is independent of X_0, it is easier and more accurate to estimate the $t_{1/2}$ value from the earlier part of the process. To test this, try calculating the

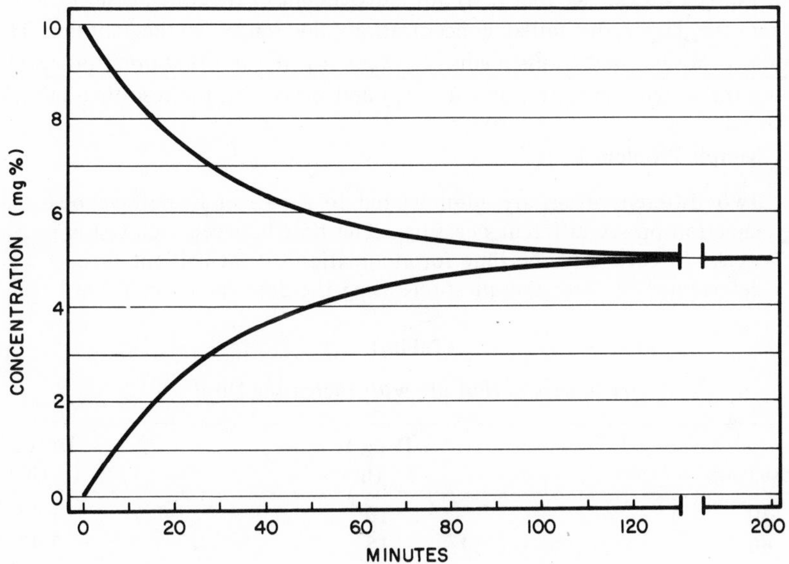

Fig. 1. Data from Sample Problem 1 in Chap. 2.

half-life as illustrated above, but using 6 mg% as the initial concentration in the A compartment and 4 mg% in the B compartment of Fig. 1.

A process which behaves according to first-order mathematics will have a uniform value for the $t_{1/2}$ throughout the entire process. This requirement can serve as a quick test to determine the adherence to first-order principles from a plot of the raw data. Although $t_{1/2}$ is commonly used, one could define the time to reach any desired fraction and this would be a constant for that process if it is indeed first-order. For example, the time for 10% loss can be defined as the time required to reach 90% of the original transferable material. In this case $t_{0.9}$ would be equal to $(\ln 0.9)/-k_1$ or

$$t_{0.9} = \frac{0.105}{k_1} \tag{4}$$

b. Zero-order. The half-life of a zero-order process is not like that just discussed for a first-order process. Applying the definition of half-life to the zero-order equation yields

$$0.5X_0 = X_0 - k_0 t_{1/2} \tag{5}$$

which rearranges to

$$t_{1/2} = \frac{0.5\ X_0}{k_0} \tag{6}$$

From Eq. (6) we can see that $t_{1/2}$ is not independent of the initial concentration. In fact, the larger the initial concentration, the longer is the half-life. This difference can be used to distinguish between a zero- and first-order process by varying the initial concentration (or dose) and measuring the resulting half-life.

Sample Problem 1

Two different drugs are administered to a patient by intravenous injection on six different occasions. The time between each test is 1 week. In each case the time for elimination of one-half the dose is determined. Answer the questions using the data shown in Table 1.

Table 1

Changes in Half-life with Increasing Dose

Dose (mg)	Drug 1 $t_{1/2}$ (hr)	Drug 2 $t_{1/2}$ (hr)
40	10	3.47
60	15	3.47
80	20	3.47

(a) What is the order of the elimination rate process of drug 1 and drug 2?
Solution: Drug 2 has a constant $t_{1/2}$, while the $t_{1/2}$ for drug 1 increases with the dose. Therefore, drug 1 must be eliminated by a zero-order process, and drug 2 by a first-order process.

(b) What is the value of the rate constant and the units of that constant for drug 1 and drug 2?
Solution: Solving Eq. (6) for k_0,

$$k_0 = \frac{0.5\ X_0}{t_{1/2}}$$

At a dose of 40 mg, drug 1 has a $t_{1/2}$ of 10 hr, so

$$k_0 = \frac{(0.5)(40\ \text{mg})}{10\ \text{hr}}$$

$$k_0 = 2\ \text{mg/hr}$$

The other doses give the same answer. The rate constant for drug 2 may be calculated from Eq. (2):

$$k_1 = \frac{0.693}{t_{1/2}}$$

$$k_1 = 0.20\ \text{hr}^{-1}$$

(c) If a dose of 10 mg were given to the same patient, how much time would be required to eliminate 2 mg in the case of drug 1 and drug 2?
Solution: For drug 1, Eq. (44) in Chap. 2 may be rearranged and solved:

$$t = \frac{X_0 - X_t}{k_0}$$

$$t = \frac{10\ \text{mg} - 8\ \text{mg}}{2\ \text{mg/hr}}$$

$$t = 1\ \text{hr}$$

In the case of drug 2, Eq. (1) may be solved for t to give

$$t = \frac{\ln (X_0/X_t)}{k_1}$$

$$t = \frac{\ln (10/8)}{0.20\ \text{hr}^{-1}}$$

$$t = 1.1\ \text{hr}$$

Practice Problem 1

Use your data and graphs from Sample Problem 6 in Chap. 2 to answer these questions.

(a) What is the half-life in experiment 1 starting at $t = 0$? Starting at $t = 5$ min?
Answer: 4.99 hr

(b) What is the half-life in experiment 2 starting at $t = 0$? Starting at $t = 30$ min?
Answer: 30 min, 15 min

2. Determination of Biological Half-life

The biological half-life may be defined using the blood concentration data as a point of reference or from the standpoint of an observed biological response. In reading the literature one must be aware of this ambiguity and determine which criterion is used by the author. The half-life based on biological response may or may not be the same as that determined from the blood. They will agree only when there is a direct relationship between the blood concentration and the biological response. For the purpose of developing this treatment of pharmacokinetics, we will define the biological half-life on the basis of blood level data.

A drug being eliminated by a first-order process will have a half-life which is constant and independent of the initial concentration or dose. This biological half-life may be defined as the time required for the body to eliminate one-half of the drug which it contains. Since we are considering elimination from the body, this half-life will be the half-life which is associated with the rate constant for overall elimination, β, according to

$$t_{1/2} = \frac{0.693}{\beta} \tag{7}$$

where $-\beta$ is the slope of the first-order plot based on the equation for a one-compartment model or the final slope of the biphasic plot based on the equation for a two-compartment model. The value of $t_{1/2}$ is *not* equal to $0.693/k_2$. This would be true only for the trivial case where drug distribution is limited to the blood and therefore $k_2 = \beta$. However, since drugs are distributed into body fluids, the overall elimination is reflected by β rather than by k_2—which was previously defined as the specific rate constant for elimination from the central compartment. A model-independent equation relating k_2 and β is [2]

$$\beta = k_2 f_p \tag{8}$$

where f_p is the fraction of drug in the blood under postdistributive conditions, relative to the total drug in the body.

In addition to dose independence, biological half-life defined in this manner should be independent of the route of administration. Figure 2 illustrates two typical blood level patterns following I.V. and oral doses of the same drug. Note that the curves become parallel in the later time periods of the graph. At this time both curves reflect the elimination of drug from the body. In the case of the I.V. dose the distribution phase has been completed prior to the parallel portion. In the case of the oral dose both distribution and absorption have been completed. Since the β phase curves are parallel, the half-lives calculated from them are equal. This result would be expected from Eq. (7). When possible, however, it is always preferable to calculate $t_{1/2}$ from data collected following intravenous administration. In order to be valid, a value of $t_{1/2}$ calculated from a dose placed in an extravascular depot must be calculated from data representing the time when *both* absorption and distribution are complete. This time may be difficult to determine, since independent data for drug in the depot are generally not available. The fact that the data yield a straight line when plotted on semilog paper does not necessarily mean that the depot is empty. This uncertainty makes the calculation of $t_{1/2}$ from such data risky.

The half-life of a drug will be affected by any factors which change β. As might be imagined, therefore, intersubject variations may be quite large. Renal insufficiency is one obvious cause of an increased half-life. Metabolic differences

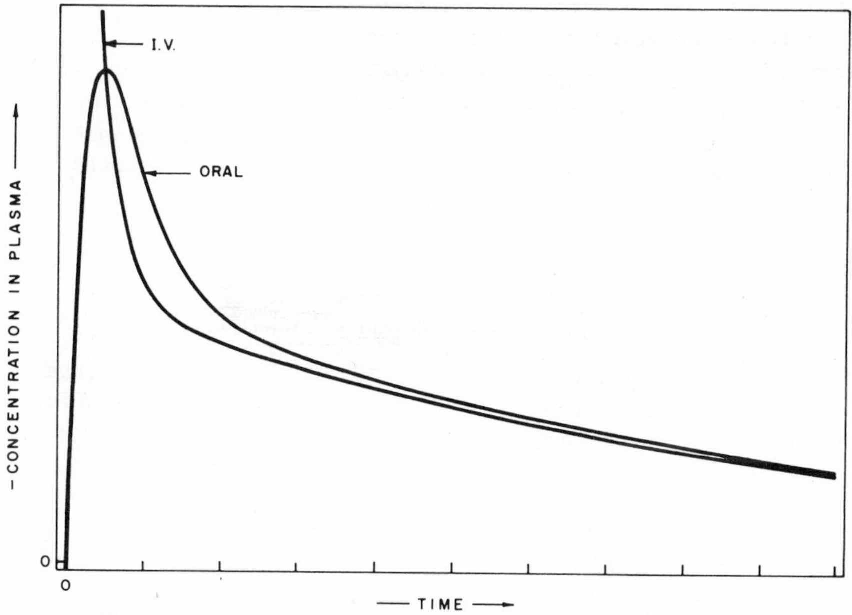

Fig. 2. Blood level curves representing equal doses of the same drug administered by two different routes (I.V. and oral). The drug behaves according to a two-compartment model with values $k_1 = k_{12} = 9$, $k_{21} = 3$, and $k_2 = 2$.

because of age or disease are also important. Changes in the pH of the urine or co-administration of drugs which stimulate or inhibit metabolism can also change the half-life. These changes all affect β by changing k_2. Ritschel [3] has published an extensive list of drugs and their half-lives, including some examples of how the changes in metabolism with age affect half-lives.

However, β may also be altered by changes in the distribution of drug, since we know from Eq. (22) in Chap. 2 that k_{12} and k_{21} are included in β. Wagner [4] has pointed out that a change in distribution rate constants with an increase in dose could change β even when k_2 is independent of the dose.

Sample Problem 2

Calculate the biological half-life from data given in each of the following in Chap. 2.

(a) Sample Problem 3.
Solution: $t_{½} = 0.693/\beta = 5.33$ hr

(b) Sample Problem 4.
Solution: $t_{½} = 4.91$ hr

(c) Practice Problem 4.
Solution: $t_{½} = 3.15$ hr

Practice Problem 2

(a) A drug was administered to a 70-kg patient by an I.V. injection of 100 mg. All of the patient's urine was collected by catheterization over a period of 30 hr. The urine samples were assayed for drug content. Calculate the biological half-life using the results as given in Table 2.

Table 2

Intact Drug Appearing in the Urine as a Function of Time Following I.V. Injection

t (hr)	Cumulative Amount of Drug in urine (mg)	t (hr)	Cumulative Amount of Drug in urine (mg)
0	0	12	91
1	18	14	94
2	33	16	96
3	45	18	97
4	55	20	98
5	64	24	100
6	70	30	100
8	80	36	100
10	87		

Answer: $t_{1/2} = 3.43$ hr

(b) What is the value for β?
Answer: $\beta = 0.20\ \text{hr}^{-1}$

B. Apparent Volume of Distribution

The apparent volume of distribution of a drug, Vd, is not literally a volume at all. That is, it should not be regarded as a particular physiological space within the body. It might be hypothetically defined as the volume of body water which would be required to contain the amount of drug in the body if it were uniformly present in the same concentration in which it is in the blood. However, all compartments which contain the drug may not have equal concentrations, so any volume calculated utilizing the drug concentration in only one compartment can be only an *apparent* volume. In the long run, it appears most useful to avoid all analogies to volumes and consider Vd simply as a proportionality factor which, when multiplied by the concentration of drug in the blood, yields the amount of drug present in the body, or

$$D_t = \text{Vd}\ P_t \tag{9}$$

where D_t and P_t represent the total amount of drug in the body and the concentration of drug in the blood at some time, t. It has been common practice to associate calculated values for Vd with known values for the volumes of body water compartments. For example, the average volumes for body water compartments are roughly (in % v/wt of body weight), plasma 5%, extracellular fluid 20%, and total body water 70%. The inadequacy of interpreting Vd values in terms of body "space" will become apparent after studying the limitations of the Vd calculations themselves. Consideration of this conceptual problem has led Benet and Ronfeld [5] to suggest that the distribution of a drug ought simply to be described by amounts in the central and tissue compartments instead of by misleading volume terms. In any case, volumes of distribution do figure prominently in the literature, so it is important to have some appreciation of the problems and inherent errors associated with the calculation of these numbers.

1. *Pre-equilibrium or One-compartment Calculations*

There are a number of ways of calculating Vd when dealing with a drug distributed by a one-compartment model, all of which yield the same value. Derivations for the equations are given in the Appendix. The Vd value, calculated from these equations, fulfills the requirement that it accurately predicts the amount of drug in the body.

From Eq. (9), it follows that

$$\text{Vd} = \frac{D_t}{P_t} \tag{10}$$

Therefore, it is necessary to know both the amount in the body and the blood concentration at the same time to calculate Vd. Using blood level data alone, this is possible only at time zero following an intravenous injection. At time zero, D is given by the size of the dose, and P is defined by B, the intercept of the semilog plot of the blood level data. In the one-compartment case, B may be said to be equal to the plasma concentration at time zero where distribution of the drug is instantaneous. This method of obtaining the volume of distribution, which we shall refer to as the *extrapolation method*, may then be expressed as

$$\mathrm{Vd} = \frac{D_0}{B} \tag{11}$$

When complete data for elimination of drug are available, it is of course possible to use Eq. (10) to calculate Vd at times other than time zero. This approach has the disadvantage of being a single-point determination. The accuracy could be increased by repeating the calculation at more than one time, but the accurate determination of blood concentrations at more than one level may present an additional problem if the concentration becomes dilute.

One method which allows repetitive calculations at a given blood concentration employs zero-order infusion. Once a constant blood level is achieved, the total amount administered can be corrected for elimination and Eq. (10) can be employed. Since the blood level (and thus T'/P') remains constant, the calculation may be repeated at more than one time interval without loss in assay sensitivity. Equation (13) also yields the value for the volume of distribution calculated during this steady state. Principles governing infusion and further discussion of such calculations are found in Sec. II.F.

Alternatively, the area under the blood level vs time curve following intravenous injection can be used to calculate Vd. Equation (12) is used for this calculation,

$$\mathrm{Vd} = \frac{D_0}{(\text{area})\beta} \tag{12}$$

where the area from time zero to infinity is employed. This equation is also usable for routes of administration other than rapid intravenous injections, since the area is independent of the route of administration if absorption of the dose is complete [2]. If absorption is incomplete but the fraction absorbed, F, is known, this may be applied as a correction to yield FD_0 in the above numerator. Methods for calculating the areas under plasma level curves are given in the Appendix (for rapid intravenous injections) and Sec. II E.2 (for any route of administration).

2. *Two-compartment Calculations*

The calculation of Vd for a two-compartment model has been the cause of considerable confusion in the literature. The methods outlined for use in the one-compartment model have also been applied to the two-compartment model. However, unlike the one-compartment case, the Vd values calculated by the various methods are not equal. This observation and the reasons behind it have been discussed at some length by several authors [6–10], and a short discussion of pertinent mathematical relationships is provided in the Appendix.

Methodology for calculating the Vd values is similar to that previously discussed. Extrapolation of the β phase of the semilog plot of plasma concentration following intravenous injection back to zero time allows the application of Eq. (11). Equation (10) may also be used, provided that the time chosen is after the establishment of a constant ratio for T'/P' (Tissue content/Plasma content), that is, during the β phase. If T'/P' is not constant, values of Vd calculated at several subsequent times will not be constant. This method of calculating Vd has been shown to be equivalent to the area method (Eq. 12) [2]. Finally, infusion data may also be used as described for the one-compartment model by employing Eq. (13).

Variation in results obtained by the above methods may be briefly summarized as follows. The values obtained by the extrapolation method and the two equivalent methods utilizing area and Eq. (10) depend on the size of k_2, but to different degrees. Only the Vd calculated from infusion data after the plasma concentration has become constant is independent of k_2. For a given two-compartment drug in the same subject, Vd calculated by extrapolation is the largest, and Vd from infusion data is the smallest volume. More important, however, only the volume of distribution calculated by means of either Eq. (10) or Eq. (12) will correctly predict the amount of drug in the body during the final, or β phase following intravenous injection of a two-compartment model drug. The extrapolation Vd (Eq. 11) overestimates the amount of drug in the body except in the trivial case at zero time, and Vd from infusion data underestimates the amount of drug except during the steady state of an infusion when it alone gives the correct answer.

An understanding of the conditions which affect the Vd allows us to explain some clinical findings which might otherwise appear anomalous. A number of drugs, including cephalexin, colistimethate, lincomycin, methicillin, and insulin, show decreased apparent volumes of distribution (calculated using areas) in patients with renal failure as compared to normal patients [11,12]. Also, administration of probenecid, an inhibitor of renal tubular secretion of organic acids, reduces the apparent volume of distribution of penicillin derivatives [12,13].

These observations are not surprising if we recognize certain facts. First, remember that the observed changes may not reflect any change in the tissues through which the drugs are distributed, since Vd does not necessarily represent a real volume at all. Second, these changes in elimination have the effect of reducing k_2 while apparently not significantly affecting k_{12} and k_{21}. The only difference between a one- and a two-compartment model is the rate of distribution relative to the rate of elimination. Therefore, decreasing k_2 while leaving k_{12} and k_{21} the same will essentially shift a two-compartment system toward a one-compartment model. As demonstrated in the Appendix, the volume of distribution of a one-compartment model is given by

$$Vd_1 = Vp\left[1 + \frac{k_{12}}{k_{21}}\right] \tag{13}$$

while the volume of distribution of a two-compartment model (area method) is described by

$$Vd_2 = Vp\left[1 + \frac{k_{12}}{k_{21} - \beta}\right] \tag{14}$$

Since β is subtracted from the denominator in Eq. (14), Vd_2 is clearly larger than Vd_1. However, when kidney failure causes a decrease in k_2, and therefore in β, Vd_2 will approach Vd_1, and the calculated apparent volume of distribution will decrease.

Sample Problem 3

A physician wishes to inject sufficient drug to achieve a plasma level equal to 0.10 mg/ml in a patient weighing 70 kg. The apparent volume of distribution for the drug is given as 18% v/w. How many milligrams of drug must be injected into the blood in order to have a plasma level of 0.10 mg/ml after distribution, assuming that 10% of the dose is excreted unchanged by the kidney and no drug is lost via biotransformation during this time, t?

Solution: The apparent volume of distribution is

$$Vd = 0.18(70\text{kg}) = 12.6 \text{ liters}$$

To achieve the desired concentration in the plasma, the amount that must be present in the body after distribution is complete is given by

$$D_t = Vd\ P_t \qquad \text{[from Eq. (10)]}$$

$$D_t = (12.6\ \text{l})(0.10\ \text{g/liter}) = 1.26\ \text{g}$$

Since 10% of the dose has been lost by this time, the dose given must be

$$D_0 = \frac{D_t}{0.90}$$

$$D_0 = 1.40\ \text{g}$$

Practice Problem 3

The pharmacokinetic parameters of a new drug are being studied. Blood level and elimination data following a 1.4-g dose were collected, with the results shown in Table 3.

Table 3

Blood and Elimination Data
Following I.V. Injection

t (hr)	Blood Conc (mg/liter)	Total Amount Eliminated (mg)
1.0	80.0	—
2.0	51.0	—
3.0	36.5	—
4.0	29.3	—
5.0	25.0	555
7.0	20.8	—
9.0	18.2	730
12.0	15.5	835
15.0	13.0	920
18.0	11.2	995

(a) What compartmental model describes this data?
Answer: Two-compartment

(b) Calculate Vd using the extrapolation method [Eq. (11)].
Answer: 47.5 liters

(c) Calculate Vd using Eq. (10).
Answer: 37 liters

(d) Given the following information,
$k_{12} = 0.40\ hr^{-1}$ $k_{21} = 0.20\ hr^{-1}$
$k_2 = 0.20\ hr^{-1}$ and $Vp = 10$ liters

what value would have been obtained for Vd if an infusion experiment had been performed?
Answer: 30 liters. Equation (13) may be used when blood levels are maintained in steady state as described in Sec. II.F.

3. *Other Factors Affecting Volume of Distribution*

In Chap. 2 we discussed equlibrium between nonequivalent compartments, and how primarily un-ionized drug or unbound drug can pass through a biological membrane. This has important consequences in the calculation of Vd since many drugs, such as erythromycin, sulfonylureas, salicylates, and coumarin anti-coagulants are bound to plasma protein. The apparent volume of distribution should be calculated on the basis of freely diffusing drug, so a correction must be made for the fraction bound. If this correction is not made, two types of error can occur. When the assay method determines only free drug, the bound drug will be counted with drug distributed to the tissues and the Vd calculated will be too large. On the other hand, if the assay is for total drug, the denominator in Eq. (10) or (11) will be too large, and the value of Vd too small. If corrections are not made for protein binding, Vd values calculated at different doses for a drug whose extent of binding varies with dose will also vary [14].

Sample Problem 4

Ten grams of sodium salicylate are given I.V.

(a) What is the Vd if B is found to be 40 mg%?

Solution

$$\text{Vd} = \frac{D_0}{B} \qquad \text{(Eq. 11)}$$

$$\text{Vd} = \frac{10 \times 10^3 \text{ mg}}{4.0 \times 10^2 \text{ mg/liter}}$$

$$\text{Vd} = 25 \text{ liters}$$

(b) What is the Vd if 20 g is given I.V and B is 55 mg%?

Solution

$$\text{Vd} = \frac{20 \times 10^3 \text{ mg}}{5.5 \times 10^2 \text{ mg/liter}}$$

$$\text{Vd} = 36 \text{ liters}$$

(c) Offer an explanation for this difference.

Solution: Total salicylate–bound and unbound–is being measured. When 20 g are given, some binding sites may have become saturated so that a smaller fraction of the total is bound. More drug is free to distribute to the tissues so that B is proportionately less. (If the extent of binding were the same as in part (a), B would equal 80 mg%). Therefore, Vd appears larger.

(d) If only *free drug* were assayed, which Vd would be larger–that in part (a) or part (b)?

Solution: Since drug bound to protein would be counted with drug distributed to tissues, and since a larger fraction of drug in (a) is bound, Vd calculated in part (a) would be larger.

Practice Problem 4

One gram of aspirin is administered to each of two subjects. Extrapolation of the first-order plots representing the final slope of the blood level curves yields the following results [14]:

Subject	*Initial* Serum Level (mg/liter)	Body Wt (kg)
A	74	83
B	123	83

(a) What is the calculated value for Vd based on this data?
Answer: Subject A, Vd = 13.5 liters
Subject B, Vd = 8.13 liters

(b) If the assays are for total salicylate in the blood, what explanation can be offered for the difference in the calculated values for Vd?
Answer: Since a large portion of salicylate in the blood is bound to serum albumin, a relatively high albumin concentration in subject B would account for the smaller Vd. Reference 14 discusses these data.

C. Clearance

1. The Meaning of Clearance

A clearance value is simply another way of expressing the rate constant for loss of drug. The rate of loss from the body (R_{ex}) at some time, t, assuming first-order elimination, is given by the equation

$$R_{ex\ t} = \beta D_t = \beta\ Vd\ P_t \tag{15}$$

Since β and Vd are both constants for a given subject and a given mode of administration, their product is a new constant with units of volume per unit time, which we will call clearance. Clearance, C, is therefore written

$$C = \frac{R_{ex\ t}}{P_t} = \frac{(\text{amount eliminated per unit time})_t}{P_t} \tag{16}$$

The relationship between C and β suggests an alternative way of calculating biological half-life. Since

$$C = \beta\ Vd = \frac{0.693\ Vd}{t_{1/2}} \tag{17}$$

then

$$t_{1/2} = \frac{0.693\ Vd}{C} \tag{18}$$

Consideration of the earlier discussion on rates of first-order processes suggests one difficulty in the determination of clearance values; the rate is constantly changing with time, so it is difficult to determine accurately. For example, a graph of amoung of drug in the body vs time will resemble Fig. 3.

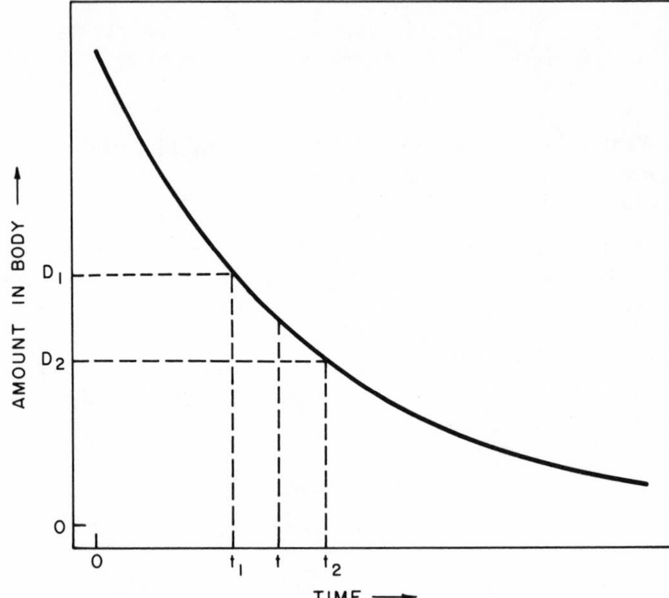

Fig. 3. Time course for the total amount of drug in the body following a rapid I.V. injection of a one-compartment model drug.

Calculation of the rate of loss at a particular time involves finding the slope of the curve at that time. This is a difficult task. The procedure usually followed involves taking two measurements quite close together and essentially linearizing the curve between them. This process is illustrated in Fig. 3, where the rate at time t would be approximated by

$$R_{ex\ t} = \frac{D_1 - D_2}{t_2 - t_1} \tag{19}$$

Determination of clearance values also requires a value for the concentration of drug in the blood. The most representative plasma value is the one corresponding to time t, the point midway between t_1 and t_2, since that point provides roughly an average value for the time period. Clearly, the longer the time interval between t_1 and t_2, the less chance that the calculated rate will be representative of the actual rate at time t, and hence the more inaccurate the clearance value.

There is a way to circumvent this problem however, through the use of a zero-order intravenous infusion. When the rate of elimination becomes equal to the rate of infusion, the plasma concentration remains constant, as discussed in the section on infusion. At this time, therefore, the denominator in Eq. (16) will be unambiguous. Also, determination of the rate of elimination will no longer involve assessment of the slope of a curved line since this rate equals the rate of infusion, which is a constant.

2. *Renal Clearance*

We have seen where drugs placed into the body will undergo distribution and elimination. Elimination is used here as a general term to include metabolism or excretion from the body by the skin, alimentary tract, lungs, or kidney. Although some volatile drugs such as anesthetics may be removed primarily by the lungs, the kidney will generally serve as the primary route for excretion. The kidney is responsible for removal of organic nonvolatile constituents, inorganics which are not retained by the body, and waste products of nitrogenous metabolism (urea, uric acid, etc.). The basic approach to determining *renal clearance* will be explained here, noting that this parameter may (in theory at least) be determined by analogous methods for any route of elimination.

Renal clearance, C_R, may be defined as that volume of plasma, in milliliters, which is cleared of a substance by the kidneys in 1 min. This may be calculated from

$$C_R = \frac{UV}{P} \tag{20}$$

where U is the concentration in the urine (mg/ml), V is the volume in milliliters of urine excreted during 1 min, and P is the concentration in the plasma (mg/ml). This is equivalent to defining C_R as (the amount excreted in 1 min)/(amount contained in 1 ml of plasma). Thus the units resulting from the solution of Eq. (20) are milliliters per minute, which agree with the definition of C_R as the volume of blood cleared in 1 min.

The functional unit of the kidney is the nephron, which is composed of glomerulus and tubule. Urinary excretion of drugs may involve any or all of the following processes:

1. Glomerular filtration
2. Active tubular secretion
3. Passive tubular resorption

The relative importance of these processes in elimination of a drug may be indicated to some extent by the clearance value obtained. Before discussing the meaning of clearance values, it is instructive to consider some tests employed for kidney function. The substances creatinine, inulin, mannitol, and sodium thiosulfate are completely *filtered by the glomeruli* and excreted in the urine. The term filtration is perhaps an unfortunate one here. Actually, water and all the dissolved material from plasma pass through the glomeruli, leaving behind only proteins and colloidal material. The filtrate is thus the same concentration as the blood itself. However, most of the water is resorbed from the tubules. The normal clearance value for such substances is thus equal to the glomerular filtrate formed per minute or 125 to 130 ml.

Creatinine clearance values are often useful for individualizing a dosage regimen for a pateint with renal impairment. Normal creatinine clearance values are in the range of 97 to 140 ml/min for men and 85 to 125 ml/min for women. Since the clearance value varies with body size, it is often normalized by multiplying the observed clearance value by the fraction (1.73/patient's surface area in m^2). The value 1.73 corresponds to an observed clearance value of 120 ml/min. In cases of severe impairment, clearance values are included as part of the patient's profile, while less serious cases more commonly include creatinine serum levels obtained as part of blood analyses. Garamycin dosing information, for example, includes a table which allows the adjustment of the time interval between doses using either creatinine serum levels or clearance values.

Low-threshold substances such as urea, uric acid, certain phosphates and sulfates, are *filtered by the glomeruli* and *passively resorbed* in the tubules. Since the resorption is passive, there is an approach to equilibrium involved and thus some of the substance will be excreted. The amount will be less than the previous case. Normally the clearance value for urea is less than 75 (approximately 73). The urea is not injected for this test, since it is already present in the blood.

High-threshold substances such as glucose, ascorbic acid, Na, K, Ca, Mg, P, Cl, and S are normally completely resorbed by *active tubular resorption*. The glucose clearance test thus has a normal value of zero.

Diodrast (TM), hippuran, and *para*-aminohippurate (PAH) are substances which are completely removed from the plasma in a single passage through the kidneys when present in blood in low concentrations. These are *actively secreted by the tubules* in addition to glomerular filtration. Thus, as long as the capacity of the active system is not exceeded, the blood will be completely cleared. The clearance vlaue (650 to 700 ml) is therefore equivalent to the plasma flow in the kidneys. When a dose of PAH sufficient to provide a 1 mg% plasma level is administered, the clearance value is equal to the plasma flow. However, a dose providing 50 mg% is capable of saturating the capacity-limited active tubular secretion. The C_R value obtained will therefore decrease. Although the clearance value is less at the dose which is above saturation, tubular secretion is nevertheless operating at maximum capacity. Thus the C_R value at the 50 mg% dose can be used as a measure of overall kidney function since it will reflect tubular secretion at maximum capacity plus glomerular filtration.

Thus we may use the renal clearance value for a given drug as a first approximation of how the kidney is excreting that particular drug. In general, a value of 130 ml would indicate *glomerular filtration*, a value greater than 130 would indicate both *filtration* and *secretion*, and a value less than 130 would then indicate *passive resorption*. It should be noted here that this is only a first approximation, since combinations can give clearance values which are misleading. However, if a value is large, such as the case of C_R = 650 ml, there is no doubt that active secretion is involved. Since this is an active transport system it will be subject to all of the properties discussed in Sec. II.D. We have already discussed the *saturation* of the system at high doses of PAH. This same principle can be responsible for a change in the apparent kinetic order of elimination and thus the apparent half-life. At low doses, filtration and secretion will be first-order and $t_{1/2} = 0.693/\beta$. However, if secretion becomes saturated due to a large dose, then elimination will be the sum of apparent zero-order secretion and first-order filtration. Thus the effect of dose on the $t_{1/2}$ will depend upon the relative contribution of secretion to the overall elimination process.

If secretion is saturated, it cannot increase any further in rate with increased dose. Filtration rate, however, can increase, since it is a function of plasma concentration. Thus at sufficiently high plasma concentrations, the elimination rate may again become apparent first-order if the primary component of the elimination process becomes filtration. Similarly, a dose which was just sufficient to saturate the secretion process would result in mixed kinetics only until the plasma level had decreased to the point where the elimination system was no longer saturated. At that time it would return to a first-order process.

This active secretion will also be subject to *competition*. That is, two drugs which are sufficiently similar to be secreted by the same active process will enter into competition for the available enzymes. It is important to realize that any drug with a large clearance value, indicating active secretion, is potentially capable of competing with other actively secreted drugs. The coadministration of two actively secreted drugs can, in effect, increase the $t_{1/2}$ for both drugs, since the total available sites for transfer are decreased in number. This factor can change the pharmacokinetic picture for a drug whose $t_{1/2}$ was established by independent studies. This could result in accumulation of drug and untoward effects from an otherwise normal dosage regimen.

Competition for tubular secretion has actually been put to therapeutic usage. The compound probenecid is actively secreted and is thus capable of competitively inhibiting the tubular secretion of other acidic compounds which are excreted by this route. It has therefore been employed as an adjuvant in penicillin therapy, where it inhibits penicillin tubular secretion and thus increases the biological half-life of the antibiotic. It also inhibits excretion (renal or hepatic) of such agents as *p*-aminosalicylic acid (PAS), *p*-aminohippuric acid (PAH), phenosulfonphthalein (PSP), pantothenic acid, 17-ketosteroids, sodium iodomethamate, and sulfobromophthalein (BSP). The PSP excretion test may be used to determine the adequacy of probenecid blood levels for penicillin therapy. The PSP renal clearance is reduced to about one-fifth the normal value when probenecid levels are sufficient to inhibit penicillin secretion. Probenecid also inhibits tubular resorption of urate. Thus serum uric acid levels are decreased, and probenecid is useful in gout and gouty arthritis.

Substances which undergo passive resorption in the tubules will be subject to the principles previously discussed under passive transport. Tubular resorption will be predominantly by passive diffusion of the uncharged species. Accordingly, the resorption will be a function of the pH of the urine and the pK_a of the drug. For example, the $t_{1/2}$ of salicylic acid may be increased by acidifying the urine with NH_4Cl and thus enhancing passive resorption of undissociated salicylic acid. Conversely, alkalinization of the urine with sodium bicarbonate will decrease the $t_{1/2}$ of salicylic acid by increasing the salicylate concentration and thus decreasing the passive resorption. This latter approach has been employed to treat cases of salicylate poisoning. Similar results have been demonstrated upon adjustment of the pH of the urine during sulfonamide excretion, where the $t_{1/2}$ was shortened from 11 to 4 hr upon alkalinization of the urine [15].

The use of infusion to study renal clearance has other advantages in addition to those discussed in the previous section. A minor clearance route may be detected by comparing urinary drug output with infusion input during steady state, whereas a minor elimination route might be overlooked in a single dose type of study. Examining clearance at several steady-state blood levels allows the recognition of capacity-limited processes.

3. Nonrenal Clearance

As has already been mentioned, compounds may be eliminated in a number of ways other than by the kidneys. However, although theoretically possible, calculation of clearance values for these for nonrenal elimination routes are seldom performed. Reasons for this are easy to understand. While collection of drug eliminated by the kidney is a simple matter, allowling relatively easy determination of the rate of renal elimination, drug eliminated by other routes is more difficult to measure. Reuning and Schanker [16] have successfully determined clearance values for biliary excretion of ouabain in rats. For most classes of drugs, the most important alternate route is metabolism. It is not our purpose to go into the mechanism and chemistry of metabolism, since the subject is complex and there have been several good reviews published on the subject [17-21]. This complexity makes clearance studies difficult. For example, if we wished to study the clearance value for elimination of a drug by formation of a certain metabolite, we would be hampered by the difficulty of collecting the metabolite as it is formed. Even if the compound were formed entirely in the liver, there is no simple, painless way to collect it. Besides this, the required enzymes are probably present in other tissues as well, making loss of drug by this route virtually impossible to follow.

Of course, if drug is lost by only one route, whether it be renal or not, the clearance value for this route is the same as the value for total clearance from the body and may be calculated as indicated for Fig. 3.

If more than one elimination pathway is present, it seems most reasonable to abandon the concept of clearance and compare the efficiencies of the various paths by comparing their rate constants, as will be discussed in the following section. Renal clearance has been in use for many years, and from that standpoint at least it is useful to be familiar with the concept, but the application of clearance to other routes does not seem to offer any advantages.

Sample Problem 5

Assume the normal glomerular filtrate is 130 ml/min. Of this about 106 ml are reabsorbed in the proximal tubule. Another 9 ml are absorbed in the thin segment. The distal tubule further reabsorbs "actively" about 14 ml of this. Assume that PAH is injected I.V. at a rate that gives a plasma level of 1 mg/100 ml. At the end of 3 min, 19.5 mg of PAH is excreted in the urine.

(a) Calculate the renal clearance for PAH.

Solution

$$C_R = \frac{\text{rate of appearance in urine}}{\text{plasma conc}}$$

$$C_R = \frac{(19.5 \text{ mg/3 min})}{(0.01 \text{ mg/ml})}$$

$$C_R = 650 \text{ ml/min}$$

(b) What is the renal plasma flow and why?

Solution: PAH is actively secreted. At low doses, such as this one, the capacity of the system is not exceeded, so the blood is completely cleared. Therefore, plasma flow equals the clearance value, or 650 ml/min.

(c) Would you expect this value to change at a PAH plasma level of 50 mg/100 ml? How would it change and why?

Solution: At this concentration the capacity-limited system would be expected to be saturated. In this case C_R will decrease, since the rate of excretion will be lower relative to the plasma concentration than it was in part (b).

Practice Problem 5

(a) A table of data is presented below for six hypothetical drugs. Assuming that no biotransformation is involved, rank the drugs in the order of decreasing $t_{1/2}$.

Drug	Vd (liters)	C_R (ml/min)
A	50	130
B	50	40
C	50	700
D	15	700
E	50	1
F	70,000	1

Answer: F > E > B > A > C > D

(b) Compare each of the drugs with A. In each case choose one or more of the following reasons as probable explanations for the difference in elimination rates.

List of Reasons

A Renal tubular reabsorption
B Renal tubular secretion
C Low Vd
D Extensive tissue binding
E Poor absorption
F Decreased glomerular filtration

Answer:

Drug	Reason
B	A, F
C	B
D	C, B
E	A, possibly F
F	A, D, possibly F

D. Rate Constants for Elimination

1. *Parallel Drug Loss*

In Chap. 2 we examined the transfer of drug from one compartment to another. The final concentration gradient was shown to be dependent upon the solvent system in each compartment and the dissociation or the binding properties of the drug. We shall now consider the case where the drug is *completely transferred* from compartment A into two compartments, B and C, as illustrated in Fig. 4. For the case in point the transfer process to each compartment will be

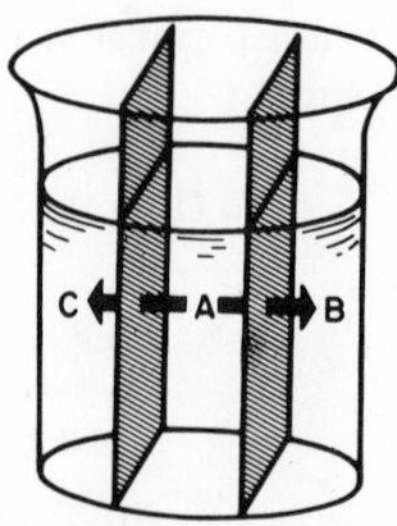

Fig. 4. Parallel first-order transfer processes. Drug placed in compartment A is simultaneously and in time completely transferred to compartments B and C.

defined as a first-order process, and the first-order rate constants will be designated as k_B and k_C for transfer to compartments B and C, respectively. This model is especially important in the pharmacokinetics of a drug eliminated from the body by more than one route, so it is necessary to develop a sound understanding of the meaning of the observed rate constant for this case. However, the kinetics associated with this model are usually surprising on first examination. The problems at the end of the section are therefore particularly useful in demonstrating the validity of the equations to be derived here.

The simultaneous transfer of drug from compartment A to B and C may be illustrated as

$$C \xleftarrow{k_C} A \xrightarrow{k_B} B \tag{21}$$

As will be demonstrated in the following derivation, the apparent first-order rate constant obtained from consideration of any compartment—A, B, or C—is the same, and is equal to the sum of k_B and k_C.

The rate of loss from A may be written

$$\frac{dX}{dt} = -(k_B + k_C)X \tag{22}$$

where X equals $(A_t - A_\infty)$. Since by definition in our present example, A_∞ equals zero, Eq. (22) becomes

$$\frac{-dA}{dt} = (k_B + k_C)A_t \tag{23}$$

Separating variables and integrating between the limits of A_0 and A_t and zero and t yields

$$\ln A_t = \ln A_0 - (k_B + k_C)t \tag{24}$$

or, in nonlogarithmic form,

$$A_t = A_0 e^{-(k_B + k_C)t} \tag{25}$$

The rate of appearance in B is given by

$$\frac{dB}{dt} = k_B A_t \tag{26}$$

or, applying Eq. (25),

$$\frac{dB}{dt} = k_B A_0 e^{-(k_B + k_C)t} \tag{27}$$

This integrates to

$$B_t = \left(\frac{k_B A_0}{k_B + k_C}\right) [1 - e^{-(k_B + k_C)t}] \tag{28}$$

between the limits of $B_0 = 0$ and B_t and zero and t. At t_∞, B_t becomes

$$B_\infty = \frac{k_B A_0}{k_B + k_C} \tag{29}$$

Substituting Eq. (28) into Eq. (27),

$$B_t = B_\infty e^{-(k_B + k_C)t} \tag{30}$$

which may be written

$$\ln(B_\infty - B_t) = \ln B_\infty - (k_B + k_C)t \tag{31}$$

A similar derivation for the rate of increase of drug in C gives

$$\ln(C_\infty - C_t) = \ln C_\infty - (k_B + k_C)t \tag{32}$$

A comparison of the form of Eqs. (24), (31), and (32) indicates that a first-order plot of data for compartment A, B, or C will have a slope of $-(k_B + k_C)$. Thus, the apparent first-order rate constant, k_a, is the sum of the parallel first-order rate constants, or

$$k_a = k_B + k_C \tag{33}$$

The individual rate constants may be determined from a knowledge of the yields and the overall rate constant, k_a. For example, Eq. (29) may be rearranged to calculate k_B according to

$$k_B = \frac{k_a B_\infty}{A_0} \tag{34}$$

and a similar equation can be written for k_C using C_∞. The ratio of B_t to C_t can be expressed using Eq. (27) and a similar equation for C_t. The resulting expression,

$$\frac{B_t}{C_t} = \frac{k_B}{k_C} \tag{35}$$

shows that the ratio of the concentration in B to that of C at any time will be the same as the ratio of the rate constants.

Although the present example involves transfer to only two compartments, the principles remain the same for simultaneous transfer to any number of parallel compartments. It should also be noted here that we have considered only the case where *transfer is complete*. If the transfer to either one or both of the compartments is not complete, the simplified approach derived above will not satisfactorily describe the resulting kinetics. Derivations for these more complex cases [22] as well more detailed derivations for the simple case presented are given in various kinetics texts.

Sample Problem 6

A drug of the type HA is dissolved in compartment A as shown in Fig. 4. The concentration of drug in compartments A and B is measured as a function of time. The results are given in Table 4.

Table 4

Concentration of Drug in Compartments A and B as a Function of Time During the Transfer Process C ← A → B

	Conc (mg%)			Conc (mg%)	
t (hr)	A	B	t (hr)	A	B
0.0	10.0	0.0	8.0	0.7	6.2
0.5	8.4	1.0	10	0.3	6.4
1.0	7.1	1.9	12	0.2	6.5
1.5	6.0	2.6	14	0.1	6.6
2.0	5.0	3.3	16	0.0	6.7
3.0	3.6	4.2	18	0.0	6.7
4.0	2.5	4.9	20	0.0	6.7
6.0	1.3	5.8	22	0.0	6.7

(a) Make a first-order plot of A data and calculate the overall rate constant, k_a. Do the same for B and C data.
Solution: For the A compartment, a semilog plot of A_t vs t has a slope equal to $-k_a$, so that

$$k_a = \frac{(\ln 10 - \ln 1.82)}{5 \text{ hr}}$$

$$k_a = 0.34 \text{ hr}^{-1}$$

Similar plots of $(B_\infty - B_t)$ and $(C_\infty - C_t)$ vs t yield the same rate constant.

(b) What is the calculated value of $t_{1/2}$ for each compartment?
Solution: For A, B, and C,

$$t_{1/2} = \frac{0.693}{0.34 \text{ hr}^{-1}}$$

$$t_{1/2} = 2.0 \text{ hr}$$

(c) What are the individual rate constants, k_B and k_C?
Solution: Using Eq. (34),

$$k_B = \frac{(0.34\ hr^{-1})(6.7\ mg\%)}{10\ mg\%}$$

$$k_B = 0.23\ hr^{-1}$$

Since $k_a = k_B + k_C$,

$$k_C = 0.34\ hr^{-1} - 0.23\ hr^{-1}$$

$$k_C = 0.11\ hr^{-1}$$

Note that

$$\frac{k_B}{k_C} = \frac{2}{1} = \frac{B_t}{C_t}$$

Practice Problem 6

A drug was administered to a 70-kg patient by an intravenous injection of 150 mg. All of the patient's urine was collected by catheterization over a period of 36 hr. The urine samples were assayed for drug content. The resulting data are found in Table 5. The drug is eliminated by metabolism and excretion. Only the unmetabolized drug was assayed in the urine.

Table 5

Intact Drug Appearing in the Urine as a Function of Time Following I.V. Injection of 150 mg

t (hr)	Cumulative Amount of Drug in urine (mg)	t (hr)	Cumulative Amount of Drug in urine (mg)
0	0	12	91
1	18	14	94
2	33	16	96
3	45	18	97
4	55	20	98
5	64	24	100
6	70	30	100
8	80	36	100
10	87		

(a) Plot the data for amount in urine as function of time on coordinate graph paper. Make the appropriate first-order plot and calculate the apparent first-order rate constant.
Answer: $k_a = 0.20\ hr^{-1}$

(b) What are the values of the apparent first-order rate constants for excretion and for metabolism?
Answer: $k_e = 0.13\ hr^{-1}$, $k_m = 0.07\ hr^{-1}$

(c) There are three compartments involved in this transfer process: the body, urine, and metabolism. In part (a) you constructed a coordinate plot of amount in the urine vs time. Complete that plot by graphing the amount remaining in the body and the cumulative amount metabolized vs time.

(d) Determine the $t_{1/2}$ from each of the three plots which you constructed in the above problem. What is the value of the apparent first-order rate constant calculated from the $t_{1/2}$?
Answer: $t_{1/2}$ in each case is 3.5 hr, $k_a = 0.20\ hr^{-1}$

Note: The symbols k_a, k_e, and k_m were used to relate this problem to the illustration given in Sample Problem 6. These will be replaced with the symbols β, β_e, and β_m to describe the kinetics of loss from the body.

2. *Metabolism and Excretion: One-compartment Model*

The rate constant β represents the overall first-order elimination constant for loss of drug from the body by all routes. For example, if drug is eliminated by urinary excretion and metabolism the one-compartment case may be written

$$U \xleftarrow{\beta_e} \boxed{\begin{matrix} B \\ \text{and} \\ T \end{matrix}} \xrightarrow{\beta_m} M \tag{36}$$

where β_m and β_e are first-order rate constants for metabolism and excretion, respectively. This corresponds to the general Eq. (21) for parallel irreversible first-order processes. Therefore, β is defined by

$$\beta = \beta_m + \beta_e \tag{37}$$

As in the case of the beaker (Fig. 4) just discussed, the fraction of dose recovered as metabolite or intact drug can be used to calculate the individual rate constants if elimination is first-order. When D_t becomes zero,

$$\beta_e = \frac{\beta U_\infty}{D_0} \tag{38}$$

and

$$\beta_m = \frac{\beta M_\infty}{D_0} \tag{39}$$

where U_∞ is the total amount excreted intact and M_∞ is the total amount metabolized. Alternatively, the constants can be calculated by substituting into Eq. (37) from

$$\frac{U_t}{M_t} = \frac{\beta_e}{\beta_m} \tag{40}$$

In general, k_2 is not known for a one-compartment model drug, so its component parts, k_e and k_m are not calculable. However, if the proper information is available, these constants too may be determined, as will be demonstrated later in Sample Problem 7.

Elimination by simultaneous first-order processes has the following characteristics:

1. The ratio of drug to metabolite is independent of time.
2. The ratio of drug to metabolite is independent of dose.
3. The percent of drug eliminated at a given time is independent of the dose.
4. The percent of drug either metabolized or excreted at a given time is independent of the dose.
5. The total fraction metabolized (or excreted) is independent of the dose.

3. *Metabolism and Excretion: Two-compartment Model*

Values for β_m and β_e may be calculated in the manner described for a one-compartment model. However, because of the existence of an observable α phase, we are also able to calculate the specific rate constant for loss from the blood, k_2, as described in Sec. II.A.2 of Chap. 2. When both metabolism and excretion take place, the two-compartment model becomes

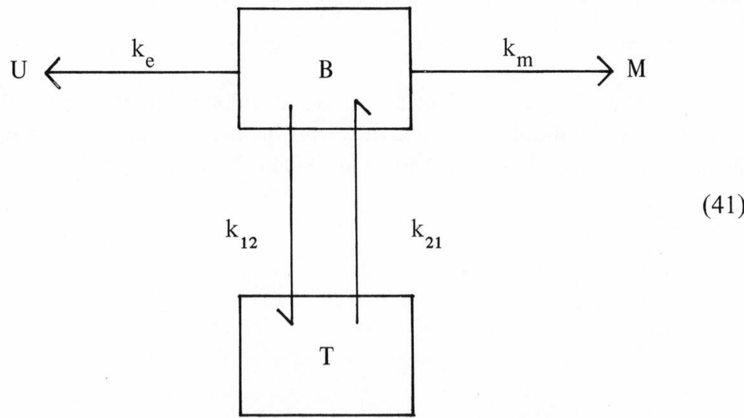

(41)

where k_e and k_m are the specific rate constants for drug loss from the blood by way of excretion and metabolism. By analogy to Eq. (33),

$$k_2 = k_e + k_m \tag{42}$$

Values for k_e and k_m may be calculated in the same way as β_e and β_m using the following equations, which correspond to Eqs. (38) through (40):

$$k_e = \frac{k_2 U_\infty}{D_0} \tag{43}$$

$$k_m = \frac{k_2 M_\infty}{D_0} \tag{44}$$

$$\frac{U_t}{M_t} = \frac{k_e}{k_m} \tag{45}$$

4. *Dose-dependent Changes in Elimination Kinetics*

a. Capacity-limited Systems. The previous discussion was limited to first-order elimination. It is also possible to encounter a capacity-limited elimination route and to saturate this system by a large dose. A more detailed coverage of the kinetics of capacity-limited systems may be found in a discussion by Levy [23].

We have already discussed one case of this type in our consideration of active secretion by the kidney. If this process (or a capacity-limited metabolic transformation) is the only method for removal of a drug, the compartmental scheme at saturation might be written

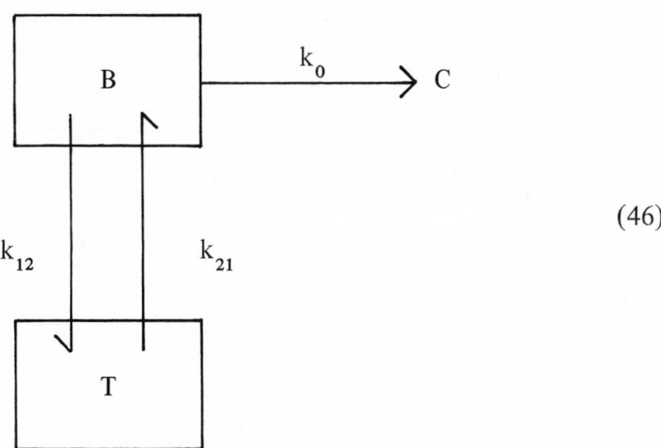

(46)

where k_0 is the apparent zero-order rate constant for loss of drug from the body. Under these conditions the biological half-life would increase with dose. Indeed, one method to test for saturation of a capacity-limited elimination process is to examine the effect of dose size on the apparent half-life.

Another possibility is that of elimination by two simultaneous routes where one is capacity-limited. An example is elimination of a drug by urinary excretion and metabolism where the capacity of the enzyme system involved in the metabolic process has been exceeded. This may be represented as

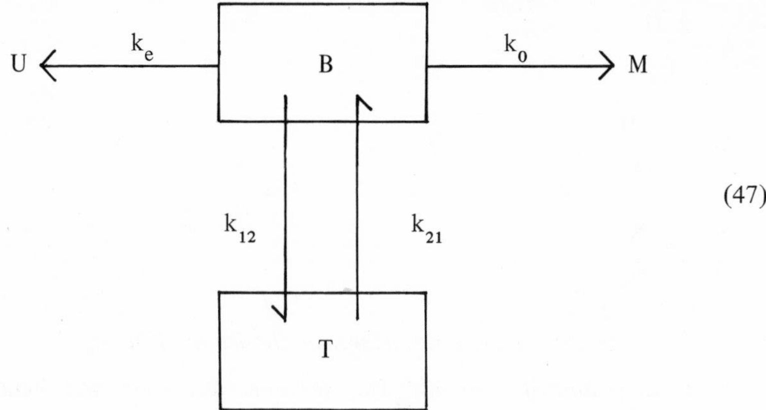

(47)

where k_0 is the zero-order rate constant for metabolism and k_e is the first-order rate constant for excretion. Figure 13a in Chap. 2 illustrated how a zero-order rate process will predominate over a first-order rate process of equal initial rate as the substrate concentration decreases. Thus simultaneous zero-order and first-order elimination processes will behave quite differently from the parallel first-order processes described earlier. Elimination described by Eq. (47) would have the following properties:

1. The ratio of metabolite to intact drug would increase with time.
2. The ratio of metabolite to intact drug at a given time would decrease with increasing dose.
3. The percent metabolized after complete elimination would decrease with increasing dose.
4. The half-life would not be dose-independent.

Levy [24] has described a related situation in which a single metabolite is formed by simultaneous zero- and first-order processes and urinary excretion is first-order.

An example of a system similar to that shown in Eq. (47) is salicylic acid elimination. Salicylic acid is eliminated both intact and as the metabolites, salicyluric acid and salicyl glucuronide. The major route of loss is through salicyluric acid formation, which is a capacity-limited process. The following characteristics have been demonstrated for this elimination [25,26]:

1. *Saturation.* We have previously discussed why a saturated rate process will

behave by apparent zero-order kinetics. It appears that the formation of salicyluric acid is capacity-limited at doses of 1 g and above. The apparent half-life for decrease in salicylic acid blood concentration following I.V. sodium salicylate administration increases with dose. The values of $t_{1/2}$ are 2.4 hr at 0.25-g doses, 6.1 hr at 1.3-g doses, and 19 hr at 10- to 20-g doses. However, since elimination has both zero- and first-order components, the $t_{1/2}$ is not described by the simple zero-order expression, $t_{1/2} = 0.5X_0/k_0$.

It was demonstrated in Chapt. 2 (Sample Problem 6) that a first-order plot of zero-order data will show a negative deviation from linearity. A semilogarithmic plot of plasma salicylate concentration following a 3-g dose of sodium salicylate curves downward for almost 30 hr.

2. *Competition.* Co-administration of *para*-aminobenzoate effectively blocks the formation of salicyluric acid. The elimination of sodium salicylate then occurs by the first-order processes of salicylic acid secretion and salicyl glucuronide formation. Thus a semilogarithmic plot of plasma concentrations following a 3-g dose of sodium salicylate together with *para*-aminobenzoate is linear.

3. *Change in fraction metabolized.* Under conditions where salicyluric acid formation is not saturated, one would expect to find elimination described by a simple first-order process, and the percent metabolized to salcyluric acid at t_∞ would be defined as

$$\% \text{ met} = \frac{100\beta_{met}}{\beta} \tag{48}$$

Thus as long as the process remains first-order, the ratio of metabolite to dose will be constant. However, if the metabolism becomes capacity-limited and thus zero-order, the fraction β_{met}/β would be expected to decrease with increasing dose. Indeed, the fraction of salicylurate decreases with increasing dose when the doses exceed about 0.5 g in adults.

b. Other Dose-dependent Kinetics. A number of drugs are eliminated from the body by an apparent first-order process, yet show an apparent decrease in the first-order rate constant for elimination with increasing dose. Among these compounds are phenylbutazone, biscoumacetate, probenecid, diphenylhydantoin, and bishydroxycoumarin [27–29]. Although the reasons for this behavior have not been determined, several mechanisms have been put forward, including substrate inhibition of metabolizing enzymes [27,28,30], and inhibition of biotransformation by metabolic products [29].

Sample Problem 7

Assume the therapeutic blood level of sulfaethylthiadiazole (SETD) is 12 mg% as total sulfa. The drug is eliminated by both urinary excretion and metabolism. The first-order biological half-life ($t_{1/2}$) is

6 hr. A single 2.0-g dose is required to reach the therapeutic blood level in a 70-kg man. The amount excreted in the urine is 180 mg when the blood has reached 12 mg%. The drug is 100% absorbed, and 90% remains in the body when the desired level is achieved.

(a) What is the first-order rate constant for total elimination (β)?
Solution

$$\beta = \frac{0.693}{t_{1/2}} = \frac{0.693}{6 \text{ hr}}$$

$$\beta = 0.116 \text{ hr}^{-1}$$

(b) What is the rate constant for excretion (β_e) and for metabolism (β_m)?
Solution: When the blood concentration reaches 12 mg%, 90% of the drug remains in the body, therefore 10%, or 200 mg, has been eliminated. At this time 180 mg is found in the urine, so 20 mg must have been metabolized. According to Eq. (40),

$$\frac{\beta_e}{\beta_m} = \frac{U_t}{M_t} = \frac{180}{20} = \frac{9}{1}$$

therefore

$$\beta_e = 9\beta_m$$

since

$$\beta = \beta_e + \beta_m = 10\beta_m$$

$$\beta_m = \frac{\beta}{10} = 0.012 \text{ hr}^{-1}$$

and

$$\beta_e = 0.104 \text{ hr}^{-1}$$

(c) What is Vd if the β phase is in effect when the desired plasma level is achieved?
Solution

$$\text{Vd} = \frac{D_t}{P_t}$$

$$\text{Vd} = \frac{(2{,}000 \text{ mg} - 200 \text{ mg})}{120 \text{ mg/liter}} = 15 \text{ liters}$$

(d) What is the amount of drug (P′, T′, U, and M) in each compartment when the blood level is 12 mg%? Assume a volume of 3.5 liters for the central compartment.
Solution: The amount in the central compartment is given by

$$P' = V_p P$$

$P' = (3.5 \text{ liters})120 \text{ mg/liter} = 420 \text{ mg}$

therefore, the tissues contain

$T' = D_t - P'$

$T' = 1{,}800 \text{ mg} - 420 \text{ mg} = 1{,}380 \text{ mg}$

U and M are given in part (b).

(e) Assuming that the drug is distributed according to a one-compartment model, what are the values for k_2, k_e, k_m, and the relative values for k_{12} and k_{21}?
Solution: In a one-compartment model k_2 may be calculated from Eq. (36) in Chap. 2,

$$k_2 = \beta\left(1 + \frac{k_{12}}{k_{21}}\right)$$

since

$$\frac{k_{12}}{k_{21}} = \frac{T'}{P'} = K$$

$$\frac{k_{12}}{k_{21}} = \frac{1{,}380}{420} = 3.3$$

then

$k_2 = (0.116 \text{ hr}^{-1})4.3 = 0.50 \text{ hr}^{-1}$

The constants k_e and k_m are determined from Eqs. (42) and (45) with the results

$k_e = 0.45 \text{ hr}^{-1}$

$k_m = 0.050 \text{ hr}^{-1}$

Practice Problem 7

A drug fitting a one-compartment open model was found to be eliminated from the plasma by the following pathways with the corresponding rate constants for loss from the plasma:

Metabolism, $\beta_m = 0.175 \text{ hr}^{-1}$
Excretion by the kidney, $\beta_e = 0.150 \text{ hr}^{-1}$
Excretion through the bile, $\beta_e' = 0.50 \text{ hr}^{-1}$
Excretion by the salivary glands, $\beta_e'' = 0.01 \text{ hr}^{-1}$

Answer the following questions from the data provided.

(a) What is the half-life of the drug?
Answer: $t_{1/2} = 0.83$ hr

(b) What would be the half-life of the drug if the metabolism of the drug were completely blocked?
Answer: $t_{1/2} = 1.05$ hr

(c) If the patient suffered from liver disease such that biliary flow were completely blocked, what would be the half-life of the drug?
Answer: $t_{1/2} = 2.07$ hr

(d) If one were to assay for the drug (not metabolites) in the urine, the feces, and the saliva, what would be the ratio of drug to be found in these biological samples? Express your answer as the ratio feces:urine:saliva.
Answer: 15:50:1

(e) If the amount of drug-metabolizing enzyme were increased such that the rate of drug metabolism were doubled, what would be the plasma half-life of the drug?
Answer: $t_{1/2} = 0.69$ hr

E. Supply Constants

1. General Model

Up to now we have considered the analysis of blood level curves obtained following rapid intravenous administration of a drug. Essentially, this simplifies our modeling by eliminating the added complexity of an absorption phase. In practice, however, dosage forms which exhibit an absorption phase are very important, and it is useful to be able to interpret the time course for drug in the blood under these conditions.

When a drug is put into a depot, such as the stomach, intestines, or muscle, it is usually absorbed by a first-order process. Of course, because of design of the dosage form, the possibility of active absorption, or the nature of the chemical itself, absorption may not appear first-order. In most cases, though, the first-order assumption fits the data well. This discussion is limited to first-order absorption. A general scheme fitting such a model is shown here:

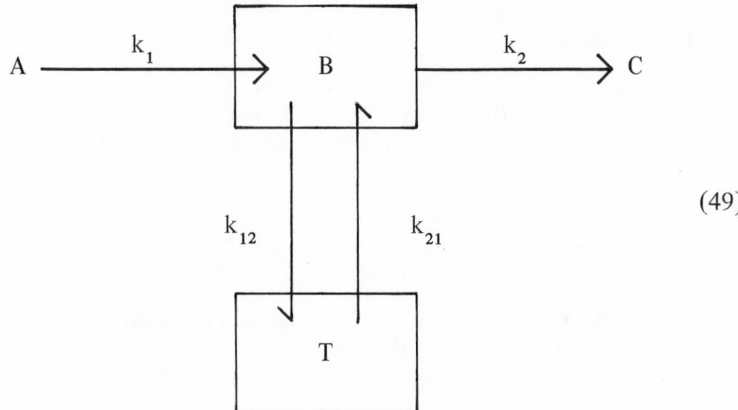

(49)

The apparent first-order rate constant for absorption from depot A may be a complex constant. In the case of a solid dosage form it can be affected not only by the ease with which the compound itself is absorbed from the depot, but also by such factors as the rate of tablet disintegration and rate of dissolution of the solid. If a prodrug, such as an ester, is administered, k_1 for the appearance of active drug in the blood may also reflect hydrolysis of the ester. Details of factors influencing k_1 will be discussed in later chapters. Blood level curves following extravasal administration are, of course, quite different than those obtained from intravenous administration, and we will now briefly discuss their qualitative interpretation.

2. *Blood Level Curves*

An alteration in any one of the rate processes shown in Eq. (49) will be reflected in the blood level curve. Thus, the plasma concentration-time profile for a drug that is described by this compartmental scheme can vary in shape because of variations in:

1. Release rate from the depot
2. Rate of metabolism
3. Rate of urinary excretion
4. Amount released from the depot
5. The distribution of drug between blood and tissues
6. Binding to various sites

Each of these variables will show a unique effect on the blood level pattern. If any or all of these variables change simultaneously, as is the case when different drugs are administered, no simple deductions regarding the relative magnitudes of the variables may be drawn by comparing the curves. That is, it is impossible simply to compare such parameters as amount absorbed or the ratio of drug in tissue to drug in plasma by comparing blood level curves for two different drugs, even when administered under identical conditions to the same subject. Methods for the comparison of different drugs are discussed in Chap. 5 in the section on penicillins. Different dosage forms of the *same drug*, however, will be compared here.

For a given drug, certain of the rate constants in Eq. (49) may be considered constant regardless of the mode of administration. These, as might be expected, are the constants that depend largely on the molecular identity of the drug. The distribution constants, k_{12} and k_{21}, are in this category. An individual, assuming his physiological condition remains stable, would not be expected to show vastly different values for k_{12} and k_{21} each time a drug is given. The elimination constant, k_2, will also remain stable if conditions such as urine pH, biological variation, and the possibility of enzyme induction are controlled. Thus the area under a blood level curve following a rapid intravenous injection is proportional to the dose (Fig. 5). Since drug is injected directly into the

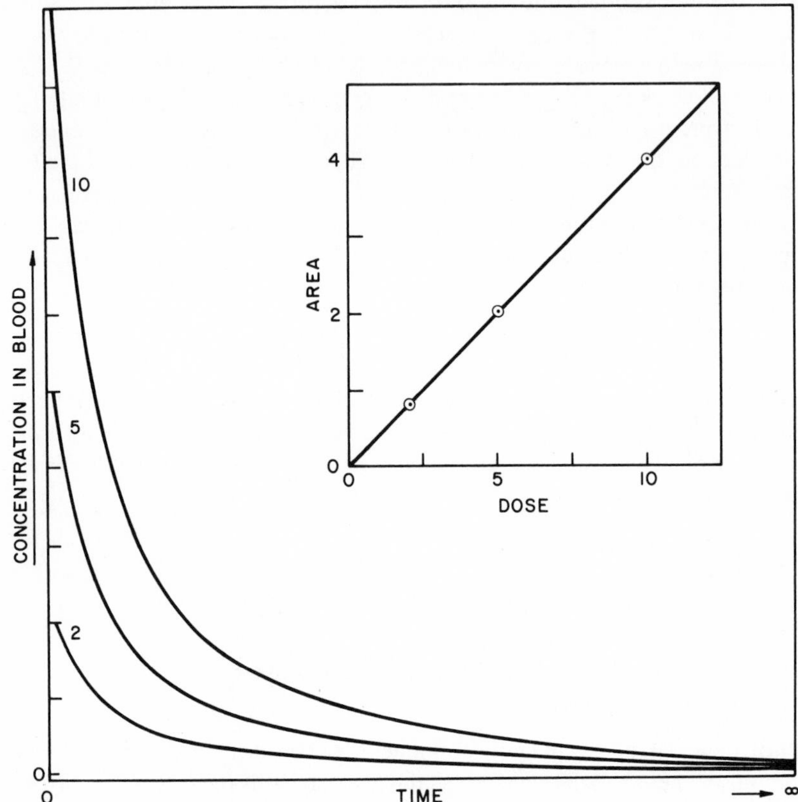

Fig. 5. Blood level curves representing rapid I.V. doses of 10, 5, and 2 for a two-compartment model drug. The insert illustrates that the area under such a curve is proportional to the administered dose.

bloodstream, only the dose size alters the curves. On the other hand, in Eq. (49) both the absorption parameters, k_1 and available dose, are easily changed by alterations in formulation or route of administration. Therefore, we will now briefly examine how changes in k_1 and the size of the dose absorbed alter blood concentration curves in order to indicate the kind of judgments possible when comparing different routes of administration, or different forms of the drug administered by the same route.

Figure 6 shows four examples of blood level patterns where only the first-order rate constant for release from the depot has been changed. This could occur if, for example, a change was made from one crystalline form of a drug to another with a different dissolution rate, or if absorption from an elixir was compared to that from a tablet. The rate constants for distribution have been held constant at $k_{12} = k_{21} = 2$ and the rate constant for elimination at 3. The

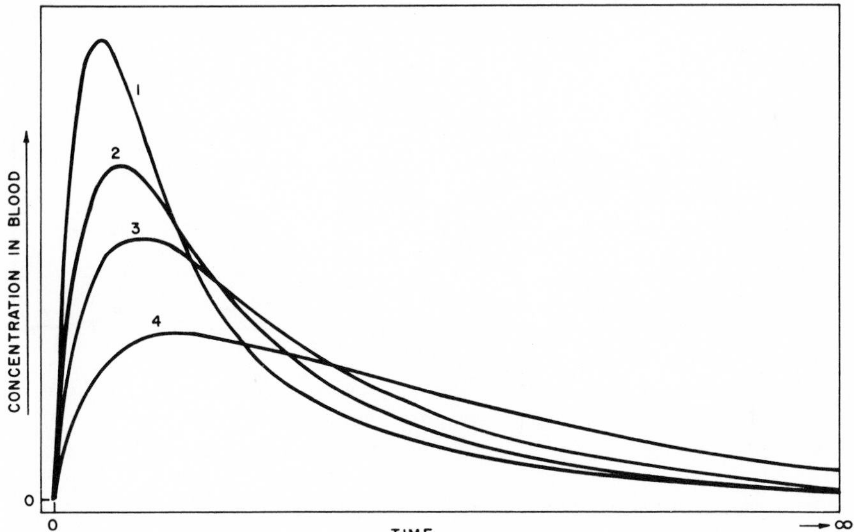

Fig. 6. The effect of the first-order rate constant for supply of drug to the blood. The values decrease from top to bottom: $k_1 = 6$ (curve 1), 3 (curve 2), 2 (curve 3), and 1 (curve 4). Other constants have been held constant: $k_{12} = k_{21} = 2$; $k_2 = 3$.

units are reciprocal time. The rate constant for release from the depot has been given the values 6 in curve 1, 3 in curve 2, 2 in curve 3, and 1 in curve 4. The following characteristics are evident. As the rate constant for supply is increased for a given drug, the peak value is increased and the time to achieve this value is decreased. In addition to this, the blood is cleared of drug sooner in the case of a high peak than it is for a lower peak.

In spite of the dramatic differences in the shapes of these curves, the area under each curve from t_0 to t_∞ is identical. In each case all of the drug placed in the depot was released into the bloodstream and only the rate of release varied. The identical areas under the curves can be used as evidence to demonstrate that the same amount of drug was released from the depot to the blood in each case. When the rate constant for supply of drug is the only rate constant subject to change, then the area under the plasma concentration vs time curve is proportional to the total amount released from the depot. Thus, increasing the rate of supply of a given drug increases the peak height, decreases the time required to reach the peak, and decreases the total time during which there is drug in the blood. It does not effect the area under the curve.

An intravenous injection is really a limiting case of this model. "Absorption" is instantaneous, so the peak occurs at zero time. Since we know that the entire dose reaches the bloodstream, we can compare the area under a rapid

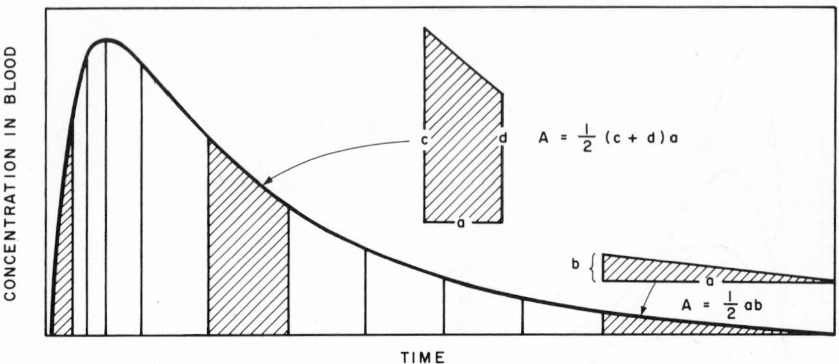

Fig. 7. The total area under a curve may be estimated by summing the areas of the trapezoids and triangles which approximately comprise it.

intravenous curve (Fig. 5) with the areas under curves obtained after the same dose by other routes to determine the amounts absorbed by these routes.

The areas may be obtained in several ways. One is by use of a planimeter. Another involves plotting data for the different routes on the same scale, then cutting out the curves and weighing them. The areas may be calculated from the weights if the weight of one unit area of the paper is known. In a third method, the area under a curve is estimated by dividing the curve into sections that approximate a series of trapazoids with a triangle at each end as shown in Fig. 7. The individual areas of the trapezoids, $a(c + d)/2$, and the triangles, $ab/2$, are summed to obtain the area under the curve. It is necessary to have the same units of concentration and time in order to compare different curves. However, it is not necessary to have the same scale. In fact, one of the advantages of the trapezoidal method is that the curves can be drawn to occupy the maximum amount of space on the graph paper, therefore improving the estimates of the lengths of the sides involved in the calculations. In the method involving cutting and weighing, a small blood level profile would be less accurate than the larger one that might be used for comparison.

The other parameter easily changed is the size of the available dose. This may change because the amount actually placed in the depot changes, or because of some physical or chemical interaction at the site of administration such as the failure of the drug to dissolve completely. Thus Fig. 8 is a typical pattern for five different doses of the same drug placed in a depot which releases drug by a first-order process. In this example the rate constants have been kept constant as follows: $k_1 = 1$, $k_{12} = k_{21} = k_2 = 2$. The dose, or the amount released from the depot, has been set at 10 in curve 1, 8 in curve 2, 6 in curve 3, 4 in curve 4, and 2 in curve 5. Since we are considering a single drug with fixed rate constants, the area under a curve is proportional to the dose. That is, the ratio of the areas under the curves, curve 1/curve 2/curve 3/curve 4/curve 5, is 10:8:6:4:2 in direct proportion to the dose released. In this example, where k_1 is the same for each curve, the peak heights are also found to be proportional to the dose released. As would be expected, the initial rate is proportional to the dose since k_1 is constant, but the product $k_1 A_0$ is decreasing with decreasing available dose, A_0. Unlike Fig. 6, the peak times for the curves in Fig. 8 are all the same and, therefore, independent of the initial dose. Since all the processes in Eq. (49) are first-order, the time for the blood concentration to reach its maximum value is dependent upon the first-order rate constants and not the initial dose. It can also be observed that the time required to clear the blood of drug is directly related to the peak height. This is in direct contrast to the curves in Figs. 5 and 6, which showed more rapid drug loss with increased peak height.

Thus, comparisons of blood level curves for the same drug may be summarized by two observations. A change in the time required to reach the peak indicates a change in k_1. A change in the area under the curve indicates a change in the amount absorbed. Application of these principles will be demonstrated in the problems which follow.

We have discussed idealized blood level curves following drug administration under controlled conditions. Most clinical studies are done with groups of people. This leads to the problem of individual variations which may cause all the rate constants to change from subject to subject. When data from these studies are to be used in comparisons such as those just discussed, it is therefore

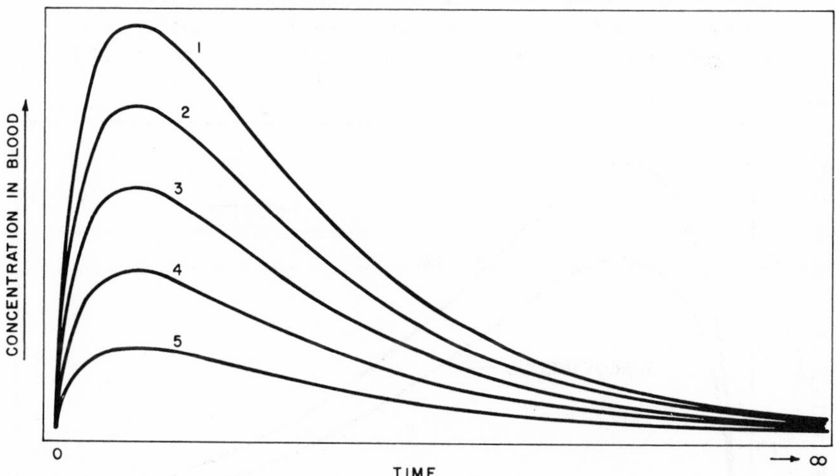

Fig. 8. Effect of the size of the available dose administered by an extravascular route. From top to bottom the relative dose is: 5 (curve 1), 4 (curve 2), 3 (curve 3), 2 (curve 4), and 1 (curve 5). Rate constants have been held constant at $k_1 = 1$ and $k_{12} = k_{21} = k_2 = 2$.

important that proper experimental design be employed so that effects of individual variation will be minimized. Wagner [31] has discussed the designs of clinical studies and their analysis. Several additional references on the subject are cited in that paper.

Sample Problem 8

While testing a new drug, a pharmacologist administered the same dose both intramuscularly and subcutaneously to his test animals. He found the ED_{50} for the intramuscular route to be about 25% lower. A study using the same experimental conditions produced the blood level curves shown in Fig. 9. Offer an explanation for the observed difference in ED_{50}.

Solution: Both curves are for the same drug. Therefore, k_{12}, k_{21}, and k_2 are held constant. The peak time is the same in both cases, indicating that k_1 is the same for both routes. However, the areas under the curves appear different. Because k_1 remains constant, we can use peak height to compare areas, and we find that subcutaneous administration shows 25% less area under the curve, indicating 25% less drug absorbed. Therefore, the change in amount absorbed will explain the difference in ED_{50}.

Practice Problem 8

Capsules of the amorphous and crystalline forms of a new drug were administered to healthy volunteers in a crossover study. Nearly all of those receiving the amorphous form showed some toxicity, while those who received equal doses of the crystals had no side effects. In

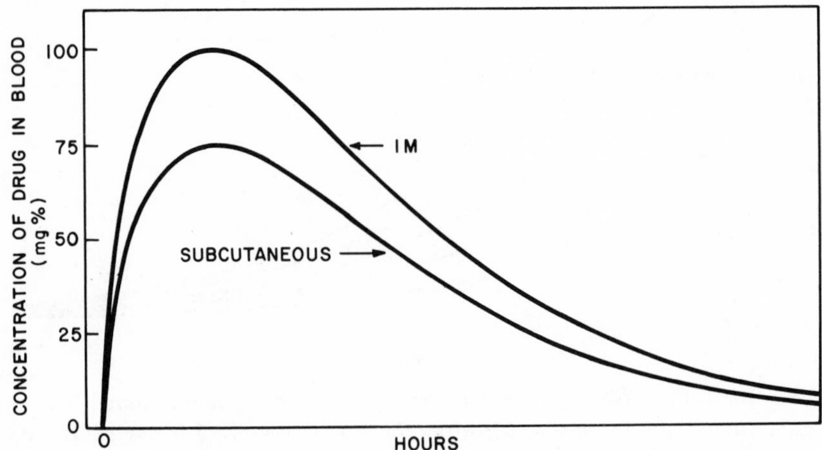

Fig. 9. Time course for drug in the blood following administration of equal doses by two different routes as described in Sample Problem 8.

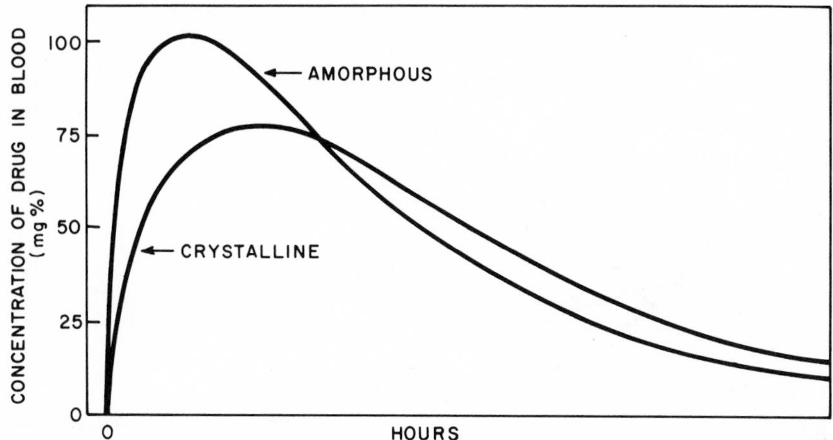

Fig. 10. Time course for drug in the blood following equal oral doses administered as the amorphous and crystalline forms as described in Practice Problem 8.

both cases all of the administered drug was recovered in the urine. Using the blood level curves shown in Fig. 10, explain the results. *Answer:* The amorphous form dissolves more rapidly, leading to a larger k_1. An increase in k_1 increases the peak height and decreases the peak time, as observed in the figure. This increase in peak height accounts for the toxic symptoms even though the same amount of drug was absorbed in each case.

3. *Calculation of Absorption Rate Constants*

a. Simple Case. In chemical kinetics, a sequence of reactions such as

$$A \xrightarrow{k_1} B \xrightarrow{k_2} C \tag{50}$$

may be handled in various ways to determine k_1 and k_2 depending on whether data are available for A, B, or C. Figure 11 shows the time course for each component for the case where the first-order constants are equal. This scheme resembles, in an overall way, Eq. (49), with B representing the total drug in the body. We will not go into the analysis of systems like Eq. 50, since this is discussed in other texts [22]. It is sufficient to say that the calculation of k_1, which is analogous to the absorption constant, is most simply done if data for A are available, since

$$\ln A_t = \ln A_0 - k_1 t \tag{51}$$

so that a plot of $\ln A_t$ vs t has a slope of $-k_1$.

Unfortunately, in pharmacokinetic studies, the amount of drug remaining in

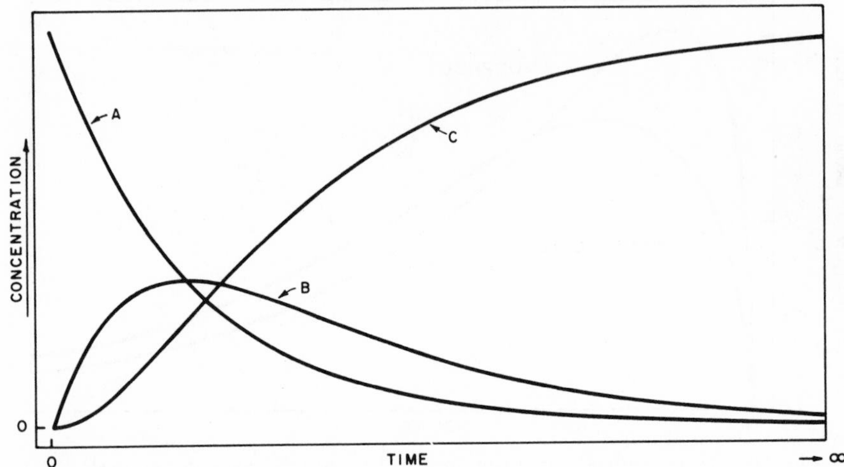

Fig. 11. Time course for each component in consecutive, irreversible first-order processes: $A \xrightarrow{k_1} B \xrightarrow{k_2} C$, where $k_1 = k_2$.

the depot is not usually available for direct measurement. Instead, data for plasma or blood concentration of the drug are most commonly collected. The methods we will discuss for the calculation of k_1 allow us to calculate a measure of the amount in the depot from blood concentration data so that this may be plotted to obtain the desired constant.

These methods, developed by Wagner and Nelson [32], and Loo and Riegelman [33], are applicable to one- and two-compartment model drugs, respectively. Other methods for calculation of absorption rates from blood or urine data have been published [34,35]. Benet and Chiang [36] have applied the techniques of numerical deconvolution to absorption rate calculations.

b. Rate-determining Step. The overall rate process, from beginning to end, is limited by the slowest step in the sequence provided that one step is sufficiently slower than the rest. This may be likened to a bucket brigade with one lethargic member. In a simple series of consecutive, irreversible first-order rate processes (Eq. 50), either step may become rate-limiting.

If the initial step is rapid, it may be possible to calculate both k_1 and k_2 from data for B or C. This is illustrated in Fig. 12, where two different time scales have been chosen to display the same data. It is obvious that data for A will always provide an estimate for k_1. However, data for B may be used to calculate k_2 by a simple first-order plot of the data shown in Fig. 12a or to calculate k_1 using the data in Fig. 12b, where the variable X_t would be defined as $(A_0 - B_t)$. This estimate for k_1 will be reasonable as long as $k_1/k_2 > 10$. The data for C can also be used to calculate k_2 by applying a first-order treatment to the data in Fig. 12a, where X_t would be defined as $(A_0 - C_t)$. A method which

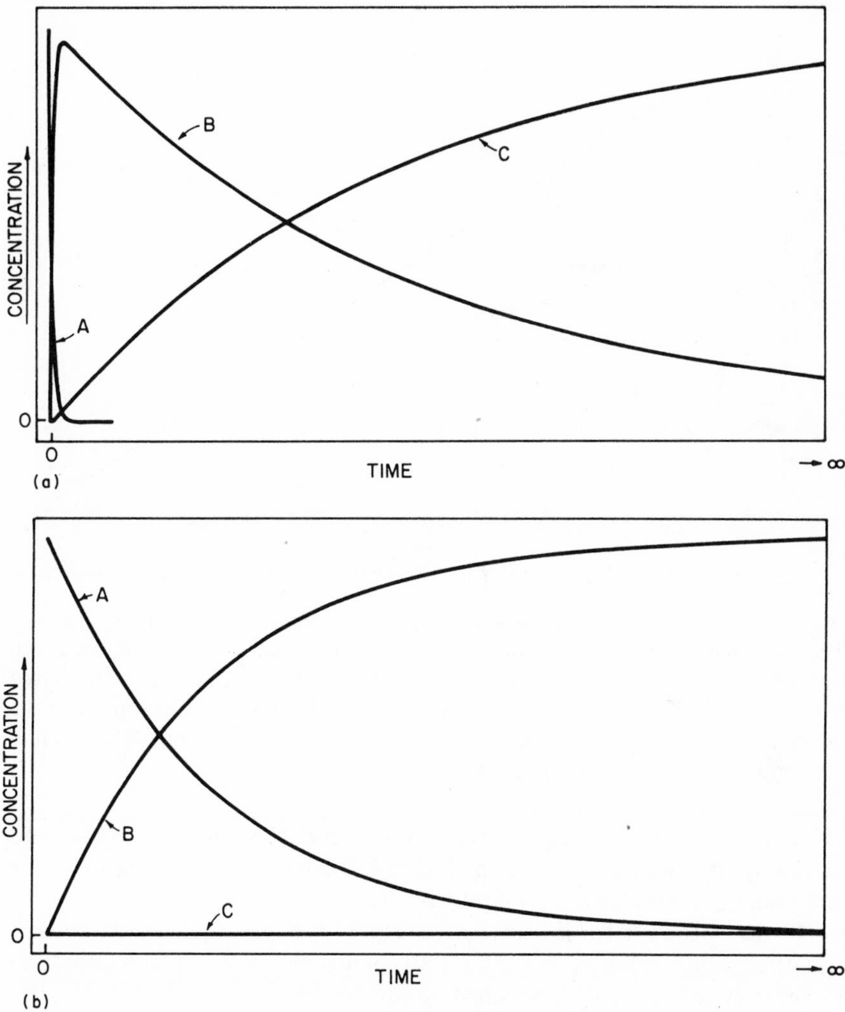

Fig. 12. Consecutive, irreversible first-order processes where the initial step is rapid. In this example for $A \xrightarrow{k_1} B \xrightarrow{k_2} C$, $k_1/k_2 = 500$. (a) This time scale illustrates primarily the second step. (b) This time scale illustrates the first step in the sequence.

can be applied to cases where $2 \leqslant k_1/k_2 \leqslant 10$ with reasonable success (±10%) is that of "feathering." This is illustrated in Fig. 13. The first-order plot for the terminal portion of the B data is extrapolated to zero time and a difference plot is made using the line and the experimental points. It is necessary that A_t be equal to zero for the plot of ln B_t vs t to yield k_2. Linearity of this plot is not

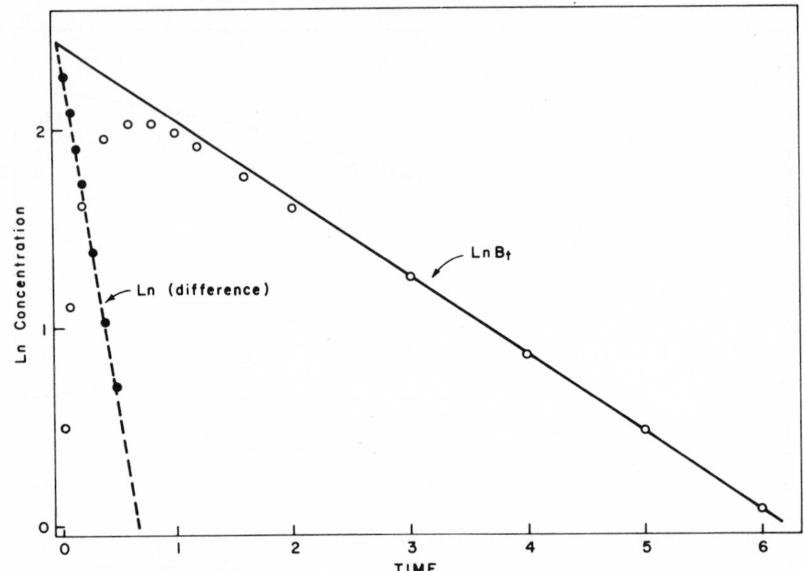

Fig. 13. "Feathering" data for concentration of B in the consecutive first-order processes $A \xrightarrow{k_1} B \xrightarrow{k_2} C$ to obtain estimates for both k_1 and k_2. The negative value for the slope of the terminal portion of ln B_t vs t will estimate k_2 provided that A_t has approached zero. The value for k_1 is estimated from the dashed line, which is a first-order plot of the natural logarithm of the difference between the experimental values and the extrapolated values (antilogarithm values from the solid line).

sufficient evidence for the acceptability of the slope. This problem was discussed previously as a warning and that biological half-life values from data following oral administration of drug may not be accurate.

If the second step is sufficiently rapid, the initial step will become rate-determining. When $k_2 \gg k_1$, Eq. (50) approaches the steady-state case since B_t becomes constant and approximately equal to zero. This is illustrated in Fig. 14, where $k_2/k_1 = 20$. It can readily be observed in this figure that data for A, B, or C all provide estimates for the slower constant, k_1. Generally one would not expect to analyze B data in the steady state, since the values would be very small and nearly constant by definition. However, it may not be necessary to have the case where B is actually in the steady state in order to obtain k_1 estimates from first-order plots for loss of B. The apparent biological $t_{1/2}$ values estimated from first-order loss from blood following four intramuscular penicillin dosage forms were found to agree more closely with the half-lives representing the absorption constants than with those for elimination following rapid intravenous injection [37]. The ratio of β/k_1 varied from 1.5 to 3.3 for the four cases, indicating a

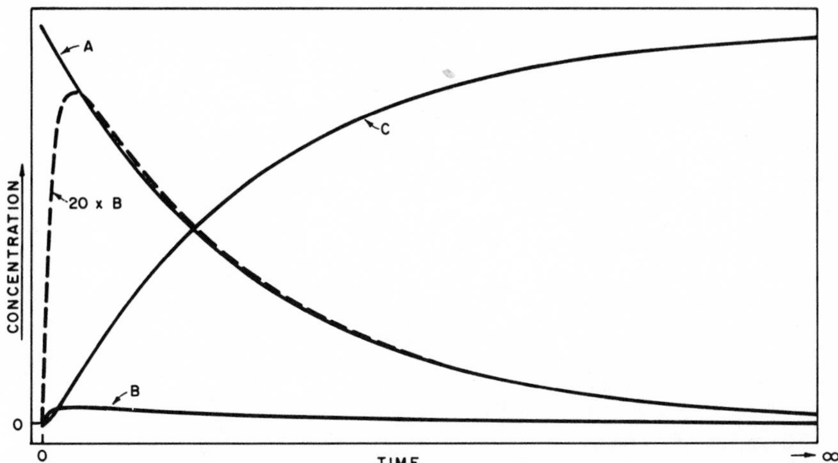

Fig. 14. Consecutive, irreversible first-order processes with rapid second step. In this example for $A \xrightarrow{k_1} B \xrightarrow{k_2} C$, $k_2/k_1 = 20$. In the steady-state case, B_t approaches zero. This figures illustrates the trend toward the steady state for the moderate ratio of $k_1/k_2 = 20$.

rapid second step though not a steady state. The cases with low ratios (1.5) provided $t_{1/2}$ estimates which were longer than either the absorption or the biological $t_{1/2}$. This would be expected, since neither step can be regarded as rate-limiting when they are nearly equal. In the general case (Fig. 11), the decrease in B is described as the net difference between its supply and loss, as can be seen from the equation

$$B_t = \left(\frac{A_0 k_1}{k_2 - k_1}\right) [e^{-k_1 t} - e^{-k_2 t}] \tag{52}$$

c. The Loo-Riegelman and Wagner-Nelson Equations. These are both applied in much the same manner. Both of these equations allow us to calculate the percent of drug remaining unabsorbed at any time. This percentage is based on the *absorbable* fraction of the dose in the case of incomplete absorption [38]. An appropriate plot (first-order or zero-order) of this data allows calculation of the absorption rate constant (k_1 or k_0). We will first look at the application of the Loo-Riegelman equation [33] to a drug described by a two-compartment open model and absorbed by a first-order rate process. The first-order rate constant for absorption will be calculated from the data in Table 6.

Table 6

Plasma Levels of Drug Following
Oral Administration of 490 mg

t (hr)	P (mg%)	t (hr)	P (mg%)
0.5	3.2	4.0	4.8
1.0	4.8	5.0	4.1
1.5	5.5	7.0	3.1
2.0	5.7	9.0	2.2
2.5	5.7	11.0	1.8
3.0	5.4	13.0	1.4

The equation to be used is

$$\left(\frac{A}{V_p}\right)_{tn} = P_{tn} + k_2 \int_{t_0}^{tn} P\,dt + T_{tn} \tag{53}$$

where $(A/V_p)_{tn}$ represents the total amount absorbed, A, at time tn, expressed in terms of V_p, the plasma volume. Concentrations of drug in plasma and tissue are given by P and T. The most convenient and simple way to explain the use of this equation is to work through an example.

A drug is found to exhibit both an α and β phase following I.V. injection. The calculated values for the rate constants are $k_{12} = 0.30$, $k_{21} = 0.40$, and $k_2 = 0.25$ (hr^{-1}). The same drug was administered orally, and the data given in Table 6 were obtained. We will now use this information to calculate the three unknown quantities in Eq. (53), T_{tn}, $k_2 \int P\,dt$, and $(A/Vp)_{tn}$. The results of our stepwise calculations are entered in Table 7.

Step 1: Calculation of tissue concentrations as a function of time. The equation to be used is

$$T_{tn} = T_{tn-1}\, e^{-k_{21}\Delta t} + \left(\frac{k_{12}}{k_{21}}\right) P_{tn-1}\, [1 - e^{-k_{21}\Delta t}] + \frac{k_{12}\Delta P\, \Delta t}{2} \tag{54}$$

This equation will be solved for each data point. In our example the first set of points is 0.5 hr, 3.2 mg%. Thus $\Delta t = 0.5$, $\Delta P = 3.2$, and tn - 1 is zero since it refers to the time of the previous data point. Thus P_{tn-1} and T_{tn-1} are also zero, since no drug is in the body at time zero. The first entry in our table under step 1 is calculated from

$$T_{0.5\ hr} = 0 + 0 + \frac{(0.3)(3.2)(0.5)}{2} = 0.24 \tag{55}$$

and the second entry from

$$T_{1.0\ hr} = 0.24e^{-0.20} + \left(\frac{0.3}{0.4}\right) 3.2(1 - e^{-0.20}) + \frac{0.3(1.6)0.5}{2}$$

$$= 0.751 \tag{56}$$

and so on. Each of the entries for T_{tn} is given in Table 7.

Step 2: Calculation of elimination as a function of time. We have now calculated the values for T_{tn}. Since we have data for P_{tn} there is only one part of Eq. (53) yet to be calculated and that is

$$k_2 \int_{t_0}^{tn} P\,dt \tag{57}$$

where the integral of P dt represents the area under the plasma time curve from time zero to time tn. This can be done most easily by use of the trapezoidal rule as illustrated in Fig. 7. Thus the curve for P vs t must be drawn and the individual areas calculated for each trapezoid (or triangle) as described by the data points. The answers are illustrated in Table 7, column 6. These are the areas of the various trapezoids. However, the integral in Eq. (57) represents the total area up to tn. Therefore each area up to and including tn must be summed to obtain the value of the integral in Eq. (57) as shown in column 7. Each of these values is then multiplied by the elimination constant, $k_2 = 0.25$, to obtain the values in column 8.

Step 3: Calculation of A/V_p. The three component parts of Eq. (53) are now calculated (columns 3, 4, and 8) and are to be summed to obtain the values given in column 9. Examination of the entries in column 9 as a function of time will reveal that A/V_p appears to approach a maximum value of about 13.6. The values of A/V_p are next converted to a percent of this maximum value according to

$$\frac{\%A}{V_p} = \frac{(100A/V_p)}{13.6} \tag{58}$$

and the results are shown in column 10. Column 11 represents the percent of drug unabsorbed as a function of time and it is calculated by subtracting column 10 from 100%. The first-order plot of percent unabsorbed vs time yields a value of 0.60 hr^{-1} for k_1.

Table 7

Answers to Stepwise Calculation for Loo-Riegelman Equation

Step 1					Step 2			Step 3		
(1)	(2)	(3)	(4)	(5)	(6)	(7)	(8)	(9)	(10)	(11)
tn	Δt	P_{tn}	ΔP	T_{tn}	Area tn − 1 *to* tn	Area t_0 *to* tn	$k_2 \times$ Col. 7	$A/V_p =$ Cols. 3 + 5 + 8	$\%A/V_p$	100% − Col. 10
0.5	0.5	3.2	3.2	0.240	0.80	0.80	0.20	3.64	26.8	73.2
1.0	0.5	4.8	1.6	0.752	2.00	2.80	0.70	6.25	46.0	54.0
1.5	0.5	5.5	0.7	1.32	2.58	5.38	1.35	8.17	60.1	39.9
2.0	0.5	5.7	0.2	1.84	2.80	8.18	2.04	9.58	70.4	29.6
2.5	0.5	5.7	0.0	2.28	2.85	11.03	2.76	10.7	78.7	21.3
3.0	0.5	5.4	-0.3	2.62	2.78	13.81	3.45	11.5	84.6	15.4
4.0	1.0	4.8	-0.6	3.00	5.10	18.91	4.73	12.5	91.9	8.1
5.0	1.0	4.1	-0.7	3.09	4.45	23.36	5.84	13.0	95.6	4.4
7.0	2.0	3.1	-1.0	2.78	7.20	30.56	7.65	13.5	99.3	0.7
9.0	2.0	2.2	-0.9	2.26	5.30	35.86	8.96	13.4	98.5	1.5
11.0	2.0	1.8	-0.4	1.80	4.00	39.86	9.96	13.6	100.0	0.0
13.0	2.0	1.4	-0.4	1.43	3.20	43.06	10.8	13.6	100.0	0.0

The calculation of k_1 for a drug distributed according to a one-compartment model is done by means of the Wagner-Nelson [32] equation:

$$\left(\frac{A}{Vd}\right)_{tn} = P_{tn} + \beta \int_{t_0}^{tn} P\,dt \qquad (59)$$

The procedure for solving this equation to obtain k_1 is basically the same as that just described.

d. First-order Loss of Drug from Depot. The rate constant calculated using Eq. (53) or (59) does not truly represent absorption if part of the drug in the depot is lost to some parallel process that competes with absorption. Examples of such processes might be chemical degradation, biotransformation by enzymes or intestinal bacteria, or transfer to a compartment other than the blood. This kind of process can be shown schematically as

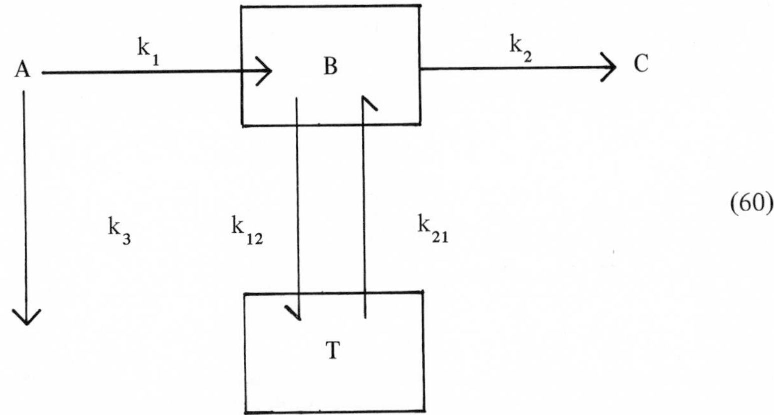

(60)

where k_3 represents the rate constant for drug loss by the competing process. In such a system, and where k_3 is a first-order rate constant, it has been shown that the rate constant calculated for absorption is the sum of k_1 and k_3 provided that these represent the only routes for loss of drug from the depot [38]. We can see that this system is similar to that discussed in Sec. II.D.1. The true rate constant for absorption may be obtained in a manner similar to that used earlier for obtaining the specific rate constants for metabolism and excretion from the apparent elimination constant. That is, adapting Eq. (34),

$$k_1 = \frac{k_a B_\infty}{D_0}$$

where k_a is the apparent rate constant for absorption and B_∞/D_0 represents the fraction absorbed. Loss of drug by a non-first-order process cannot be treated in this simple manner, however.

Thus, we recognize a potential problem in that false impressions of rapid absorption may result from a competing process such as rapid hydrolysis. Studies employing the Wagner-Nelson or Loo-Riegelman method should therefore include a calculation of the fraction of dose absorbed. If the drug is well absorbed, the absorption rate constant calculated should represent a good estimate of the actual value. If absorption is poor, the reason must be established before a physical meaning can be assigned to the apparent rate constant [38].

F. Intravenous Infusion

A constant intravenous infusion delivers a fixed amount of drug per unit time to the bloodstream. This represents a zero-order rate process. This kind of administration may be depicted by

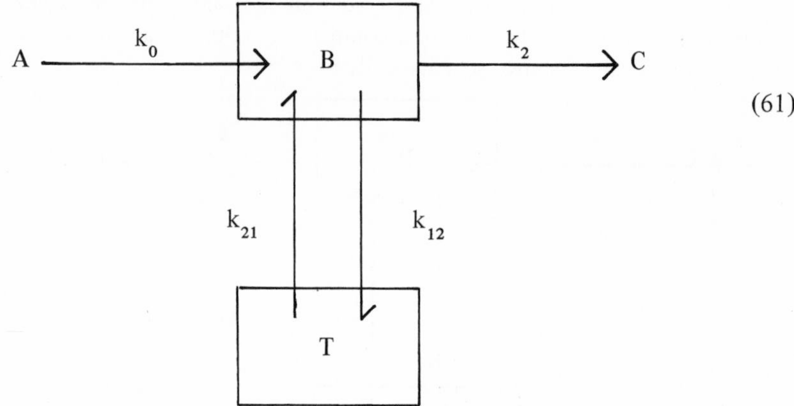

(61)

where k_0 is the zero-order rate constant for supply from the intravenous solution. Infusion allows the maintenance of a constant drug concentration in both blood and tissues. This can be used to advantage in designing pharmacokinetic experiments, since the steady-state body concentration provides a convenient device for accurate calculation of such parameters as clearance values or for obtaining data under capacity-limited and non-capacity-limited conditions. The influence of mode of administration on distribution may be quite significant, however, and should be taken into account when evaluating experimental data.

Figure 15 illustrates some typical blood level curves for a variety of infusion rates. After the infusion has been in effect for roughly five half-lives, the plasma level becomes constant. This stage will be referred to as the infusion steady state. At infusion steady state, as is shown in Appendix B,

$$k_0 = k_2 P_{inf} V_p = k_2 P'_{inf} \tag{62}$$

or the rate at which drug enters the body is equal to the rate at which it is removed. Rearranging Eq. (62), the plasma concentration at steady state is given by

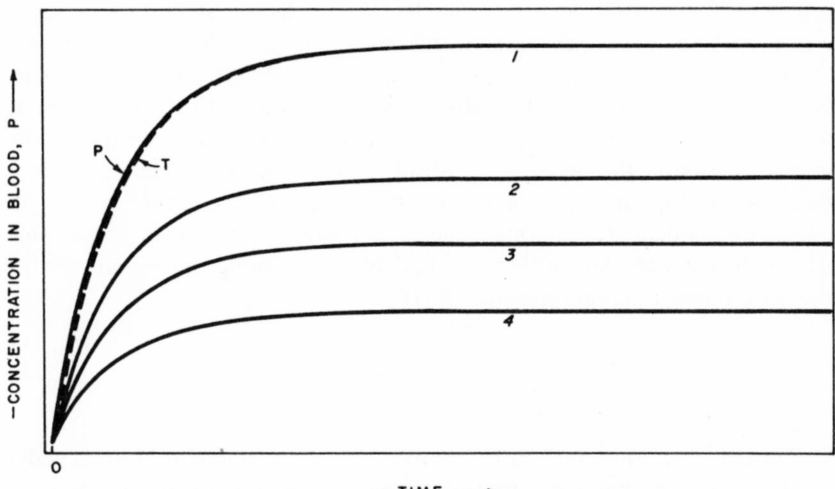

Fig. 15. Steady-state blood levels achieved by constant-rate intravenous infusion of drug distributed according to a two-compartment model. The steady-state levels (P_{inf}) are proportional to the infusion rates (k_0), which are (from top to bottom): 10 (curve 1), 6.6 (curve 2), 5 (curve 3), and 3.3 (curve 4). The values for the constants are $k_{12} = k_{21} = 10$, $k_2 = 1$. The steady-state ratio for the *amount* in the tissue relative to plasma is therefore $T'/P' = K = (k_{12}/k_{21}) = 1$ as shown in curve 1.

$$P_{inf} = \frac{k_0}{k_2 Vp} \qquad (63)$$

The elimination rate constant, k_2, is defined as first-order, and therefore is independent of blood concentration. Also, the volume of the central compartment, Vp, is postulated to be constant and independent of dose. Under these conditions, P_{inf} is proportional to the infusion rate.

Examination of Fig. 15 also indicates that the time to reach the maximum plasma concentration is independent of the infusion rate. It is dependent only on the $t_{1/2}$ of the drug. Approximately 95% of the steady-state value is reached after four half-lives and 99% after five half-lives.

Probably the single most important characteristic of a constant intravenous infusion is that at the steady state, a two-compartment drug behaves as a one-compartment drug. That is, for any drug, $T'/P' = k_{12}/k_{21}$, as demonstrated in Appendix B. This has several important implications which we will now examine.

First, as noted in Sec. II.B.2, the apparent volume of distribution calculated at the steady state is smaller than that obtained by the other methods if the drug in question fits a two-compartment model. It is, in fact, described by the same equation as Vd for a one-compartment model drug. In Sec. II.B.1 we have already referred to one method for determining Vd at the steady state, this being the collection of all elimination products during the infusion. This information is used to correct the amount infused for the drug lost in order to obtain the amount of drug in the body at the steady state. A variant of this procedure would be to stop the infusion during the steady state and then collect all elimination products to determine the drug content of the body at the time infusion had ceased. Still a third method for determining the amount in the body uses only plasma concentration [9,10]:

$$D_{inf} = D_0 \left(1 - \frac{\int_0^t P\,dt}{\int_0^\infty P\,dt} \right) \tag{64}$$

The integrals from time zero to t and from zero to ∞ represent the areas under the plasma level vs time curve from time zero to time t, when the infusion was stopped, and from zero until all drug was eliminated from the body. In each case, the value obtained for drug content in the body may be applied in Eq. (10) to find Vd_{inf}.

Second, β at the steady state for a two-compartment model drug is described by the equation for β for a one-compartment model. Since the supply rate equals the rate of loss, and β is defined as the overall rate constant for elimination,

$$k_0 = \beta_{inf} D_{inf} = \beta_{inf} P_{inf} Vd_{inf} \tag{65}$$

Combining with Eq. (63),

$$\beta_{inf}\, Vd_{inf} = k_2 Vp \tag{66}$$

Since $Vd_{inf} = Vp(k_{12} + k_{21})/k_{21}$ [Eq. (13)]

$$\beta_{inf} = \frac{k_2 k_{21}}{k_{12} + k_{21}} \tag{67}$$

which is equivalent to Eq. (38) in Chap. 2.

The value for β calculated from single-dose data is smaller than β_{inf} if the drug is described by a two-compartment model. This is because

$$\beta = k_2 f_p \tag{68}$$

for any model [27] in which f_p becomes constant, and, as will be discussed shortly, the fraction of drug in the central compartment, f_p, is less at infusion steady state that after a rapid injection for a multicompartment drug. It might therefore seem that the use of the usual β in Eq. (65) to calculate the infusion rate necessary to maintain a certain plasma volume would lead to an underestimation of the required k_0. However, the important term in (65) is the product of β and the volume of distribution. The product β Vd, calculated from a rapid intravenous dose, will equal k_2 Vp (as in Eq. 66). So as long as the values used were both determined by the same method the k_0 calculated will be correct.

Third, drug distribution in a two-compartment system is different during an infusion than after a single dose. As shown in the Appendix in Eq. (39a), the tissue-to-plasma ratio during the β phase after a single dose is given by

$$\left(\frac{T'}{P'}\right)_\beta = \frac{k_{12}}{k_{21} - \beta} \qquad (69)$$

Comparing this to the ratio at the steady state of an infusion, $(T'/P')_{inf} = k_{12}/k_{21}$, it is clear that

$$\left(\frac{T'}{P'}\right)_\beta > \left(\frac{T'}{P'}\right)_{inf} \qquad (70)$$

so that of the total drug in the body, the fraction present in the tissues is greater following a rapid intravenous injection than during an infusion. Gibaldi [10] reports a 1.7-fold difference in these ratios for aspirin, and the possibility of a two- to threefold difference for penicillin G. Therefore, at equal plasma concentrations, the amount of drug in the peripheral compartment might be quite different for one mode of administration as compared to the other. This change in distribution may elicit different degrees of clinical response.

Some drugs, because of limited solubility, irritation, and so on, are not suitable for rapid intravenous injection. In these cases, therefore, the values of the pharmacokinetic parameters cannot be obtained in the usual manner. Methods have been devised [39,40], however, for obtaining the various rate constants and the apparent volume of distribution from blood concentration curves obtained after cessation of the infusion. It should be noted that the parameters obtained in this way, including β and Vd, are the same as those obtained after rapid administration.

Sample Problem 9

A drug was given by intravenous injection and the following rate constants were determined: $k_{12} = 0.80\ hr^{-1}$, $k_{21} = 0.60\ hr^{-1}$, $k_2 = 0.40\ hr^{-1}$, and $\beta = 0.14\ hr^{-1}$. What is T'/P' after a single dose and during an infusion?

Solution: Since $k_{12} + k_{21} = 3.5/\ k_2$, this appears to be a two-compartment model. Therefore, after an injection $(T'/P')_\beta$ is given by Eq. (69):

$$\left(\frac{T'}{P'}\right)_\beta = 0.80/0.46$$

$$\left(\frac{T'}{P'}\right)_\beta = 1.7$$

During the steady state of an infusion,

$$\left(\frac{T'}{P'}\right)_{inf} = \frac{0.80}{0.60}$$

$$\left(\frac{T'}{P'}\right)_{inf} = 1.3$$

Practice Problem 9

Following rapid I.V. injection, the parameters for a group of related drugs were obtained as shown in Table 8.

Table 8

Pharmacokinetic Parameters

Drug	$t_{1/2}$ (hr)	Vd (%V/W)
W	1.0	12.9
X	0.7	13.6
Y	0.5	16.4
Z	0.4	18.6

(a) In each case, what rate of infusion is needed to maintain a plasma concentration of 10 mg% in a 70-kg man?
Answer: W, 630 mg/hr; X, 950 mg/hr; Y, 1,600 mg/hr; Z, 2,250 mg/hr

(b) After the infusion is started, in what order will they reach their steady-state concentration in the blood (first to last)?
Answer: Z, Y, X, W

REFERENCES

1. J. K. Seydel, Sulfonamides, Structure-Activity Relationships and Mode of Action, *J. Pharm. Sci.*, *57*, 1455 (1968).
2. M. Gibaldi, R. Nagashima, and G. Levy, Relationship Between Drug Concentration in Plasma or Serum and Amount of Drug in the Body, *J. Pharm. Sci.*, *58*, 193 (1969).
3. W. A. Ritschel, Biological Half-lives of Drugs, *Drug Intel. Clin. Pharm.*, *4*, 332 (1970).
4. J. G. Wagner, Pharmacokinetics, in *Annual Reviews of Pharmacology*, Vol. 8, (H. W. Elliot, ed.), Annual Reviews, Inc., Palo Alto, Calif., 1968, pp. 85-86.

5. L. Z. Benet and R. A. Ronfeld, Volume Terms in Pharmacokinetics, *J. Pharm. Sci., 58*, 639 (1969).
6. R. Dominguez, Kinetics of Elimination, Absorption and Volume of Distribution in the Organism, in *Medical Physics,* Vol. II (O. Glasser, ed.), Year Book Publishers, Chicago, Ill., 1950, pp. 476–489.
7. J. G. Wagner and J. I. Northram. Estimation of Volume of Distribution and Half-life of a Compound After Rapid Intravenous Injection, *J. Pharm. Sci., 56*, 529 (1967).
8. D. S. Riggs, *The Mathematical Approach to Physiological Problems*, Williams and Wilkins Co., Baltimore, Md., 1963, pp. 193–214.
9. S. Riegelman, J. Loo, and M. Rowland, Concept of a Volume of Distribution and Possible Errors in Evaluation of this Parameter, *J. Pharm. Sci., 57*, 128 (1968).
10. M. Gibaldi, Effect of Mode of Administration on Drug Distribution in a Two-compartment Open System, *J. Pharm. Sci., 58*, 327 (1969).
11. M. Gibaldi and D. Perrier, Drug Distribution and Renal Failure, *J. Clin. Pharmacol., 12*, 201 (1972).
12. M. Gibaldi and D. Perrier, Drug Elimination and Apparent Volume of Distribution in Multicompartment Systems, *J. Pharm. Sci., 61*, 952 (1972).
13. M. Gibaldi and M. Schwartz, Apparent Effect of Probenecid on the Distribution of Penicillins in Man, *Clin. Pharmacol. Ther., 9*, 345 (1968).
14. L. Hollister and G. Levy, Some Aspects of Salicylate Distribution and Metabolism in Man, *J. Pharm. Sci., 54*, 1126 (1965).
15. H. B. Kostenbauder, J. B. Portnoff, and J. V. Swintosky, Control of Urine pH and Its Effect on Sulfaethidole Excretion in Humans, *J. Pharm. Sci., 51*, 1084 (1962).
16. R. H. Reuning and L. S. Schanker, Effect of Carbon Tetrachloride-induced Liver Damage on Hepatic Transport of Ouabain in the Rat, *J. Pharmacol. Exp. Therap., 78*, 589 (1971).
17. H. Remmer, The Role of the Liver in Drug Metabolism, *Am. J. Med., 49*, 617 (1970).
18. R. L. Smith, The Biliary Excretion and Enterohepatic Circulation of Drugs and Other Organic Compounds, *Fortschr. Arzneim.-Forsch., 9*, 299 (1966).
19. L. S. Schanker, Secretion of Organic Compounds in Bile, in *Handbook of Physiology–Alimentary Canal*, American Physiological Society, Washington, D.C., 1968, pp. 2433–2449.
20. R. R. Scheline, Drug Metabolism by Intestinal Microorganisms, *J. Pharm. Sci., 57*, 2021 (1968).
21. D. A. P. Evans, Individual Variations of Drug Metabolism as a Factor in Drug Toxicity, *Ann N.Y. Acad. Sci., 123*, 178 (1965).
22. C. Capellos and B. H. J. Bielski, *Kinetic Systems, Mathematical Description of Chemical Kinetics in Solution*, Wiley-Interscience, New York, 1972, pp. 69–71, 73–75.
23. G. Levy, Dose Dependent Effects in Pharmacokinetics, in *Importance of Fundamental Principles in Drug Evaluation* (D. H. Tedeschi and R. E. Tedeschi, eds.), Raven Press, New York, 1968, pp. 141–172.
24. G. Levy, Possibility of Simultaneous Zero- and First-order Kinetics in the

In Vivo Formation of a Single Drug Metabolite, *J. Pharm. Sci., 55*, 989 (1966).

25. G. Levy, Pharmacokinetics of Salicylate Elimination in Man, *J. Pharm. Sci., 54*, 959 (1965).
26. G. Levy, Evidence for Nonfirst-order Kinetics of Salicylate Elimination–A Rebuttal, *J. Pharm. Sci., 56*, 1044 (1967).
27. R. Nagashima, G. Levy, and R. A. O'Reilly, Comparative Pharmacokinetics of Coumarin Anticoagulants IV. Application of a Three-Compartmental Model to the Analysis of the Dose-dependent Kinetics of Bishydroxycoumarin Elimination, *J. Pharm. Sci., 57*, 1888 (1968).
28. P. G. Dayton, S. A. Cucinell, M. Weiss, and J. M. Perel, Dose Dependence of Drug Plasma Level Decline in Dogs, *J. Pharmacol. Exp. Therap., 158*, 305 (1967).
29. G. Levy, Hydroxylated Metabolites as Inhibitors of Drug Biotransformation and Their Possible Role in Dose Dependent Elimination Kinetics, Abstracts, A.Ph.A. Academy of Pharmaceutical Sciences 13th National Meeting, Chicago, Ill., *2*, 179 (1972).
30. R. Nagashima, G. Levy, and E. J. Sarcione, Comparative Pharmacokinetics of Coumarin Anticoagulants III. Factors Affecting the Distribution and Elimination of Bishydroxycoumarin (BHC) in Isolated Liver Perfusion Studies, *J. Pharm. Sci., 57*, 1881 (1968).
31. J. G. Wagner, Design of Clinical Studies to Assess Physiological Availability, *Drug Inf. Bull.*, Jan./June, *45* (1969).
32. J. Wagner and E. Nelson, Per Cent Absorbed Time Plots Derived from Blood Level and/or Urinary Excretion Data, *J. Pharm. Sci., 52*, 610 (1963).
33. J. C. K. Loo and S. Riegelman, New Method for Calculating the Intrinsic Absorption Rate of Drugs, *J. Pharm. Sci., 57*, 918 (1968).
34. R. Dominguez and E. Pomerene, Calculation of the Rate of Absorption of Exogenous Creatinine, *Proc. Soc. Exp. Biol. Med., 60*, 173 (1945).
35. E. Nelson and I. Schaldemose, Urinary Excretion Kinetics for Evaluation of Drug Absorption I. Solution Rate Limited and Non-solution Rate Limited Absorption, *J. Am. Pharm. Assoc. Sci. Ed., 49*, 437 (1960).
36. L. Z. Benet and C-W. N. Chiang, The Use and Application of Deconvolution Methods in Pharmacokinetics, Abstracts, A.Ph.A. Academy of Pharmaceutical Sciences 13th National Meeting, Chicago, Ill., *2*, 169 (1972).
37. J. T. Doluisio, J. C. LaPiana, and L. W. Dittert, Pharmacokinetics of Ampicillin Trihydrate, Sodium Ampicillin and Sodium Dicloxacillin Following Intramuscular Injection, *J. Pharm. Sci., 60*, 715 (1971).
38. R. E. Notari, J. L. DeYoung, and R. H. Reuning, Effect of Parallel First-order Drug Loss from Site of Administration on Calculated Values for Absorption Rate Constants, *J. Pharm. Sci., 61*, 135 (1972).
39. M. Gibaldi, Estimation of the Pharmacokinetic Parameters of the Two-compartment Open Model from Post-infusion Plasma Concentration Data, *J. Pharm. Sci., 58*, 1133 (1969).
40. J. C. K. Loo and S. Riegelman, Assessment of Pharmacokinetic Constants from Postinfusion Blood Curves Obtained After I.V. Infusion, *J. Pharm. Sci., 59*, 53 (1970).

Chapter 4

BIOPHARMACEUTICS: CLINICAL APPLICATIONS OF PHARMACOKINETIC PARAMETERS

I. INTRODUCTION

A. Biopharmaceutics and Therapy

In the broadest sense of the word, biopharmaceutics may be said to deal with the problem of controlling the therapeutic effect of a drug when it is being administered to the patient. The degree of success achieved by the use of a drug product may be limited by the patient's diet, the co-administration of other drugs, inert ingredients in the dosage form, the dosage regimen, the route of administration, the physical or chemical state of the drug within the dosage form, or the improper choice or use of a particular dosage form of the drug. The safe and effective use of medicinal agents is based upon their degree of predictability with regard to the overall interaction between the patient and the drug at the time of use. The partial list of variables mentioned above are potentially capable of influencing the time profile for the drug concentration at the active site. Unsatisfactory therapeutic effects may thus result from a decrease in the total amount of drug released from the depot into the bloodstream or from the rate at which the drug transfer process takes place. In order to achieve optimum results with a therapeutic agent, the factors affecting its bioavailability time profile and its distribution–elimination pattern must be defined and clinically controlled. Thus it is suggested here that the rational choice and administration of a drug product cannot be separated from the biopharmaceutical properties of a given drug. This approach to the rational use of drug products is a natural outcome of the use of pharmacokinetic parameters in the design and evaluation of dosage forms. For if the developer has indeed examined the critical factors involving the bioavailability of the drug from the dosage form, then it is an exercise in futility if the clinician ignores these principles when the product is employed in therapy.

B. The Drug and the Dosage Form

It would be wise at this point to clarify some of the terms which might at first appear disarmingly obvious to the reader. This chapter does not deal in any way with the choice of a chemotherapeutic agent. Pharmacokinetic aspects of that decision are found in Chap. 5. Information dealing with particular therapeutic considerations might best be found under the realm of pharmacology. This chapter concerns dosage-form design and the clinical use of that product once the specific drug has been chosen. Many drugs are available in a variety of products and dosage forms. Which form should be employed in a particular case and how is it best used? Biopharmaceutics addresses itself to that question. In the narrowest sense of the word, biopharmaceutics may be defined as the effect of the dosage form and its administration on the biological effects of the drug. In this case the term dosage form is not limited to such categories as capsules, tablets, elixirs, and so on. We consider the drug to be the basic chemical structure of the chemotherapeutic agent. Everything else that is done by way of modification of that chemical entity in order to put it to clinical use is included in our definition of dosage form. Thus dosage form considerations for a given drug include:

1. Particle size of the drug
2. Chemical nature of the drug, such as salt, free acid or base, ester, complex, and so on.
3. Physical state of the drug, such as crystalline, amorphous, hydrate, polymorph, and so on.
4. Inert ingredients, such as diluents, buffers, disintegrating agents, excipients, and so on.
5. The type of dosage form in the more traditional sense, such as tablets, enteric coated tablets, suppositories, syrups, and so on.

Thus there exists a rather wide spectrum of choices in order for pharmaceutical product development to arrive at a marketed dosage form of a given drug.

The clinician is faced with still greater problems in drug usage in addition to those associated with the choice of a route of administration and a particular dosage form for that route. Patients often take several drugs simultaneously. The effects of co-administration of other agents along with the possible complicating factors of diet and the influence of the disease state on the absorption and elimination of the drug all make the final predictability of biological response a monumental problem. This is not to infer, however, that this challenge should receive anything less than our utmost attention. It is only by addressing our efforts to this important phase of rational therapy that any progress can be made in that direction.

C. The Scope of the Chapter

This chapter contains very little new basic material. It is primarily composed of applications of the principles covered in Chaps. 2 and 3. In that respect it is an applied presentation. The application of pharmacokinetics to dosage-form design, evaluation, and use should be of interest to those involved in product development as well as to those involved in clinical pharmacy. The examples chosen for this section are taken from the literature, and the pertinent references are given. However, it is not the objective of this presentation to review the literature in the field. The cases chosen were used merely as illustrations. The number of examples is by no means exhaustive, and many other samples could have been used to illustrate the same points. The primary goal of this chapter is to place the principles of pharmacokinetics in a framework of practicality or utility with respect to those involved in the use, design, or testing of dosage forms.

II. BLOOD LEVEL CURVES

A. Compartmental Analysis

Compartmental schemes are generally made by fitting kinetic models to blood and urine time courses. The concentration-time profile for drug in the blood and tissues is thus illustrated as the net result of several rate processes which are influenced by many physicochemical in vivo factors. The control of these factors and the resultant pharmacokinetic pattern is of ultimate importance if one is to control clinical results.

An alteration in any one of the rate processes shown in Scheme I will be reflected in the blood level curve. Thus, the plasma concentration-time profile for a drug described by this compartmental model can vary in shape because of

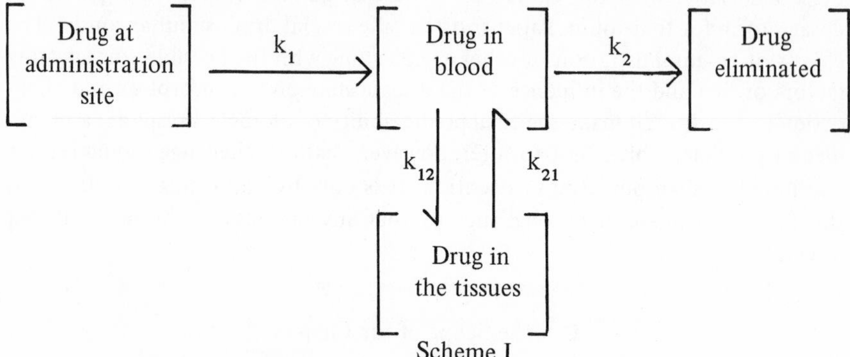

Scheme I

variations in: (a) absorption rate constant (k_1), (b) rate of metabolism, (c) rate of urinary excretion, (d) amount available from the site of administration, (e) the distribution of drug between blood and tissues. Each of these variables will show a unique effect on the blood level pattern. These patterns will be considered individually in the following sections.

B. Comparing Different Curves for One Drug

First, let us consider how one might obtain different blood level patterns from administration of the same drug. As noted in Chap. 3, either k_1 or the bioavailable dose (or both) may vary. This case may be illustrated by using different routes of administration or by administering different forms of the same drug by one route (e.g., salt, free acid or base, amorphous, crystalline, etc.). Since we are considering one given drug, the rate constants for elimination, k_2, and distribution, k_{12} and k_{21}, will remain constant. As the rate constant for supply is increased for a given drug, the peak value is increased and the time to achieve this value is decreased. See Fig. 6, Chap. 3 for an example.

In spite of the dramatic differences in the shapes of such curves, the area under each curve from t_0 to t_∞ is identical provided that equal amounts of the drug were released into the bloodstream and only the rate of release varied. The identical areas under the curves can be used to demonstrate that equal doses of the drug were supplied from the depot. When the rate constant for supply of drug from the depot to the blood is the only rate constant subject to change, then the area under the plasma concentration-vs-time curves is proportional to the total amount available to the blood. Thus, increasing the rate of supply of a given drug increases the peak height and the speed with which the peak height is attained while decreasing the total time during which there is drug in the blood. It does not affect the area under the curve.

The amount which arrives in the bloodstream from the depot may vary due to some physical or chemical interaction of the drug at the site of administration or due to variation in the dose administered. Figure 8 of Chap. 3 is a typical pattern for five different doses of the same drug. In this example absorption rate constants have been kept constant. Since we are considering a single drug with fixed rate constants, the areas under the curves are proportional to the dose. That is, the ratio of the areas under those curves is in direct proportion to the bioavailable dose.

C. Comparing Different Drugs

By way of contrast, let us now examine the blood level curves when only the rate constant for elimination is changed. Figure 1 illustrates four examples where the absorption rate constant and the distribution constants k_{12} and k_{21} are held constant. The rate constant for total elimination by all routes, k_2, has been set at 1 in curve 1, 2 in curve 2, 4 in curve 3, and 10 in curve 4. Thus, the rate constant for elimination has been varied through a factor of ten. Since the rate of output of drug from the body is increased in going from curve 1 to curve 4, the blood level peak decreases. Also, the time required to clear the blood of drug

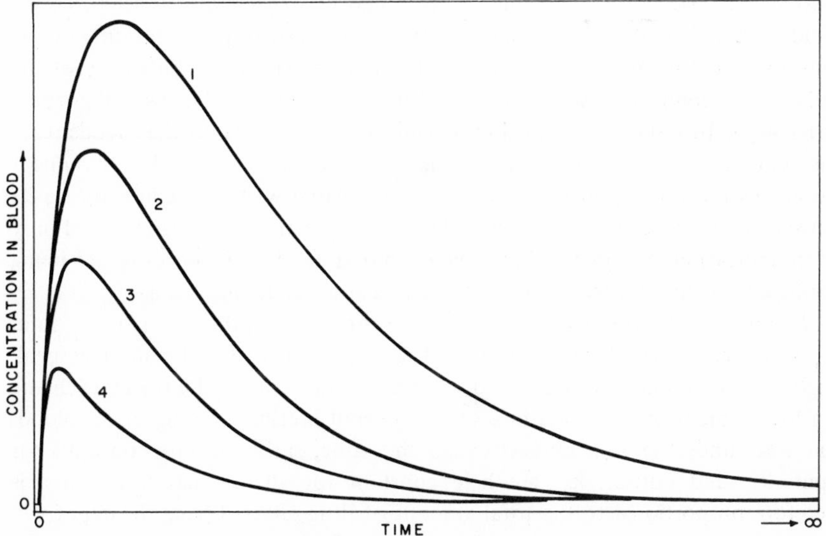

Fig. 1. Effect of increasing the elimination rate constant. The values for k_2 in Scheme I (from top to bottom) are 1 (curve 1), 2 (curve 2), 4 (curve 3) and 10 (curve 4). Other rate constants are held constant at $k_1 = 1$ and $k_{12} = k_{21} = 2$.

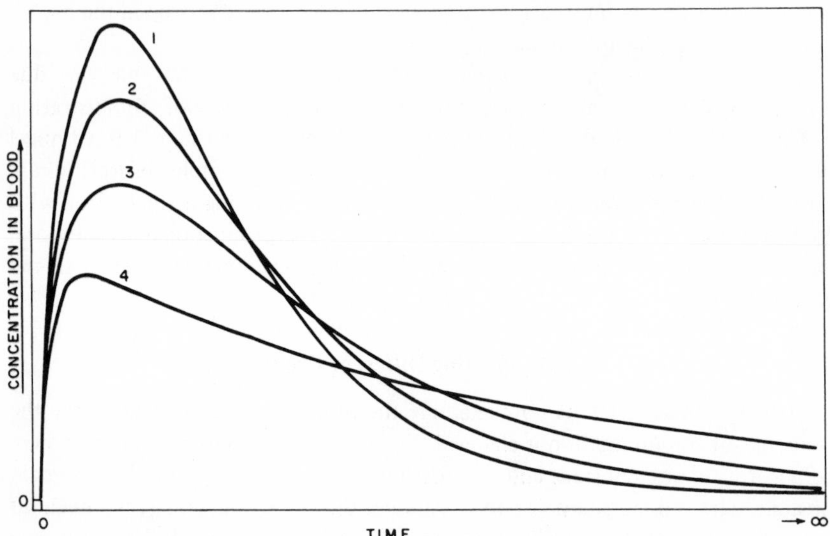

Fig. 2. Effect of distribution on time course for drug in blood. The rate constants k_{12} and k_{21} have been given the values (from top to bottom): 1, 4 (curve 1); 2, 3 (curve 2); 3, 2 (curve 3); and 4, 1 (curve 4). Other rate constants are held constant at $k_1 = k_2 = 1$.

content decreases with increasing k_2, as would be expected. This set of curves could reflect four different drugs with the same distribution constants or the same drug in four different subjects with some variation in the ability of the biological system to dispose of the drug (e.g., kidney damage or enzyme deficiency). In either case, the bioavailable dose delivered to the bloodstream was kept the same in all four cases. It is therefore obvious that the areas under the curves are not proportional to the dose released when the elimination rate constant is not held constant. Thus, the areas under the curves can be used only as an indication of bioavailability when blood levels for one drug are being compared and the elimination rate constant is not undergoing change.

Figure 2 shows the resulting blood level curves where the values for k_{12} and k_{21} were varied. The higher the ratio of k_{21}/k_{12}, the higher the observed peak height. Since elimination occurs from the blood rather than the tissues (Scheme I) a higher blood level results in a shorter overall lifetime of drug in the blood. The areas under all four curves remain the same, since the rate constants for input, k_1, and output, k_2, are held constant for all four cases. The area is therefore proportional to the total amount of drug released from the depot. No simple trend describing the time for reaching the peak height is evident, since curves 1, 2, and 3 are about equal, whereas curve 4 reaches its peak in roughly one-half the time of the others. In comparison to k_1 and k_2, the time to reach the peak is relatively insensitive to changes in the values of k_{12} and k_{21}.

D. Relationship to Biological Response

The previous section has described the effect of changing several rate processes in Scheme I upon the shape of blood level curves. We are concerned with blood level patterns because generally only the blood and urine compartments are accessible, and the concentration of intact drug and metabilites are therefore determined in these compartments. Figure 3 illustrates the fraction of the initial dose in each compartment in Scheme I following an extravascular administration of drug. A figure such as this could be constructed from actual biological data representing assays for blood and urine. By fitting these data to the model in Scheme I, one can then generate curves for the tissue and the fraction remaining at the site of administration. This represents the general approach of pharmacokinetics, where the concern is to account for the drug within the body at all times and to relate this distribution to the pharmacological responses. The approach, therefore, allows one to distinguish between differences in intrinsic activities of drugs and differences in their ability to reach the site of action.

Let us begin with the assumption that the intensity of the pharmacological activity is a function of the concentration of drug at the site of action. We will also be realistic in our assumption and state that the site of action is either unknown or, if known, inaccessible to the analyst except by sacrifice of the subject. That is, we cannot directly determine a dose-response curve based upon the concentration of drug which is actually at the site of action. Assuming that this site of action is not in the blood itself, Scheme I shows that drug in the blood diffuses reversibly into the tissues where the site is located. This is not to

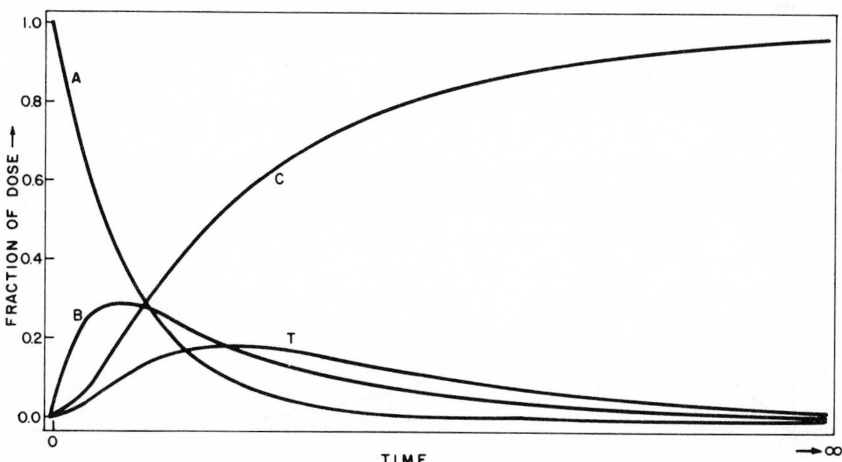

Fig. 3. The fraction of the dose in each compartment of Scheme I as a function of time. In this illustration the rate constants have the values $k_1 = k_2 = 3$ and $k_{12} = k_{21} = 2$.

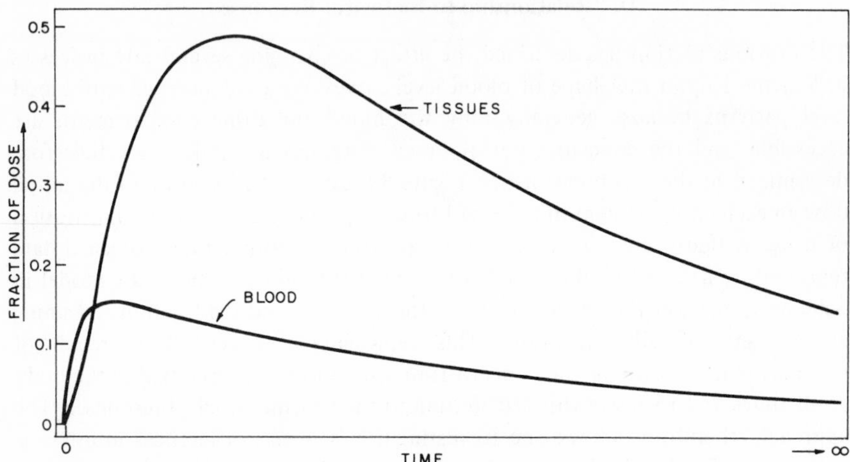

Fig. 4. The fraction of the dose in the blood and tissue compartments of Scheme I as a function of time. This corresponds to curve 4 in Fig. 2, where $k_1 = k_2 = k_{21} = 1$ and $k_{12} = 4$.

say that the site is assumed here to be in a particular tissue, but only that it is somewhere outside of the bloodstream. It follows, then, that the concentration at the site corresponds to some concentration in the blood. This is illustrated in Figs. 4 and 5. These figures serve to illustrate how the distribution of a drug can affect its tissue concentration and thus its concentration at the site. A

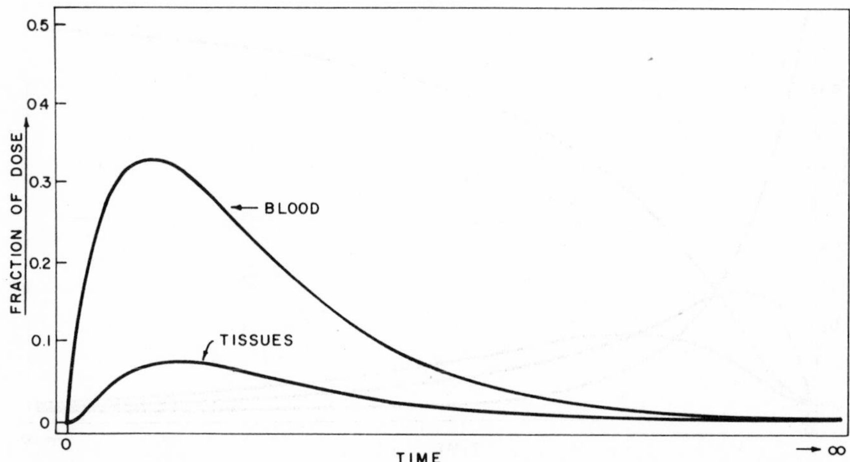

Fig. 5. The fraction of the dose in the blood and tissue compartments of Scheme I as a function of time. This corresponds to curve 1 in Fig. 2, where $k_1 = k_2 = k_{12} = 1$ and $k_{21} = 4$.

pharmacological test without the knowledge of this difference might attribute the increased biological activity of the drug in Fig. 4 to its receptor site interaction. Recognizing that it is not the concentration in the blood per se that is responsible for the pharmacological activity, it may still be possible to define dose responses based on blood levels which have some relationship to the concentration at the site of action.

Since the concentration in the blood is readily accessible, it is often convenient as well as appropriate to relate blood concentration and response. These criteria being satisfied, one can define a number of characteristics related to the dosage regimen. Consider, as an example, the three blood level curves given in Fig. 6, all of which have been constructed based on Scheme I, using the same dosage and elimination rate constant for all three cases. We can thus define several parameters based on the blood concentration, which will allow us to compare these curves.

1. Minimum Effective Dose.

The minimum effective dose may be defined as the minimum dose required to achieve the desired therapeutic effect. Assuming that this represents a minimum effective concentration at the site of action, the corresponding blood concentration can be determined by appropriate dose-response experiments. In this way a

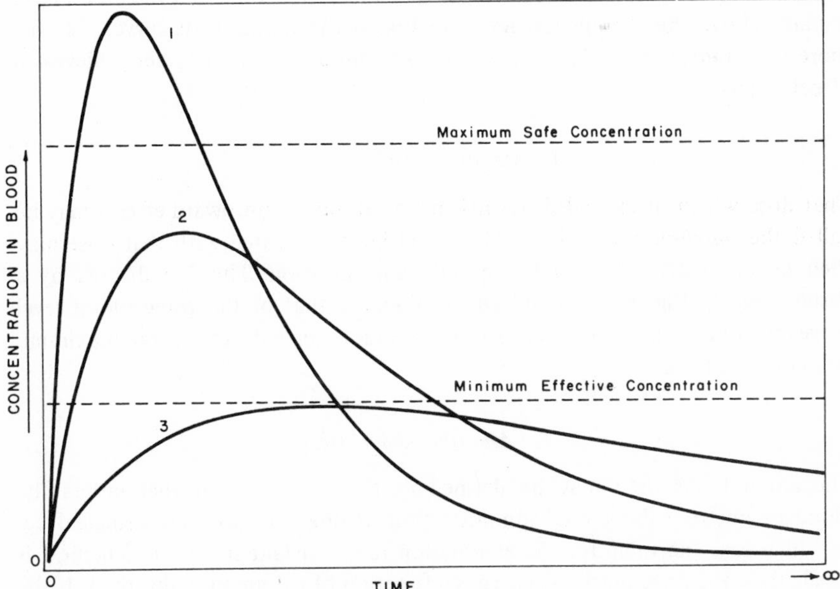

Fig. 6. Three time profiles for drug in blood following equal extravascular doses where elimination (k_2) is identical in all three cases.

minimum effective blood concentration can be defined as that concentration corresponding to the desired therapeutic effect. In Fig. 6 the minimum effective concentration is indicated by a dashed line. Thus, we can observe that curves 1 and 2 achieve therapeutic results, while curve 3 dose not. Since the bioavailable doses and elimination rate constants are equal in all three cases, either the absorption rate constant or the distribution of the drugs (or both) have been altered. Thus, curves 1, 2, and 3 might represent administration of three forms of the same drug or the same forms from three administration sites where the absorption rate has affected the blood level pattern. Once the minimum effective concentration has been defined, it is possible to define additional parameters on this basis.

2. *Onset.*

The onset may now be defined as the amount of time required to achieve the minimum effective concentration following administration of the dosage form. Thus, we can observe in Fig. 6 that the onset of curve 1 is less than curve 2 and that the onset of curve 3 is nonexistent as it never achieves an effective level. The onset of curve 2 is approximately three times longer than that of curve 1.

3. *Duration.*

The duration of action may be defined as the length of time that the blood level remains above the therapeutic level. In Fig. 6 the duration of curve 2 is 30% more than that of curve 1, and curve 3 has no duration since it never achieves an effective level.

4. *Maximum Safe Dose.*

That dose which, if exceeded, results in side effects or untoward effects may be called the *maximum safe dose*. The blood level associated with that dose may then be defined as the maximum safe concentration. This is indicated by a dashed line in Fig. 6. Thus, it can be observed that of the three blood level curves illustrated in Fig. 6, curve 1 is not desirable since it exceeds the maximum safe concentration.

5. *Amount Absorbed.*

The amount absorbed may be defined as the total amount that enters the bloodstream from the site of administration. If one is considering a single drug, in which case the value for the elimination rate constant shown in Scheme I is fixed, then the area under the curve is a function of the amount absorbed. If the amount absorbed in each case is equal and the absorption rate constant varies, then the areas under the curves will be equal. In this case the shape of the curves would be a reflection of the differences between the absorption rate constants rather than the amount absorbed.

Although it may not be readily apparent in Fig. 6 (because all of curves 2 and 3 are not shown), each curve has the same area. Each dose of the drug was absorbed 100% in creating this figure and k_2 was held constant. Thus, a drug may be absorbed 100% and still be inactive as in the case of curve 3. Alternatively, it may show complete absorption and fast onset but decreased duration and increased side effects such as in curve 1. Figure 6 is hypothetical, but it could easily apply to three different formulations of tablets taken orally by humans. A striking similarity to this figure has been shown by Breimer [1], who administered 600 mg of hexobarbital to humans (in order of reference to curves 1, 2, and 3 in Fig. 6) as: sodium salt orally in capsules, free acid orally in tablets, and the sodium salt in rectal suppositories.

E. Caution in Comparing Curves

While plots such as Fig. 6 can be used to compare the relative availability of a given drug from several dosage forms, such plots cannot be indiscriminately used to compare different drugs. One has only to consider Scheme I to realize the many factors which can affect the blood pattern when more than one drug is considered. For example, we can list the following parameters which can result in alteration of the appearances of blood level curves from two drugs:

1. Differences in supply rate or amount
2. Different rates of metabolism
3. Different rates of excretion
4. Different rates of distribution
5. Different distribution pattern or differences in their relative volumes of distribution
6. Differences in binding phenomena

In this chapter we will consider the first factor. All of the remaining factors in the above list will be considered in Chap. 5. Indeed, the study of these factors and of their significance in the design and evaluation of drugs and drug products serves as the justification for studying pharmacokinetics.

III. ABSORPTION OF DRUGS FROM THE GASTROINTESTINAL TRACT

A. Absorption Processes

1. Passive Diffusion Through the Gastrointestinal Wall

Drugs pass from the gastrointestinal (g.i.) tract into the bloodstream primarily by passive diffusion. Few drugs are actively absorbed, and these will be discussed later. The absorption of drugs by passive transport will thus be a function of the concentration gradient between the gastrointestinal tract and the blood. A drug moves from the gastrointestinal tract into the bloodstream because diffusion occurs from a region of high concentration to that of a lower concentration. This point has been dramatically illustrated by the demonstration that drugs administered parenterally are secreted into the gastric juice [2]. Although we are accustomed to thinking about drugs passing from the stomach into the blood, this experiment reminds us that passive transport is described by the principles of physical chemistry and that the rate and direction of mass transport from one side of a membrane to the other is due entirely to the concentration gradient of the diffusing species.

Since this gradient refers to the diffusing species only, we must define what kind of chemical entities can in fact permeate this membrane. The gastrointestinal membrane is composed of a lipoidal sheet covered on both sides by protein, oriented perpendicularly to the cell surface and having frequent water-filled pores of about 4 Å in radius. There are relatively few substances capable of passing from the g.i. tract into the blood by the pore route. Small atoms such as K^+ and Cl^- will fit through these openings, and they may be carried through the membrane by water passing through the pores—creating what is sometimes called solvent drag. Drugs, however, are generally large molecules with molecular weights in excess of 100. They are therefore too large to permeate these pores. Since the membrane is lipoidal in nature, it is believed that drugs undergo a partitioning process from the aqueous gastrointestinal fluids into the oleaginous membrane. After diffusion through the membrane, they then partition from the membrane into the aqueous blood and tissue fluids. This concept of absorption by an oil/water partitioning process is generally attributed to Hobgen et al. [3] about 1957. In general we will assume that drugs are passively absorbed and that their absorption is related to their ability to leave the aqueous fluids of the gastrointestinal tract, partition into the g.i. membrane, and finally into the blood. For the purpose of our discussions we will use the following model for the g.i. membrane. We shall think of the membrane as being composed of a continuous layer of mineral oil with a number of small water-filled channels of a size much smaller than the drugs themselves. This is not meant to be a physiological model, but rather an oversimplified reference state that will prove helpful in making predictions regarding the permeability of organic molecules.

2. *pH-partition Theory*

Figures 1, 4, and 5 in Chap. 2 are actually illustrations of drug transfer by passive diffusion in agreement with the pH-partition theory. It might be helpful to the reader to reread those sections in Chap. 2 before proceeding with the present chapter.

In its simplest terms this theory can be described as follows. Keeping our model of the g.i. membrane in mind, one would predict that uncharged drug molecules would permeate this membrane with more facility than charged species. That is, neutral species would be expected to be more soluble in mineral oil than ionic species. If a drug can exist in two forms, such as HA and A^- or RNH_2 and RNH_3^+, one would expect the absorption process to occur predominantly through the neutral form. Although the pH-partition theory is generally attributed to Schanker [4], there has been evidence for such behavior in the literature for some time [5]. An intriguing demonstration of this principle was carried out by Travell in 1940 [6]. When the pH of the stomach of experimental animals was kept low, there were no toxic effects from large doses of alkaloids. However, when the stomach contents were made alkaline, the animals died rapidly. Thus the gastrointestinal membrane was shown to be permeable to the neutral form of the alkaloid and relatively impermeable to the ionic species.

$$\frac{RNH_3^+}{\text{Not absorbed}} \quad \underset{H^+}{\overset{OH^-}{\rightleftharpoons}} \quad \frac{RNH_2}{\text{Absorbed}} \tag{1}$$

There is probably general agreement that a drug will be absorbed primarily as the neutral form if it is capable of existing as two species. There is another facet to the pH-partition theory, however, that seems to be qualitatively correct although not always quantitatively accurate. This principle is concerned with the prediction of relative rates or amounts of absorption by comparing the partition coefficients of the drugs in question. The apparent partition coefficient, K_{app}, may be expressed as the ratio of the equilibrium concentration of drug that is distributed between two immiscible solvents,

$$K_{app} = \left(\frac{\text{Concentration in solvent 1}}{\text{Concentration in solvent 2}}\right)_{equil} \tag{2}$$

There is no convention regarding which solvent appears in the numerator or the denominator. In considering drug absorption, the partition coefficient is often expressed in terms of the ratio of the concentration in the nonaqueous phase to that in the aqueous phase. For our model membrane the coefficient K_{app} might be expressed as the ratio of the drug concentration in mineral oil to the drug concentration in water, where the system involving an oil–water interface has been allowed to achieve equilibrium. Equation (2) would adequately describe a system where the drug exists as a monomer in both the aqueous and the oleaginous phase. It is important to realize that the partition coefficient will be constant only when it truly reflects the species that is in equilibrium between the phases. This is similar to our considerations regarding Fick's law and the concentration gradient of the species common to both sides of the barrier. The true partition coefficient, then, is the ratio of the concentration of the species common to both solvents. For example, if the drug undergoes dimerization in the oil phase so that

$$D_{H_2O} \rightleftharpoons D_{oil} + D_{oil} \rightleftharpoons (D_{oil})_2 \quad (3)$$

the partition coefficient reflecting the equilibrium concentration ratios of the monomeric species,

$$K = \frac{D_{oil}}{D_{H_2O}} \quad (4)$$

would be a constant whereas the apparent partition coefficient, K_{app}, defined in Eq. (2) would vary with total drug concentration since the association constant, K_a, is defined by

$$K_a = \frac{(D_{oil})_2}{(D_{oil})^2} \quad (5)$$

and therefore the apparent partition coefficient becomes

$$K_{app} = K(1 + 2K_a D_{oil}) \quad (6)$$

There have been a significant number of attempts to correlate the relative partition coefficients between nonaqueous solvents and water with the relative absorbability from the gastrointestinal tract for certain series of drugs such as barbituates, sulfonamides, and so on. Although there is an apparent relationship between g.i. absorption and partition coefficients of drugs in such solvent systems as chloroform/water, it is by no means a completely reliable concept from a quantitative standpoint. For the purpose of the present chapter we will accept the premise that increasing the oil/water partition coefficient of a given drug will increase its gastrointestinal absorption, although we will not presume that there is necessarily a linear relationship between the absorption values and the K values.

Earlier the problem of establishing a meaningful number for the partition coefficient of a drug relative to its actual distributive behavior between the g.i. membrane and the aqueous g.i. fluids was discussed. This may not be the only obstacle to establishing a dependable method for predicting absorption of drugs based on their partition coefficients. One problem may reside in the fact that the partition coefficient is an equilibrium value and the membrane concentration of drug may never be in an equilibrium state but rather in a steady state due to loss of drug at the systemic side. We cannot even be entirely predictive regarding the types of organic molecules which are capable of being absorbed. Although one may predict that a molecule existing as both an ion and a neutral species will be primarily absorbed in the noncharged form, there are many quaternary drugs which exist only as cations that are still absorbed. In spite of the limitations outlined here we can still make some practical use of the pH-partition theory, as will be demonstrated throughout this chapter.

3. *Active Transport Through the Gastrointestinal Wall*

Most drugs are absorbed by passive diffusion and their transport is therefore characterized by the factors outlined in Chap. 2. However, some drugs are absorbed by active transport mechanisms. The characteristics of such a transport system were also described in Chap. 2. The carrier system may be an enzyme or some other component of the g.i. wall, and each carrier is generally concentrated in a specific segment of the g.i. tract. The substrate for that carrier will be preferentially absorbed in the location of highest carrier density. For example, more riboflavin is absorbed from the proximal portion of the small intestine than from the large intestine or upper intestine. Some studies have indicated better vitamin B_{12} absorption in the lower small intestine. Drugs such as 5-fluorouracil and 5-bromouracil are actively absorbed—presumably in the same manner as uracil itself, which is absorbed by the pyrimidine transport system. Several substances which are essential to the body, such as vitamins, minerals such as iron, bile salts, amino acids, and monosaccharides, are actively absorbed. In some cases the level of activity of the carrier system has been thought to reflect directly the body's immediate need for the particular substrate. Drugs absorbed by active mechanisms most likely compete with the natural substrates for the active site in the transport system.

B. Absorption of Drugs from Solutions

1. *Rate-determining Step*

The fastest rate of absorption by the oral route can generally be achieved by administering a solution of the drug. Thus if one is concerned primarily with onset of action, the drug would best be administered in the form of an elixir, syrup, or aqueous solution. For a neutral drug the rate-determining step would simply be the passive transfer of drug from the g.i. fluids through the g.i. wall to the systemic circulation. In this case the process should be relatively independent of the position in the g.i. tract, since we have limited the example to passive absorption of a neutral drug. Many drugs are either general acids or general bases and are therefore influenced by the environment or the g.i. fluids. This is discussed next.

2. *pH and Gastrointestinal Absorption Sites*

Figure 7 is a schematic representation of part of the digestive tract. As noted in the figure, there is a gradual decrease in acidity in moving from the stomach to the lower intestine. The stomach varies in pH from 1 to 3.5, but pH 1 to 2.5 is probably the most common range. Stomach pH is affected by foods and can be clinically altered by administration of antacids. By comparison, the intestinal pH is relatively independent of such foreign influences. The duodenum has a pH of 5 to 6 and the lower ileum approaches a pH of 8.

This difference in pH of the g.i. fluids can be a key factor in determining the primary site of absorption of a drug from an orally administered solution. We have already discussed the absorption of a drug that can exist in both a charged and an uncharged form. According to the pH-partition theory the primary mode of absorption will be by passive diffusion of the neutral species. If we consider all drugs as acids (in the protonated form), we can generalize their dissociation by considering two groups. The groups may be represented

$$\underset{\text{Absorbable form}}{HA} \rightleftharpoons H^+ + \underset{\text{Nonabsorbable form}}{A^-} \tag{7a}$$

and

$$\underset{\text{Nonabsorbable form}}{R_3NH^+} \rightleftharpoons \underset{\text{Absorbable form}}{R_3N} + H^+ \tag{7b}$$

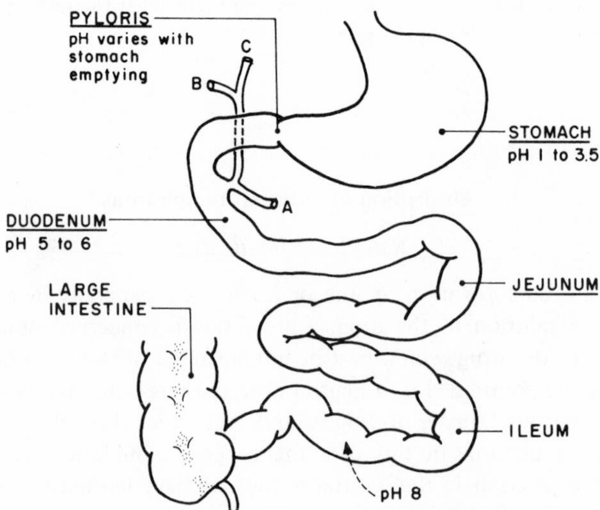

Fig. 7. Diagram illustrating the pH of various regions in the gastrointestinal tract.

where HA represents carboxylic acids, sulfonamides, imides, phenols, and so on, and R_3NH^+ represents all amines such as alkyl amines, phenylalkylamines, alkanolamines, pyridines, quinolines, imidazoles, piperidines, indoles, and phenothiazines. The only word of caution is to remember that the protonated form is *neutral for acidic compounds* (HA) and *charged for basic amines*. Thus the Henderson-Hasselbalch equation can be employed to calculate the relative amount of the charged form from the pK_a of the drug (HA or RNH_3^+) and the pH of the environment.

Since the rate-determining step in g.i. absorption of drugs that are orally administered in solution is partitioning of the neutral species, the preferred site for absorption would be expected to be that area of the g.i. tract where the neutral species is at its maximum. If we consider the ingestion of a weak acid, HA, of pK_a in the range 4 to 5 for example, we would expect this drug to exist primarily in the neutral form in the stomach at pH 1 to 3.5. Thus we would predict that the drug would be absorbed primarily from the stomach. It is likely that we will be correct in this case at least in a semiquantitative sense. When the solution of drug is ingested, it will first arrive in the stomach. Since the neutral species will predominate, absorption would be expected to occur. This is not to say that absorption from the intestines cannot take place. If the drug solution passes into the intestines, its absorption may not be limited by pH considerations alone. Absorption may still occur in spite of the fact that a drug of type HA with a pK_a of 4 would be predominantly charged throughout the intestines. The reason for this behavior lies in the anatomy of the intestinal tract. The intestinal tract is extremely long. In addition to its length, it is composed of large numbers of villi which serve to increase the overall surface area of the intestines. When drug is exposed to this long tract of great area, it becomes relatively easy for absorption to occur across the thin, 25-μm epithelial layer which also has 6,000 ml/min of blood plasma circulating on the systemic side—thus maintaining a high concentration gradient. Thus the intestine is anatomically well adapted for absorption of drugs and other substances.

Our predictions for R_3N types of drugs will be a little more successful. Since the stomach is relatively small, a drug that exists in the charged form, R_3NH^+, will probably not be well absorbed from the stomach. Using the same pK_a value of 4 for the protonated amine, we would predict that absorption from the stomach would be poor since the drug would exist almost entirely in the protonated (and in this case charged) form in the stomach. Once the drug passed into the intestines, it would be in the neutral form and would be expected to show good absorption by the intestinal route.

It should be recognized here that we have referred to absorption in a rather undefined manner. That is, we have not differentiated between absorption rate and amount absorbed. The large intestinal surface may in certain cases result in complete absorption at a rather slow rate. As previously discussed, the time that there is necessarily a quantitative relationship between the absorption values and the K values.

profile may be all important clinically. We will discuss this aspect further under the section on solid dosage forms. It might also be mentioned here that a drug absorbed primarily from the intestines could have stomach emptying time as its rate-determining step. Since this would be more pronounced with a solid dosage form, it will also be discussed in that section.

C. Absorption of Drugs from Solid Dosage Forms

1. Rate-determining Step

In the previous discussions the absorption process began the instant the drug arrived at the site for absorption. This is not the case when a drug is administered in a solid dosage form. In order for a drug to be absorbed, it must first be in solution. Let us consider the absorption of an acidic drug, HA, from a tablet. The usual steps involved in the absorption process are represented in Fig. 8. Once the tablet is swallowed, it normally undergoes disintegration, dissolution, and finally absorption as illustrated in the figure.

It is important to realize the difference between disintegration and dissolution. Disintegration is simply the coming apart of the compressed tablet into primary particles. By including certain disintegrating agents in the formula, one can produce a tablet that will literally explode when simply dropped into a glass of water. While disintegration is a prerequisite for absorption and fast

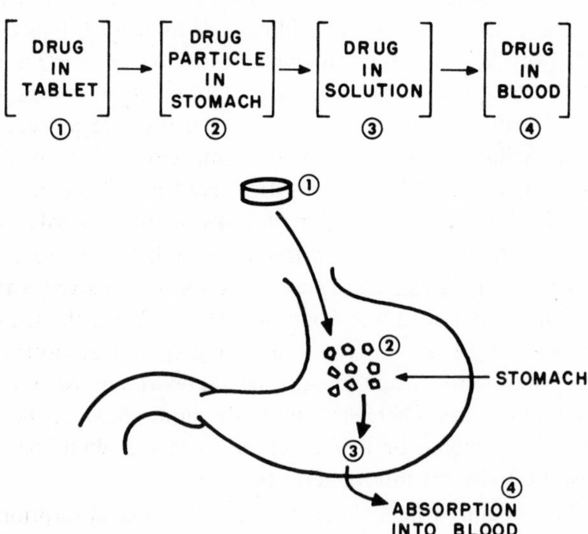

Fig. 8. Illustration of the usual steps involved in the absorption of a drug after the oral administration of a tablet.

disintegration certainly enhances a speedy onset, it does not ensure that absorption will occur. If the drug particles do not dissolve after disintegration takes place, then the drug will never reach the bloodstream. This would be no different from swallowing the ancient "perpetual pill" of gold which was retrieved for continuous use throughout a man's lifetime and passed along with the family inheritance. It is easily recognized that such treatment never resulted in blood levels of gold. Yet people are often prone to accept a disintegration test as evidence for a fast onset of the drug. A negative disintegration test is certainly evidence of a poor tablet, for if the first step does not occur, dissolution will be difficult and absorption may never take place. Fast disintegration will certainly aid in predicting uniform behavior from the tablets, but it will not, in itself, ensure efficacy.

We will assume that the proper technology has been employed to allow rapid disintegration of the tablet on ingestion. This brings us to the second step in Fig. 8, that of dissolution. It is likely that this will represent the rate-determining step in the absorption of a drug from a tablet. We are considering the rate of appearance of drug in the blood for a well-absorbed general acid, HA, taken orally in a tablet. In our scheme we have represented this process as having three major steps. (Diffusion has not been included for simplicity.) The drug can appear in the bloodstream at a rate no faster than the slowest step. This may be likened to a bucket brigade, in which the rate of arrival of buckets at the delivery end will be no faster than the rate of the slowest person in the line. Thus if disintegration has been adequately designed and the drug is readily absorbed from solution, then the rate-limiting step will be dissolution. We may expect dissolution to be generally rate-determining in the absorption of drugs from tablets and especially when the drug is poorly soluble.

2. *Controlling Absorption Rate from Solid Dosage Forms*

Under conditions of fast disintegration and well-absorbed drug, the dissolution rate of the drug particles themselves will limit the rate of appearance of drug in the blood. These conditions may be considered as generally applicable. That is, one can usually increase absorption rate by increasing the rate of dissolution. Since dissolution rate is the limiting factor, it follows that to control dissolution rate is to control absorption. This is the ultimate goal in any product development: to control the behavior of that product when it is in use in the clinic. In the case of solid dosage forms it is therefore necessary to examine the methods of controlling dissolution rate. Let us begin by examining the factors that influence the dissolution rate of a drug. By choosing those factors that can be controlled either by the design or use of the product, we should be able to control the dissolution rate of drug and ultimately absorption.

For the purpose of this discussion it is convenient to examine a modified form of the Noyes-Whitney dissolution rate law given as

$$\frac{dC}{dt} = \frac{kDS}{Vh}(C_s - C) \tag{8}$$

Although this expression appears complex, we will make it extremely simple in just a moment. First let us define the terms. The rate we are considering, dC/dt, is the rate of increase in C, the concentration of drug in a bulk solution in which dissolution of the solid particles is taking place. The constants are defined as follows: k ≡ proportionality constant; D ≡ diffusion coefficient of the drug in the solvent; S ≡ surface area of undissolved solid; V ≡ volume of the solution; h ≡ thickness of the diffusion layer around a particle; and C_s ≡ solubility of the drug in the solvent. The rate-controlling step in this process can be a function of agitation in that dissolution rate into the diffusion layer may be slower than diffusion to the bulk solution under high rates of stirring and vice versa. However, it is not necessary to examine the mechanism at a molecular level in order to understand the application of these principles to the design and use of solid dosage forms. If we consider a given drug under well-defined conditions of use (such as controlled liquid intake), we may assume that D, V, and h are relatively constant values that are not conveniently altered to any dramatic degree by the product formulation. Thus we can easily reduce Eq. (8) to:

$$\frac{dC}{dt} = k'S(C_s - C) \tag{9}$$

If we further assume that dissolution is rate-limiting to the point that the accumulation of drug in the g.i. fluids is negligible relative to the solubility of the drug itself, or $C_s \gg C$, then

$$(\text{Dissolution rate}) \propto (\text{Surface area})(\text{Solubility}) \tag{10}$$

and we are now in a position to examine some clinical applications of this law.

Equation (10) states that the variables to be controlled by the formula are simply the surface area and the solubility of the drug. These two variables can be altered by the following techniques:

1. Control solubility of a weak acid or base by buffering the entire dissolution medium, the "microenvironment" or the diffusion layer surrounding a particle.
2. Control the solubility of the drug through choice of the physical state such as crystal form, its hydrate, its amorphous form, and so on.
3. Determine the surface area of the drug through control of particle size.

We shall consider each of these factors individually with examples.

a. Controlling Solubility Through Stomach Buffering. It would be well to keep in mind that we are dealing with *solubility* as a means of increasing or decreasing *dissolution rate*. The difference between these terms should be clear in the reader's mind before proceeding. Equation (10) illustrates the fact that they are different although related. (It should be noted here that there are exceptions to the generality that dissolution rate is proportional to solubility, but they are sufficiently rare that we will assume there is generally a relationship.) Solubility is a thermodynamic parameter; that is, it represents the concentration of a solution of drug at equilibrium with undissolved solute. Dissolution rate is a kinetic term that describes how fast the drug dissolves in the medium. We are now considering increasing or decreasing the total solubility, C_s, of a drug in the g.i. fluids in order to affect the rate of dissolution and thus the rate of absorption.

The total solubility, S_T, of a weak acid increases with pH according to the equation

$$S_T = S_0(1 + 10^{pH - pK_a}) \tag{11}$$

where S_0 is the intrinsic solubility of the undissociated form and is therefore a constant that is independent of pH. This equation is valid at pH values below that pH at which the solution becomes saturated by the ionic species [7]. Thus, in the region where Eq. (11) applies, the total solubility of a weak acid will increase as the pH of the solvent is increased due to increased formation of the anion, A^-. An obvious approach to the problem of increasing dissolution rate would be to co-administer an antacid with a weak acid drug, HA. It was previously pointed out that the stomach pH can be buffered toward alkalinity. Thus the total solubility of the drug would increase in accordance with Eq. (11), and the dissolution rate would be enhanced as described in Eq. (10). The alert reader may immediately question the wisdom of converting a weakly acidic drug to its charged form in order to enhance absorption. However, the principle can be documented by considering some studies done on aspirin [8]. When aspirin was dissolved in water in the presence of buffers and administered orally, the onset for salicylate blood levels was found to be faster than those obtained by swallowing plain and buffered aspirin tablets in spite of the fact that the pH of the stomach was raised to 7 in the case of the solution. One must keep in mind that two different rate-limiting steps are being compared here. In the case of the buffered solution the dissolution step has already taken place before swallowing. Absorption occurs primarily through the uncharged form of aspirin, but this is in rapid equilibrium with a reserve of the charged form. In the case of the tablets, the rate-limiting factor is that of dissolution. One explanation for the difference in absorption rates is that dissolution of aspirin at pH 1 to 3.5 is slower than partitioning of aspirin from a solution of pH 7 into the g.i. membrane. This is partially due to the fact that the total amount of aspirin in solution is much greater at pH 7 than at pH 1 to 3.5, as can be seen from Eq. (11). In general, we will assume that speeding up dissolution rate will result in increased absorption in spite of the problem associated with the effect of pH on the concentration of absorbable species. Adjusting the pH of the entire gastric fluid content will not often be the approach used for increasing dissolution rate.

b. Adjusting the pH of the Microenvironment. A method more frequently employed is that of controlling the pH in the solution surrounding the undissolved particles of drug. In the case of an acidic drug this may be accomplished by including such agents as sodium bicarbonate, sodium citrate, magnesium oxide, magnesium carbonate, and so on. The amount of these agents in a typical buffered tablet is by no means sufficient to alter the pH of the stomach contents. For example, a typical buffered aspirin tablet contains magnesium carbonate 0.1 g and aluminum dihydroxyaminoacetate 0.05 g. Another contains 0.15 g of magnesium and aluminum hydroxide. A typical antacid dose of magnesium carbonate is 0.6 g, aluminum dihydroxyaminoacetate is 1 g and magnesium and aluminum hydroxide (combined) is 0.8 to 1.6 g. It is obvious that these agents are not included with the intent of raising the pH of the stomach. In fact, it has been determined that the pH of the stomach remains unchanged by buffered aspirin. Yet it has been demonstrated that the dissolution rate and the absorption rate of aspirin is increased in buffered tablets as compared to plain aspirin [8-10].

This might be thought of as raising the pH of the microenvironment, since the pH of the bulk solution is not changed but dissolution rate is increased. Thus the area immediately surrounding the aspirin particles may be elevated in pH due to the proximity of the buffer components of the dosage form itself.

c. Salts of Weak Acids or Weak Bases. When a weak acid is dissolved in water, the pH may be approximated from

$$\mathrm{pH} = \frac{1}{2}(\mathrm{pK_a} - \log C) \tag{12}$$

where C is the total concentration of the acid in the solution [7]. If a salt of a strong base and a weak acid is dissolved in water, the pH may be approximated from

$$\mathrm{pH} = \frac{1}{2}(\mathrm{pK_w} + \mathrm{pK_a} + \log C) \tag{13}$$

Thus for moderately concentrated solutions, the pH of a solution of the salt of a weak acid and a strong base will be higher than that of a solution of the same weak acid. Consider 1 M solutions using an acid of $\mathrm{pK_a}$ 4 as a convenient example. Since the log of 1 is zero and the $\mathrm{pK_w}$ for water is 14, we can easily calculate that the pH of a 1 M solution of the acid will be 2 and the pH of a 1 M solution of its sodium or potassium salt will be 9.0. We can now easily understand why salts are more soluble than the free acids. They are not more soluble in the literal sense of the word, since the solubility in both cases is described by Eq. (11). We can expect a higher total solubility in the case of a salt due to the buffering of the solvent to a higher pH by the strong base cation. In the example just discussed the pH was estimated as 7.0 units higher for the salt than for the acid.

Consider what difference in dissolution rate might be observed in the preparation of two solutions, an acid and its sodium salt, each in a beaker of water. As the free acid dissolves, the pH of the water would be lowered and the total solubility would approach the value of S_0 in Eq. (11). However, as its sodium salt dissolves, the pH would be increased and the total solubility, S_T, would also increase. If we were to measure the rate of dissolution, we would find that the sodium salt is dissolving at a much faster rate. This is easily understood by examining Eq. (10) for the case where the surface area for the acid and its salt are equal so that

$$\frac{dC}{dt} \propto C_s \propto S_T \tag{14}$$

Since we are speaking of one acid, the value for S_0 is constant in both beakers. The ratio of the dissolution rates will be equal to the ratio of the total solubilities as indicated in Eq. (14). This ratio may be expressed as

$$\frac{S_T}{S'_T} = \frac{(1 + 10^{pH-pK_a})}{(1 + 10^{pH'-pK_a})} \tag{15}$$

where S'_T and pH′ are the values for the free acid, and S_T and pH are the values for the sodium salt. For the sake of illustration let us assume that an acid of pK_a 3 had a pH of 2 at saturation while its salt produced a pH of 6. The ratio S_T/S'_T would thus be 910. If all the other variables are held constant, then Eq. (14) would predict that the dissolution rate for the salt of the acid would be 910 times faster than the free acid.

So far we have discussed dissolution rates in beakers of water. How significant are these calculations in vivo? Certainly the salt form of an acidic drug would not be expected to buffer the pH of the gastric fluids. We have already examined the large difference between an average dose of an antacid and the dosage contained in a typical buffered aspirin tablet. The salt form of the active ingredient would generally be even smaller than the amounts of antacids in a buffered tablet. It is easily recognized that this salt would not affect the pH of gastric juice.

There are a large number of examples illustrating the fact that the sodium or potassium salts of weak acid drugs are more rapidly absorbed than the free acid itself when both are administered orally in tablets. A few examples are sodium and potassium salts of penicillins and sodium salts of barbiturates, sulfonamides, and salicylates [11]. If the pH of the stomach is unchanged by these salts, how can the increase in absorption rate be rationalized?

We can assume that each particle of undissolved drug is surrounded by a thin zone of saturated solution which may be called the diffusion layer. The thought here is that dissolved drug diffuses from this zone into the bulk solution and thus leaves a nonsaturated space in the diffusion layer. As this occurs, more drug is dissolved from the particle into the layer. Thus the diffusion layer remains at a steady-state concentration that would approach the saturation solubility of the drug in the area immediately adjacent to the solid. We might diagram this as

$$\begin{bmatrix}\text{Drug in}\\ \text{solid state}\end{bmatrix} \rightleftharpoons \begin{bmatrix}\text{Drug in}\\ \text{diffusion layer}\end{bmatrix} \xrightarrow{\text{Diffusion}} \begin{bmatrix}\text{Drug in}\\ \text{bulk solution}\end{bmatrix} \quad (16)$$

The migration of drug from the layer surrounding the particle into the bulk solution would take place due to the concentration gradient in a manner similar to that illustrated in Fig. 1, Chap. 2 and the discussion on Fick's law. However, the g.i. fluids are poorly represented by a beaker of solvent at rest. Agitation would occur constantly, and the movement of drug into the bulk solution would be due primarily to this mixing rather than the diffusibility of the drug itself, which would achieve relatively slow distribution in the example shown in Fig. 1.

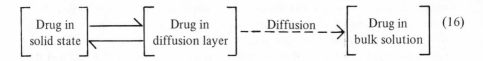

The model shown in Eq. (16) has two areas where drug exists in solution. This, of course, is diagrammatic, since a continuous concentration gradient would exist between the solution near the particle and that in the bulk. In terms of the model, we have assumed that the diffusion layer is in the steady state and that it is a saturated solution of the drug. If the pH of this layer were increased, then one would expect the solubility of a weak acid to increase. A sodium or potassium salt of a weak acid would be expected to have a diffusion layer of higher pH than that of the free acid. In spite of the fact that the bulk solution will have the same pH in both cases, the salt will have a faster dissolution rate. If we consider the dissolution rate of an acidic drug in the stomach at pH 1 to 3, it is immediately obvious that the total solubility in the bulk solution is rather limited. The question is then reduced simply to which form will saturate this gastric fluid first, the acid or the salt. Since the salt form has a higher pH in the diffusion layer, the dissolution of the particle will take place faster. If absorption is fast, we may assume that the bulk solution will also be in a near steady state and that the particle which dissolves faster into its diffusion layer will result in faster absorption. Thus it is a general observation that the sodium or potassium salts of acidic drugs are absorbed faster. It should be apparent here that one might expect reprecipitation of the free acid to occur in the bulk solution if the pH is several units lower than that surrounding the particle, since total solubility is described by Eq. (11). Several writers have expressed the opinion that this precipitation would result in very fine crystals with a resultant increase in surface area as compared to the free acid form itself. While this may or may not represent an additional advantage of the salt form, it does not negate the fact that a saturated solution of free acid in stomach fluids occurs faster beginning with the salt form.

The discussions to this point have centered around increasing the rate of absorption of weak acids. There are somewhat analogous examples for weak base drugs, R_3N. As we have previously discussed, these drugs would be expected to be absorbed from the intestines. Since they must first pass through the stomach, there is an opportunity for rapid dissolution in acidic medium as the total solubility of a base increases when it is protonated to form the charged species. However, the variability in stomach emptying time precludes any dependability in predicting that dissolution will take place in the stomach before the tablet is passed into the intestines. For this reason several basic drugs are administered in the protonated forms as chloride or other salts. This approach generally ensures that stomach emptying and not dissolution rate will be rate-determining. A few examples of such drugs are tetracyclines, antihistamines, phenylalkylamines such as amphetamine and ephedrine, and most alkaloids [12].

Thus the absorption rate of both acidic and basic drugs from solid dosage forms may be increased by administration of their salts. As shown in Fig. 6, increasing the absorption rate would be expected to increase the onset and peak blood level but decrease the duration. For example, the shortest duration for a given dosage would result from an I.V. injection. If onset and peak height are the most significant parameters for a given drug therapy, then rapid absorption should be the goal in the development of that solid dosage form. However, it may be a therapeutic advantage to have a lower peak level and a longer duration. To be more specific, we might consider the hypothetical problem of developing an oral tablet for control of blood sugar level or an oral hypoglycemic agent. If the drug is quickly absorbed, a fast dissolution rate would result in a high blood level and a possible temporary state of hypoglycemia to the patient. The very short duration would result in frequent dosing in order to control blood sugar. The onset of action would not be so critical here, since the treatment would be a chronic one and not subject to the same considerations as treating a systemic infection with an antibiotic where onset and peak height might be paramount. Since the patient will continue to take the hypoglycemic agent, a more constant blood level of longer duration may be deemed more ideal. A case in point may be that of tolbutamide and tolbutamide sodium. It has been reported that the sodium salt gives a very fast, strong, but short-acting effect on the lowering of blood sugar levels, whereas the control with the free acid was more suitable for therapy [13]. The commercial tablets are in the free acid form. Thus the control of dissolution rate can be tailored to the specific needs of the disease under treatment. From the standpoint of optimum clinical effectiveness, there is an ideal dosage regimen for every drug.

Sample Problem 1

Three formulations for aspirin tablets were prepared and their bioavailability was tested in ten subjects. The formulations were described as: (A) tablets, (B) buffered tablets, and (C) buffered tablets of micronized aspirin. Results are given in Fig. 9. Assuming

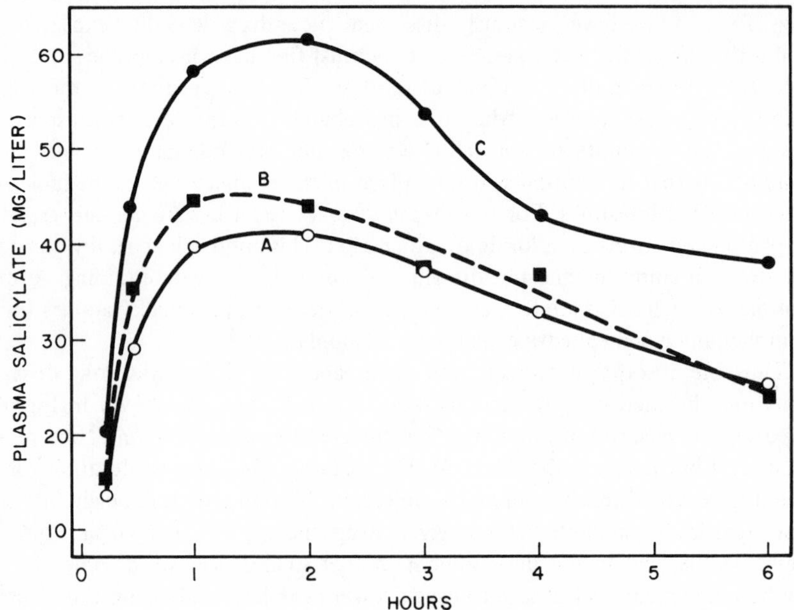

Fig. 9. Average total plasma salicylate levels following ingestion of three commercial types of aspirin tablets by ten patients. Curve A represents aspirin tablets, B is buffered aspirin tablets, and C is buffered tablets of micronized aspirin.

that tablets A and B give similar results (the difference being due to biological variation), what is the percent increase of aspirin absorbed from product C?

Solution: A rough estimate can be obtained from the peak heights which occur at about 2 hr. It would appear that approximately 50% more is absorbed from product C. However, in such an evaluation of products it is necessary to know the dose. Product C contains 7.5 grains of aspirin per tablet while products A and B contain 5 grains. If the comparison was made on equal numbers of tablets (rather than equal doses), the 50% increase would be attributed to 50% more aspirin administered. The time course for aspirin per se is also masked by the fact that this figure represents total salicylate in blood. Unfortunately, it is not difficult to observe such presentations in our advertising media.

Practice Problem 1

(a) What is the concentration in moles per liter of the diffusion layer surrounding penicillin G potassium if the pH of the layer equals 8? (The pK_a of penicillin G is 2.76.)
Answer: 0.174 moles/liter

(b) What is the *solubility* of penicillin G (not the potassium salt) at a pH sufficiently low to allow only the nondissociated form? [Hint: Use your answer from part (a) and Eq. (11). Consider the diffusion layer to be saturated.]
Answer: 1×10^{-6} moles/liter

(c) Consider the initial rates of absorption of penicillin G potassium and penicillin G from identical solid dosage forms. Calculate the value which you would predict for the ratio of the rates where Ratio = R_1/R_2 and R_1 = Rate of absorption from pencillin G potassium, R_2 = Rate of absorption from penicillin G. [Assume the solubilities that you calculated in parts (a) and (b).]
Answer: 1.74×10^5

Practice Problem 2

(a) Calculate the pH of a 4×10^{-3} M solution of sodium sulfathiazole. (The pK_a of sulfathiazole is 7.1.)
Answer: 9.35

(b) Calculate the pH of 4×10^{-3} M solution of sulfathiazole.
Answer: 4.75

(c) Assuming that the diffusion layer in the case of (a) has the pH which you calculated and that of (b) has the pH which you calculated, calculate the *total* solubility of sodium sulfathiazole and of sulfathiazole in their respective stagnant layers. The intrinsic solubility is given above, 4×10^{-3} M.
Answer: Sodium sulf = 0.716 moles/liters; sulfathiazole = 0.004 moles/liter

(d) Given in similar tablets (e.g., same binders, disintegration, etc.), which would be absorbed faster? Explain your choice.
Answer: The sodium salt

Practice Problem 3

(a) Explain, using equations, why the rate of dissolution of sodium phenobarbital is faster than that of phenobarbital.

(b) Why would you expect to find a difference in absorption between sodium phenobarbital tablets and phenobarbital

tablets but not between enteric-coated sodium phenobarbital tablets and enteric-coated phenobarbital tablets?
Answer: See discussion in text regarding absorption from tablets.

Practice Problem 4

(a) Consider the absorption following oral administration of an elixir containing two drugs: Drug A = RCOOH and Drug B = RNH_2. *Given*: the pH of the stomach is 2. Which would you expect to be better absorbed from the stomach, and why?
Answer: Drug A; see text for discussion.

(b) Write the rate expression for the absorption of each.
Answer: (Rate absorption of Drug A) = k_1 [RCOOH]; (Rate absorption of drug B) = k_1' [RNH_2]

(c) What kinetic order are these rates?
Answer: First-order

(d) *Given:* The pK_a of drug A is 2; the pK_a of protonated drug B is 3; the dose of each drug is 1 g; the volume of gastric juice is 100 ml. Write the expression for *initial* rate of absorption substituting the concentration of the absorbable species in grams per 100 milliliters for each case.
Answer: (Rate absorption of drug A)$_0$ = k_1(0.5 g/100 ml); (Rate absorption of drug B)$_0$ = k_1' (0.09 g/100 ml)

Practice Problem 5

(a) Consider transport from blood (pH 7.4) to stomach (pH 2.0) following I.V. injection. Which would appear to a larger extent in the stomach, phenobarbital (pK_a = 7.4) or morphine (pK_a = 7.9, aminium) and why?
Answer: Morphine (consider uncharged form in blood and stomach)

(b) Explain why the rate of absorption of prednisone, prednisolone, testosterone, and androsterone esters given orally in sesame oil solutions was greater than the corresponding aqueous suspensions.
Answer: Change in rate-limiting step

(c) Explain why the absorption rate of tetracyclines was increased by reducing the particle size, but the absorption rate of tetracycline hydrochloride was not affected by the same treatment.
Answer: Dissolution was not rate-limiting for the hydrochloride. Why?

(d) Consider this data:

	Percent Absorbed by Oral Route
Hexamethonium chloride (Methium, Bistrium)	5
Pentolinium tartrate (Ansolysen)	4
Mecamylamine hydrochloride (Inversine)	50

Why are hexamethonium chloride and pentolinium tartrate poorly absorbed compared with mecamylamine hydrochloride? Why is the apparent volume of distribution of drugs such as hexamethonium chloride and pentolinium tartrate only about 7 to 21%? Why are drugs such as hexamethonium chloride and pentolinium tartrate particularly dangerous by oral administration? Would you expect to find any difference in absorption from tablets of mecamylamine and mecamylamine hydrochloride and why?

Answer: Hint: Mecamylamine hydrochloride is not a quaternary, but the others are.

(e) A commercial for buffered aspirin states that two of the buffered tablets deliver almost twice as much acetylsalicylic acid as two of the plain aspirin tablets. If the aspirin is completely absorbed in both cases, what is the meaning of the statement?

(f) It has been stated by Hogben et al. that acids with a pK_a below 2 and bases with a pK_a above 9 are poorly absorbed when taken orally. Do you agree or disagree and why?

(g) Heparin is marketed only as an injection (Depo-Heparin, Upjohn; Panheprin, Abbott; etc.) because the weak acid, heparin, is not absorbed at a pH above 4, thus limiting oral availability. Esterification has been shown to result in absorption at pH 5, 6, and 7. Offer an explanation for this difference in g.i. absorption.

d. Physical State of the Drug. Polymorphism is the ability of a drug to crystallize as more than one distinct crystal species [14]. These forms can differ in such properties as melting point, density, X-ray diffraction, hardness, infrared spectra and, most important to this discussion, solubility. Thus while the solution phase will have only one form of the dissolved drug, the solid phase can contain two or more forms. Only one form will ultimately be stable, and if the solution is allowed to stand it will approach an equilibrium containing a single type of solid. If this transformation is sufficiently slow, the thermodynamically unstable polymorph is called *metastable*. The most stable polymorph usually has the highest melting point and the lowest solubility. The amorphous form is always more soluble than the crystalline form. Since the dissolution rate is proportional to the solubility and the drug must be dissolved in order to be absorbed, the conversion from a metastable to a stable form can represent a real problem in bioavailability.

A well-publicized example of this phenomenon is that of novobiocin in suspension [14]. The amorphous form of novobiocin is readily absorbed and therefore therapeutically effective, whereas the crystalline form is not. At 25°C in 0.1 N HCl, the amorphous form was found to be ten times more soluble than the crystalline form. In novobiocin aqueous suspensions the following equilibrium,

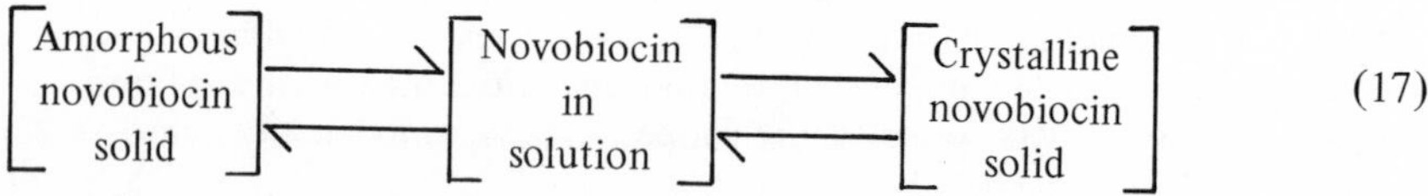

(17)

will slowly convert to the more stable crystalline precipitate, with decreasing oral effectiveness to the point where the therapeutic effect is finally lost entirely. Aqueous suspensions of amorphous novobiocin can be stabilized against conversion to the inactive crystalline form for sufficient periods of time to be clinically useful by including such agents as methylcellulose, PVP, sodium alginate, or propylene glycol algin.

Novobiocin represents only one example. There are many drugs which could have been chosen to document the importance of this principle, among them chloramphenicol palmitate, cortisone acetate, sulfathiazole, methylprednisolone, hydrocortisone, prednisolone, and perhaps even aspirin (where a 50% difference in dissolution rate between two polymorphs has been reported). Poole et al. [15] have demonstrated that the solubility of anhydrous ampicillin is 20% higher than the trihydrate, and this resulted in both an increased rate and amount of drug absorbed after oral administration of suspensions and capsules to humans.

The above examples should serve to illustrate that the bioavailability of a drug from a solid dosage form can be increased by proper control of the physical state of the drug. It should also serve to point out the fact that a product can assay for 100% potency yet be clinically inactive due to the use of the wrong polymorphic form of the drug.

e. Determining Drug Surface Area Through Control of Particle Size. Equation (10) contains two variables that can be controlled in the development of solid dosage forms: surface and solubility. We have not yet discussed any examples of surface effects on therapy. One might immediately consider the advantages of presenting a large surface area by using very finely powdered drug in order to enhance the dissolution rate. While we are prone to think in terms of fast absorption, we tend to overlook the fact that controlled absorption or an ideal absorption pattern for each individual drug should be the goal of modern product development. Two examples have been chosen to illustrate this point further. In one case we will review the rationale behind a microcrystalline product and in the other case a macrocrystalline product.

Griseofulvin is a white, thermostable powder or needlelike crystals with a solubility in water between 1 and 10 μg/ml. When given orally, griseofulvin often exhibits irregular absorption due to its limited solubility [16]. Once absorbed, however, griseofulvin is distributed into tissues, fat, skeletal muscle, and keratin and is also bound to protein in the bloodstream. Tissue levels parallel blood levels, and the apparent biological half-life is of the order of 18 to 24 hr following oral administration. The most common reason for clinical failure with griseofulvin therapy is poor absorption. Since absorption is the limiting factor for effective griseofulvin therapy, several methods for increasing dissolution rate were examined. Sodium lauryl sulfate was deemed insignificant in multiple-dose therapy. Marvel et al. [16] and Kraml et al. [17] demonstrated that 0.5 g of microcrystalline griseofulvin produced blood levels equal to or higher than 1.0-g doses of regular griseofulvin. Since griseofulvin is fat-soluble, high-fat diets were also examined. It was shown by Crounse [18] that 1 g of microcrystalline griseofulvin gave blood levels roughly twice as high as those from regular griseofulvin in fasting patients and that a high-fat diet more than doubled the levels from the microcrystalline material. The average serum levels from microcrystalline griseofulvin doses of 0.5 g can be expected to be equal to or better than those obtained from 1.0 g of the regular form. It should be kept in mind that the potential danger from administration of a drug increases as the percent absorption decreases. If a drug is only 5% absorbed, for example, the patient is swallowing 20 doses. If for some reason erratically high absorption takes place, there is chance for toxic symptoms. The advantage of microcrystalline griseofulvin seems to be quite clear. Evidence has led Blank [19] to conclude that there is no reason at the present time to employ any form of griseofulvin other than the microcrystalline form since it produces higher blood levels and, weight for weight, is more effective than the original form. We might also add that high-fat diet would seem to be a rational adjunct.

There are other examples of micronized drugs, such as sulfadiazine, sulfaethylthiadiazole, aspirin, tetracycline, and so on. However, this does not imply that micropulverization of drugs for solid dosage forms is a general panacea. Let us examine the rationale behind at least one exception, nitrofurantoin.

Nitrofurantoin has a solubility of about 200 mg/liter at a pH of 7. The usual dose is about 50-100 mg taken four times a day. Since it is a weak acid and the volume of stomach fluid is about 100 ml, one would not expect an entire dose to dissolve easily. However, it would appear that about 36% of the amount ingested in the form of fine crystals (10 μm/range) is absorbed [20]. An unspecified percent incidence of nausea and vomiting has been reported in patients taking nitrofurantoin. It was thought that these side effects might be linked to the rate of absorption. As illustrated in Fig. 6, rapid absorption can result in peak blood levels approaching those associated with side effects. In the present case unabsorbed drug in solution in contact with the surface of the gastrointestinal tract might also cause some irritation, contributing to the nausea and vomiting. In either case the proper control of dissolution rate would be expected to decrease the untoward response. Graphs representing excretion of nitrofurantoin for various particle sizes were similar in appearance to those in Fig. 6 in Chap. 3, indicating that the rate constant for release from the depot was a function of particle size. The effect of crystal size on the rate and amount absorbed was studied by determining the percent excreted as a function of time. Data indicate that the blood level peak height as well as total amount absorbed decreased with increasing crystal size. However, it was possible to choose a large crystal size (80–200 mesh) that represented about 31% absorption, which was considered to be roughly equivalent to the originally marketed crystals (10 μm) which are 35% absorbed. The macrocrystals gave lower peak blood levels as reflected by the maximum amount excreted in a fixed time interval, which was 20% for the fine crystals and about 15% for the macrocrystals. Capsules of macrocrystals were used clinically in 112 patients who experienced nausea and vomiting with the tablets (fine crystals), and 89 (79%) tolerated the macrocrystals. Twenty-two of these were rechallenged with the tablets and 86% of these again experienced nausea and/or vomiting. Thus the use of large crystals, in this case, reduced the side effects without significant reduction in the percentage of absorption. It should be noted here that total absorption is not a valid criterion for therapeutic equivalency. Nitrofurantoin is indicated for the treatment of genitourinary tract infections. The therapeutic equivalency claimed for Macrodantin is based on equivalent urinary concentrations [21] and effectiveness in treating urinary tract infections as measured by clinical and biological criteria [22].

D. Factors Decreasing Absorption from the Gastrointestinal Tract

1. Stability

Drugs may be unstable to gastric acid or enzymes present in the g.i. tract. Hydrolysis in the stomach fluids is rather a common occurrence. If a drug undergoes hydrolysis in the g.i. tract, it becomes involved in parallel rate processes as discussed in Chap. 3. This may be represented by

$$\begin{bmatrix}\text{Drug}\\ \text{in blood}\end{bmatrix} \xleftarrow{\quad k_1 \quad} \begin{bmatrix}\text{Drug in}\\ \text{g.i. fluids}\end{bmatrix} \xrightarrow{\quad k'_1 \quad} \begin{bmatrix}\text{Drug}\\ \text{degradation}\\ \text{products}\end{bmatrix} \qquad (18)$$

and the apparent first-order rate constant, k_{app}, may be defined by

$$k_{app} = k_1 + k'_1 \tag{19}$$

It should be recalled that the ratio of the rate constants will define the ratio of the competing rate processes so that

$$\frac{k'_1}{k_1} = \frac{P'}{P} \tag{20}$$

where P′ is the degradation product and P is the drug in the blood. What does this mean in terms of absorption? Let us suppose that k'_1/k_1 was 2. That is, the rate of degradation of the drug was twice as fact as its absorption. For every molecule of drug absorbed, two molecules would undergo degradation. Thus the maximum absorption would be 33%.

We will consider the problem of hydrolysis in the gastric fluids under two categories: drugs absorbed in the stomach and drugs absorbed in the intestines. The second category will be considered separately, since it presents the problem of getting the drug through the stomach without degradation.

a. Hydrolysis of Weak Acid Drugs in Gastric Juices. A good example of this problem is that of the penicillins. The carboxylic acid group of the basic structure, named 6-aminopenicillanic acid, has a pK_a in the range 2–3. As would be expected, absorption from the stomach is significant. The primary difference in the structure of the penicillins is in the substituent group on the amide. This group is largely responsible for the observed differences in gastric stability, enzyme stability, Vd, and protein binding [23,24].

Instability to gastric acid represents the major limitation in oral effectiveness. One of the major limitations in systemic activity is instability to penicillinase, an enzyme produced by microorganisms (especially staphylococci). The β-lactam ring is extremely susceptible to hydrolysis with resultant loss in activity.

Schwartz [23] has reviewed the stability of various penicillins at pH 1.3, 35°C. The half-lives for hydrolysis are summarized in Table 1.

Table 1

Penicillin	$t_{1/2}$ (min)
Methicillin	2.3
Penicillin G	3.5
Phenethicillin	68
α-Methoxybenzyl	77
Oxacillin	160
Penicillin V	160
α-Chlorobenzyl	300
Ampicillin	660

It is obvious from this table why methicillin is available only in injectable form. It is perhaps less obvious why the same is not true for penicillin G. As an injectable, methicillin has the advantage of being the most stable to penicillinase along with oxacillin and cloxacillin. Penicillin G is the least stable, and the rest lie between these extremes.

In order to calculate the percent hydrolysis of a penicillin relative to its absorption, it is necessary to have a value for the absorption rate constant. Methods for calculating the values of the absorption constant from blood level data were presented in Chap. 3. One can easily estimate the hydrolysis which would be expected to occur in the absence of parallel absorption, and it is significant. The following problem serves to illustrate this point.

Practice Problem 6

For the purpose of solving this problem we will approximate the $t_{1/2}$ for hydrolysis by using those given in the above table. These estimates will serve to compare the stability of penicillin G to V under conditions of pH 1.3, 35°C, which is closer to that of the stomach than to orange juice. The present example is meant to simplify the calculations by eliminating absorption from the problem.

(a) A mother wishes to crush penicillin G tablets in orange juice and administer them to a child. If the process takes 2 min, how much penicillin will the child swallow? (Answer in percent of dose.) What if the process takes 5 min?
Answer: 67% (2 min); 37% (5 min)

(b) What answers would you get for part (a) if penicillin V were employed?
Answer: 99% (2 min); 98% (5 min)

(c) Consider the case where the tablets are mixed with juice at 8 a.m. and used throughout the day. For each penicillin listed, how much active drug would remain at 6 p.m.?
Answer: Meth (0); G (0); Pheneth (0.2%); α-methoxy (0.5%); oxa (7.6%); V (7.6 %); α-chlorobenzyl (25%); and amp (53%)

(d) Why is it recommended that all penicillin G oral tablets (including buffered) be taken on an empty stomach at least 3 hr after meals, yet no such statement is found in prescribing information for penicillin V?
Answer: Should be taken when stomach is least acidic.

b. Drugs Unstable in the Stomach and Absorbed in the Intestines. Weakly basic drugs would be expected to be absorbed primarily in the intestines, while neutral drugs would be absorbed throughout the g.i. tract. If such drugs are not stable in stomach fluids, they may be protected from degradation by preventing their dissolution in the stomach. This approach is opposite to the mechanisms that might be employed for a weak acid, which would not be expected to show good absorption from the intestines. An acid-labile, weakly basic, or neutral drug can exhibit increased oral absorption when its dissolution takes place in the intestines but not in the stomach. Some specific examples of drug products that serve to illustrate methods for accomplishing delayed dissolution behavior are discussed below.

The antibiotic, erythromycin, provides a good example of an acid unstable drug that is available in a number of different tablet and capsule formulations. Erythromycin is most stable at pH 6-8 and is rapidly destroyed at pH values less than 4. The protonated form of the erythromycin base has a pK_a of approximately 8.9. Thus erythromycin would be primarily in the protonated form throughout the g.i. tract. (Figure 7 illustrates the pH range involved.) One would therefore expect the oral absorption of erythromycin to be poor or perhaps irregular at best. Intestinal absorption should be better than absorption from the stomach. Thus the g.i. absorption may be increased if erythromycin can be protected from the gastric fluids. Three different approaches have been employed in this case. The most obvious solution is to use enteric coating. This simple approach is not without its problems, however. In addition to the fact that certain types of enteric coatings become unacceptable upon aging [25], Wagner [26] has discussed the "all-or-none effect" in using enteric-coated tablets. The average time for passing an enteric-coated tablet from the stomach to the intestines has been reported as 3.61 hr and 2.63 hr [25]. However, a time average obtained from a group of individuals can be a misleading figure when one is considering a single tablet swallowed by one patient. In the latter case the tablet may leave the stomach right away, or it may remain in the stomach for anywhere from 0 to 12 hr [26]. This presents the potential for a patient experiencing periods of no medication or receiving a double dose on an intermittent dosage regimen. However, if the drug is divided into many small particles, then the passing of the particles within a given patient will be randomized and the effect will be a gradual and more predictable emptying. In the case of erythromycin, this effect has been achieved by development of prodrugs.

Two types of erythromycin that are in common usage are erthromycin stearate and erythromycin estolate. These forms are available in addition to enteric-coated tablets of erythromycin free base. The erythromycin stearate is a salt of the tertiary aliphatic amine of erythromycin and stearic acid. Although the coated tablet of the stearate disintegrates rapidly in the stomach, the salt does not dissolve readily and its degradation is thus retarded. Once in the intestine, however, the salt dissociates, yielding free erythromycin base to be absorbed at a pH more favorable to its stability. Since disintegration occurs in the stomach, the passing of the drug is more predictable as a divided powder.

A prodrug of erythromycin is represented by the lauryl sulfate salt of erythromycin propionate ester. These modifications promote oral absorption in two ways. Salts of weak carboxylic acids and erythromycin base tend to dissolve in human gastric juice and lose antibiotic activity quickly. Lauryl sulfuric acid is a sufficiently strong acid to resist displacement by gastric juice. Thus the estolate remains undissolved and retains its potency in acid for long periods of time [27]. In addition to protection from stomach acids by the lauryl sulfate salt, the intestinal absorption of the propionyl ester is enhanced by its solubility in oil and its pK_a of 6.9, which is two units below that of the free base—thus allowing more uncharged drug in the intestines [27,28]. Once in the blood, the propionyl ester would hydrolyze to yield the free erythromycin. The half-life for hydrolysis in human serum at pH 7.5–7.8 has been reported to be 93 min [29].

There have been conflicting opinions with regard to the advantages of obtaining high blood levels of the propionyl ester prodrug as opposed to the lower levels of drug obtained by administration of the stearate salt. Stephens [30] has reported that the levels in humans after the fifth dose contained 20–35% free base and 65–80% ester, which gives a higher net average of free base than that obtained from the salt. Part of the confusion regarding the advantage of the ester can be attributed to assay procedures and the question of bioactivity of the prodrug itself. Since the in vitro half-life for hydrolysis of the ester is 0.5 hr at pH 8, increasing to 5.0 hr at pH 5 [31], it has been suggested that hydrolysis would occur in buffered culture media during microbial assays with a resultant increase in activity due to the free form.

Thus the estolate has shown higher blood levels than the stearate in fasting patients and with controlled food intake, and the sulfonate ester appears to be more stable and better absorbed as a prodrug [32]. It should also be noted that the estolate (and not the free base, stearate, or ethylsuccinate) can infrequently result in a reversible cholestatic hepatitis that may be idiosyncratic in nature and has been found to subside upon switching to an alternate form of erythromycin [33].

Methenamine represents an example of a prodrug that is converted to ammonia plus the antibacterial agent formaldehyde in acidic media at pH 5.5 or less. The formaldehyde that is released in this manner in the urine provides the basis for the utility of methenamine in treating urinary tract infections. However, this same mechanism can act to destroy methenamine in the stomach. It has been stated that approximately 10–30% of orally administered methenamine is prematurely converted in the stomach but that enteric-coated preparations will avoid this problem [34]. An interesting approach to the combined problem of instability in gastric juice coupled with the necessity for acidic urine is that of enteric-coated methenamine mandelate. This is a salt of the methanamine base and mandelic acid. The mandelic acid aids in acidification of the urine, while the enteric coating protects the methenamine from conversion in the stomach. It should be remembered that foods or other substances, such as $NaHCO_3$, which would buffer the urine toward alkaline pH would result in decreased effectiveness of methenamine.

2. *Complexation*

The problem of decreasing the absorption of drugs by complexation with other agents in the gastrointestinal tract has been widely publicized through the examples of tetracyclines and heavy metals [35,36]. Aluminum hydroxide gels, milk, and milk products have been co-administered with tetracyclines to decrease nausea and vomiting. The complexation of tetracyclines by aluminum, calcium, and so on, might decrease such symptoms, since the complex becomes inactive and unable to penetrate biological membranes. Since tetracyclines sometimes upset the normal g.i. flora, complexation might result in decreased g.i. distress, but the same results would be obtained by not administering the tetracyclines. The following example will illustrate that this is not a facetious remark.

Practice Problem 7: Decrease in g.i. Absorption due to Complexation

In Chap. 3 it was stated that the total amount of drug absorbed was proportional to the area under the blood level-time profile. Methods for comparing the relative areas were described in Sec. II.E. of Chap. 3. Examine the data in Table 2 and then answer the questions.

Table 2

Effect of Heavy Metal Complexation on Absorption of Declomycin in Human Subjects[a] Following 300 mg Taken Orally

	Average[b] Serum Concentrations Declomycin (μg/ml)			
Time (hr)	8 hr Fasting	Meal Without Dairy Products	With 8 oz. of Whole Milk	With 20 ml Amphojel
0	0.0	0.0	0.0	0.0
1	0.7	1.0	0.1	0.2
2	1.1	1.2	0.3	0.3
3	1.4	1.7	0.4	0.4
4	2.1	2.0	0.4	0.5
5	2.0	–	0.4	0.5
6	1.8	2.1	0.4	0.5
12	1.4	1.8	0.3	0.4
18	–	–	0.2	0.3
24	0.8	1.1	0.1	0.2

48	0.4	0.7	0.0	0.1
72	0.2	0.3		0.0
96	0.1	0.2		

[a] Data taken from figures in Ref. 36.
[b] Six volunteers in fasting group and four in others.

(a) What percent absorption takes place when declomycin is taken orally with 8 oz of milk as compared with an equal dose taken after 8 hr of fasting?
Answer: 13% (by the cut-and-weigh method)

(b) What percent absorption occurs when coadministered with aluminum hydroxide gel, 20 ml?
Answer: 22%

(c) What is the effect of taking declomycin during a meal that contains no dairy products?
Answer: Appears to have increased (140%); see discussion in Ref. 36.

3. *Formulation*

It is common knowledge that factors such as inert ingredients, manufacturing processes, the form of the drug, and many other formulation variables can markedly influence both bioavailability and the time release pattern from the dosage form. Several reviews have summarized observed differences in bioavailability [37]. In the earlier discussion (Fig. 8) it was suggested that tablet disintegration should not limit bioavailability, since competent technology would normally ensure fast disintegration. This remark should not be misconstrued to imply that disintegration can never be a problem. In order to illustrate formulation effects as well as to emphaisze the importance of dependable technology, an example has been chosen in which one might not expect disintegration to be a problem. The example is one of a capsule, and the disintegration of the capsule mass might better be termed deaggregation or dispersion. This would be analogous to the processes outlined for a tablet, since absorption from a capsule would proceed according to

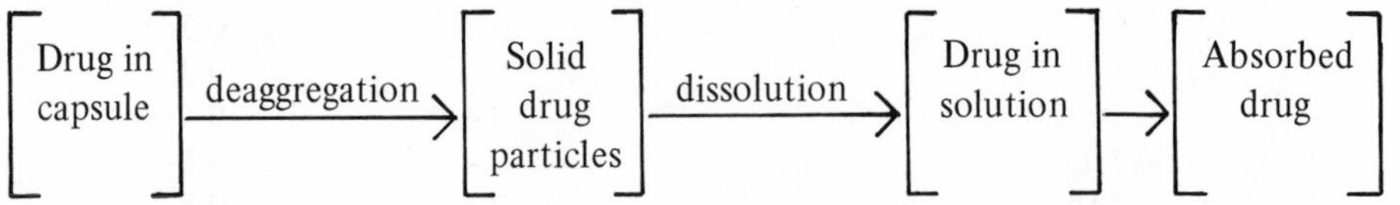

The problem of slow deaggregation limiting the absorption of a drug from a capsule can be well illustrated by the antibiotic chloramphenicol. Four commercial lots of chloramphenicol capsules produced by different manufacturers were compared with respect to their deaggregation rates, dissolution

rates, particle size, analysis of fill, labeled strength, and absorption profiles in human subjects [38]. These studies emphasize the importance of pharmaceutical formulation in controlling the bioavailability of chloramphenicol from capsules. Although all four products contained equivalent quantities of chloramphenicol, their blood level curves were dramatically different. A qualitative correlation was found to exist between the absorption of chloramphenicol and the deaggregation rates of the capsules. In one case the deaggregation rate was so slow that the capsule mass still maintained its capsulelike shape after 3 hr in simulated gastric fluid even though the gelatin capsule had dissolved. The dramatic differences in the absorption rates are demonstrated in Practice Problem 8. In a later study, 14 oral preparations of chloramphenicol were compared [39].

Practice Problem 8: Decrease in g.i. Absorption Due to Formulation

In Practice Problem 7 the relative amounts of drug absorbed were compared by comparing the weights of the curves. Another method for determining the relative areas under a series of curves was illustrated in Fig. 7 of Chap. 3. The area under a curve may be estimated by the trapezoidal rule. The individual areas of the trapezoids, a(c + d)/2, and the triangles, ab/2, are summed to obtain the area under the curve. It is necessary to have the same units of concentration and time in order to compare different curves. However, it is not necessary to have the same scale. In fact, one of the advantages of the trapezoidal method is that the curves can be drawn to occupy the maximum amount of space on the graph paper, and the estimates of the length of the sides involved in the calculations are therefore improved. In the method involving cutting and weighing, a small blood level profile would be less accurate than the larger one that might be used for comparison. The data in Table 3 illustrate the chloromycetin case just discussed. Use the trapezoidal method for estimating areas under the curves, as illustrated in Fig. 7 of Chap. 3. Then answer the questions regarding chloromycetin absorption.

Table 3

Average Plasma Levels for Groups of Ten Human Subjects Receiving 0.5-g Oral Doses of Chloramphenicol in Capsules[a]

Time	Mean plasma levels (μg/ml)			
(hr)	Capsule A	Capsule B	Capsule C	Capsule D
0.0	0.0	0.0	0.0	0.0
0.5	5.8	1.1	1.4	0.6
1.0	9.4	2.4	3.9	1.3
2.0	9.1	4.5	5.7	2.2
4.0	6.7	4.7	5.2	2.2

6.0	5.2	3.4	3.6	2.1
8.0	3.8	2.5	2.6	1.8
12.0	2.3	1.1	1.4	1.0
24.0	0.6	0.2	0.2	0.3

[a]Data taken from Table V in Ref. 38b.

(a) If capsule A is used as the standard of reference, what is the percent of chloromycetin absorbed from capsule D?
Answer: 35%

(b) What relative percent absorption takes place from capsules B and C as compared with capsule A?
Answer: 52% (B); 61% (C)

(c) Why is it not possible to calculate the absolute percent absorption rather than the relative percent absorption from this table, and why type of data would be required to calculate the absolute percent absorption?
Answer: An intravenous dose is required.

Bioavailability from capsules has been erroneously taken for granted. The data in the Practice Problem 8 illustrate the hazard in assuming that untested products are all bioequivalent. Over 200 million chloramphenicol capsules which passed the usual federal regulations were recalled from eight different sources due to poor absorption and decreased bioavailability [40]. Barr et al. [40] demonstrated significant differences in the absorption characteristics of three commercially available tetracyclines during both single- and multiple-dose administration. Wagner et al. [41] demonstrated that a commercially available enteric-coated tablet of aminosalicylic acid gave "zero" plasma levels in eight subjects following oral administration. Whole tablets and tablet fragments were recovered in the feces. Wagner [42] has cautioned against the falacious assumption that products are all bioequivalent until shown otherwise. There is no basis to assume that every lot untested in man is bioequivalent.

IV. CONTINUOUS BLOOD AND TISSUE LEVELS IN THERAPY

A. Constant Intravenous Infusion

The use of constant intravenous infusion in pharmacokinetic analyses has been discussed in Chap. 3. The same approach can be used to maintain constant therapeutic levels of drugs in a hospitalized patient. This type of administration is most commonly employed with anti-infective agents, such as antibiotics, although heparin, lidocaine, procaine, pentobarbital, thiamylal, methoxyhexital, nutrients, electrolytes, vitamins, anticancer agents, steroids, and several other drugs are administered by intravenous infusion. Examples of steady-state blood and tissue levels achieved through constant intrevenous infusion of a drug distributed according to a two-compartment open model were shown in Chap. 3, Fig. 15. Similar curves would be obtained for the one-compartment case. That figure illustrates how the infusion rate determines the steady-state blood level for a given drug. If a constant rate of infusion is used for several different drugs, the resulting steady-state blood levels may be influenced by the biological half-life, volume of distribution, protein binding, and so on. Standiford et al. [43] have examined the steady-state blood levels for several antibiotics using fixed infusion rates. Of the seven antibiotics examined, carbenicillin gave the highest blood levels. The high concentrations of carbenicillin in the blood were attributed to its long biological half-life and small volume of distribution.

In the case of a one-compartment model drug it is rather simple to calculate the rate of infusion necessary to maintain a given therapeutic level. The first, and most obvious, parameter needed is that of the desired steady-state blood level. The minimum desired blood level for an antibiotic is often referred to as the minimum inhibitory concentration (M.I.C.). Once the desired steady-state plasma level as been chosen, one can calculate the amount of drug in the body under steady-state conditions from

$$D_{inf} = (\text{Amount in body})_{ss} = P_{inf}\,Vd \tag{22}$$

where P_{inf} is the steady-state plasma level and Vd is the apparent volume of distribution. When the plasma level is constant, its rate of change is zero and therefore

$$(\text{Rate of drug input to plasma}) = (\text{Rate of drug output}) \tag{23}$$

or the rate in equals the rate out. Thus if we calculate the rate out of the body under steady-state conditions, we will have defined the rate that must be used for the intravenous infusion, k_0:

$$k_0 = \beta P_{inf}\,Vd = k_2 P_{inf}\,Vp \tag{24}$$

Practice Problem 9: Calculation of Intravenous Infusion Rates for Typical Antibiotics

The data in Table 4 are to be used to answer the questions by assuming a one-compartment model.

Table 4

Mean Values of Pharmacokinetic Parameters for Several Antibiotics in Human Subjects[a]

Pharmacokinetic Parameters:	$t_{1/2}$ (hr)		Vd	C_R
Antibiotics	Normal	Uremic	(liters)	(ml/min)
Carbenicillin	1.0	15.0	9.0	86
Ampicillin	0.8	8.0	25[b]	210
Dicloxacillin	0.7	1.0	9.4	114
Cloxacillin	0.6	0.8	10.8	162
Nafcillin	0.55	1.2	27.0	160
Penicillin G	0.5	3.0	24[b]	386
Oxacillin	0.4	1.0	13.0	190

[a] Data taken from Ref. 43.
[b] Corrected for difference in the reported infusion rates.

(a) A physician wishes to maintain a carbenicillin plasma level of 15 mg% for a 10-hr period. If a liter of intravenous solution is to be constantly infused over this time period, how much carbenicillin must be dissolved in the solution?
Answer: 9.35 g

(b) If the calibration of the intravenous injection delivers 10 drops/ml, how many drops per minute must be infused into the patient?
Answer: 17 drops/min

(c) How much more oxacillin would have to be dissolved in a liter to be used for intravenous infusion in order to accomplish the same result as defined in part (a)? How would you explain this difference?
Answer: 24.4 g more

(d) Assuming that nonrenal mechanisms are solely responsible for elimination in uremic patients, calculate the fraction of β due to urinary excretion for carbenicillin, dicloxacillin, and cloxacillin. How would you explain why the normal half-life of carbenicillin is longer than dicloxacillin or cloxacillin?
Answer: Carbenicillin (0.93); dicloxacillin (0.30); cloxacillin (0.25)

(e) Using the renal clearance values, what estimates might be made regarding the mechanism by which the kidneys eliminate carbenicillin and penicillin G? Which one would you expect to be most affected by probenicid and why?
Answer: Penicillin G is actively secreted, since $C_R \gg 130$.

(f) How much carbenicillin should be administered in an I.V. "stat" dose to achieve an immediate onset?
Answer: 1.35 g

A point which is sometimes a source of confusion to the student centers about the question of how any plasma level can be achieved if the output rate is equal to the input rate. It must be remembered that this equality is true only at the steady-state blood level. Our input rate (the infusion) is zero-order. The elimination of drug from the body is a first-order process. Equation (24) describes a single rate at the steady-state, but the rate is less than this at all times prior to the steady state. At time zero, for example, the elimination rate is zero but the infusion rate remains the same. Thus input is faster than output at all times preceding the steady state.

A rapid intravenous injection (or "loading dose") may be used to eliminate the onset period. This will be more important as the $t_{1/2}$ of the drug increases, since the calculated input rate will also decrease. For example, the time for carbenicillin to reach the steady state will be greater than 1.4 hr, since it will take 1.4 hr for the intravenous infusion to release 1.35 g and the body will delay onset further due to simultaneous elimination. The time to reach steady state is roughly four to five times the $t_{1/2}$. If a drug had a $t_{1/2}$ of 7 hr, it would require more than 35 hr to reach the desired blood level. In Practice Problem 9 it would not reach that level, since we were dealing with a 10-hr infusion. Except for drugs that have very short half-lives, it might be considered a general rule than an initial I.V. dose is advantageous. One can estimate the onset time in the manner just discussed to decide whether or not the initial dose is appropriate. It should be re-emphasized here that the actual onset time is always longer than the time it takes for the infusion to release the steady-state amount in the body, since elimination is occurring simultaneously with infusion.

B. Sustained-release Oral Dosage Forms

1. Definitions

There are several types of oral dosage forms that are designed to increase the duration of therapeutic action of the drug contained therein. In many cases these products are similar in appearance to the sustained-release preparations. Often the descriptive phrases accompanying the products do not accurately define the mechanism controlling the release pattern. General terms such as timed release, time release, extended action, or long-acting may or may not be meant to indicate that the formulation is a sustained release preparation. Unfortunately, there are no standard definitions or classifications. The following distinction will be used as a starting point, and later more precise terminology and definitions will be given to sustained release dosage forms. In general, oral long-acting solid dosage forms may be divided into three major groups:

a. Repeat-action Tablets. Repeat-action tablets are designed to release one dose immediately and a second dose after some period of time has elapsed. Some products contain a third dose, which is released some time after the second dose. The release of a subsequent dose is delayed by use of either a time barrier or an enteric coating. Basically these products save the patient a swallow or perhaps two. They can mean the difference between a continuous night of sleep and having to arise for medication. However, they are not designed for steady-state therapy. This dosage form results in the usual "peak-and-valley" type of blood level pattern, as illustrated in Fig. 10 shown later in Sec. V. The primary advantage is that additional doses are provided without the necessity of further administration of another tablet. Blood levels are the same as obtained with intermittent therapy rather than continuous.

b. Sustained-release Dosage Forms. Sustained-release dosage forms provide an initial therapeutic dose that is available upon administration of the product followed by a gradual release of medication over a prolonged period of time. The goal of this type of dosage form is to achieve a therapeutic blood level quickly and then maintain that level with the prolonged-release dose. Ideally, the resultant blood levels would be continuously maintained in the therapeutic range without the intermittent "peak-and-valley" effect of a normal dosage regimen.

c. Prolonged-action Preparations. Prolonged-action preparations provide slow release of a drug at a rate which will provide a longer duration of action in comparison to the normal single dose. They may differ from sustained-release products only in that no initial dose is included in the prolonged-action formulation.

2. Advantages and Disadvantages

The advantages generally claimed for sustained-action products may include improved therapy, patient convenience, and/or economy. Improved therapy claims are based upon the advantage of continuous therapeutic blood levels as opposed to an intermittent or "peak-and-valley" pattern. While continuous blood levels are not necessarily ideal for all drugs and disease states, there are certainly conditions in which clinical or therapeutic advantage can be realized. Typical examples are those cases where depletion of the drug from the body or low blood levels would result in symptom breakthrough; such as might be encountered with antihistamines, tranquilizers, sedatives, anorectic agents, antitussives, ataractics, antispasmodics, and so on. It is possible under certain conditions to obtain definitive therapeutic advantage from sustained-release products.

Patient convenience may represent a common reason for using a sustained-release product, although perhaps it will not always represent the most rational reason for the choice. It has also been argued that sustained-release forms help to eliminate the possibility of forgotten doses, since the patient may take one morning and night rather than three or four times a day during what may be a busy schedule. We have already mentioned the advantage of not waking a sick person during sleeping periods.

Economy may be involved from one of two points of view. Sometimes the sustained-release form may provide a less expensive approach to equivalent therapy even though the dosage form is more expensive than the normal one. That is, a daily treatment may cost less. Economy may also be the result of decreased cost of nursing time for the administration of drugs in institutions.

The primary disadvantage is probably the loss of flexibility in dosage. One dose is designed to last 8-12 hr, and the release pattern cannot be altered to accommodate individual needs of the patient. In addition, if the patient experiences some undesirable effect, such as drowsiness from an antihistamine, he cannot adjust his regimen as readily as with a dosage regimen of every 3 or 4 hr, where he could skip a dose intentionally. Although it may be more economical to take a drug in a sustained-release dosage form, there are many examples where it is more costly due to the technology involved in producing the formulation. Because these products are rather sophisticated and complex, one might suggest that it would be unwise to employ sustained-release forms of rather toxic or potent drugs because of the increased hazard involved in administering the large doses used in a long-acting preparation. However, this should be considered by pharmacy research and development, and it will therefore be mentioned again in Sec. IV.5.a regarding appropriate candidates for sustained-release dosage forms.

3. Sustained-release Theory

There are several models that could be employed in considering the theory governing the design of a sustained-release oral dosage form. The simplest model will be discussed here, and exceptions to it will be delineated as they arise in the next section. This model is analogous to the I.V. infusion with an initial rapid I.V. injection or "loading dose." The only difference here is that both the initial and sustained dose have an absorption step before entering the blood. Thus the model may be written

$$\begin{array}{ccccc} I & \xrightarrow{k_1} & & & \\ & & B & \xrightarrow{k_2} & C \\ S & \xrightarrow{k_0} & k_{12}\downarrow\uparrow k_{21} & & \\ & & T & & \end{array} \tag{25}$$

where I is the immediate dose; S is the sustained-release dose; and B, T, and C represent the blood, tissues, and elimination. It is assumed that the I dose is rapidly absorbed following oral administration, with a first-order rate constant, k_1, being the absorption constant, and that the zero-order release from the S compartment is rate-determining and equal to k_0. Thus the I compartment is designed to achieve a rapid therapeutic blood level, and the S compartment is meant to maintain it in accordance with Eq. (23). The rate of elimination is calculated in the same way it was done in the I.V.-infusion case by using Eq. (24).

Practice Problem 10: Calculation of Specifications for Oral Sustained-release Tablets

A sustained-release tablet having an outer dose of immediately available drug and an inner slow-release core is to be formulated. The desired blood level is 0.4 mg%, and the distribution volume in a 70-kg man is 50 liters. It is found that the drug is quickly and completely absorbed upon oral administration and that 200 mg is sufficient to provide a therapeutic blood level. The biological half-life is 4 hr. If 200 mg is placed into the outer shell, how much drug must be placed in the sustained-release core to maintain a therapeutic blood level for 12 hr?
Answer: 415 mg

Practice Problem 11

A prolonged-action formulation of sulfaethidole is to be designed. The optimum blood level range is 8–16 mg%. The average biological half-life is 8 hr. A 1.5-g dose administered to a 90-kg man yields a blood level of 6 mg% after 3 hr; the total amount eliminated during this time is 300 mg. At what rate must the drug be supplied in order to maintain a 12 mg% blood level, and how much must be placed in the tablet to result in a 12-hr duration?
Answer: Rate = k_0 = 209 mg/hr; 2.51/g

Practice Problem 12

A first-order plot for plasma levels of drug as a function of time in hours gave slopes of −2.8 and −0.18. How much drug must be placed in the S compartment to maintain the blood level for 8 hr, if the I compartment contains 0.40 g, and this amount produces a therapeutic level without significant loss of drug?
Answer: 576 mg

4. *Product Design and Typical Examples*

One assumption that has been stated is that the sustained-release portion of the dosage form must have a release rate that is slower than absorption. That is, it must be the rate-limiting step in absorption. Earlier, the slowest step in the absorption from tablets has been generalized as being dissolution. If the sustained-release form is to control the absorption, then it must limit the dissolution rate. Thus the normal absorption pattern,

$$A \xrightarrow[\text{Dissolution}]{\text{RDS}} \quad \Vert \longrightarrow B \qquad (26)$$

g.i. wall

must be altered by the design of some physical barrier, which may be represented as

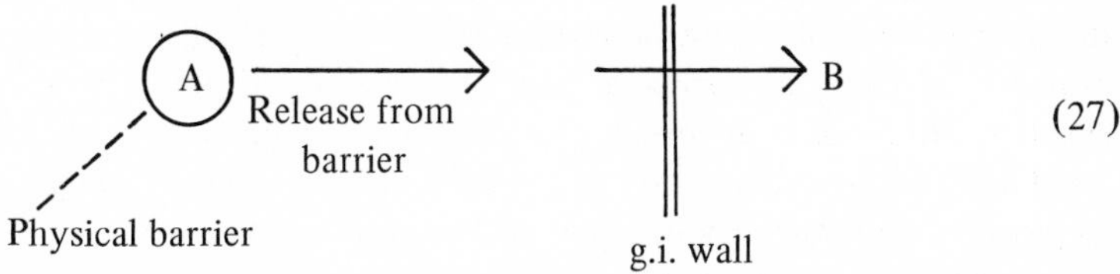

(27)

There are many methods by which the physical barrier is built into the oral dosage form. Included among them are coatings, embedding in a wax–fat matrix, incorporating into a porous plastic base, binding to ion-exchange resins, complexing with colloidal material, microencapsulation, and so on. The details of the manufacturing processes are not of concern for this discussion. However, the type of mechanism employed for the sustained-release products is important, since it governs the rational use of the products. For that reason we will attempt to survey the commonly used structures for sustained-release oral dosage forms. The titles used here are by no means standard and, in some cases may not be found outside of this text. It is believed, however, that these descriptive categories will be very helpful in providing a "handle" to aid those involved in clinical practice in remembering the types of sustained-release dosage forms and in classifying newer products as they are introduced into practice.

a. Slow-erosion Core with Initial Dose. The drug is incorporated into a tablet with insoluble materials usually of high-molecular-weight fats and waxes. This tablet *does not* disintegrate, but instead maintains its geometric shape throughout the g.i. tract. The drug release is due to surface erosion from the intact tablet. The initial dose may be in a pan-coated or press-coated outer shell or in another layer in the case of a laminated tablet. These may be illustrated as

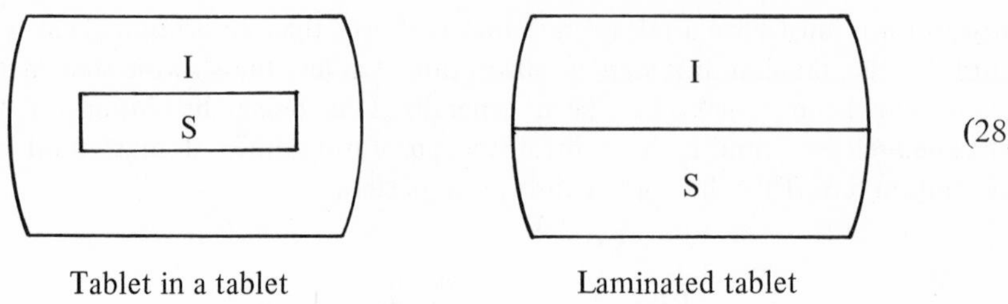

Tablet in a tablet Laminated tablet

The principle of this dosage form can be explained using Eq. (10). As demonstrated in Eq. (23), the sustained release rate must be zero-order, which is, of course, a constant rate. Since the solubility term in Eq. (10) may be considered constant for a given drug, the overall rate may be made constant by maintaining a constant surface area. Naturally, the surface cannot be constant in the absolute sense, since the dosage form will become smaller on erosion. However, the tablets are designed to approach a constant value as closely as possible. Thus the geometric shape of the S compartment is chosen so as to give the least possible decrease in surface area as the core undergoes erosion. For example, a cylinder having a large diameter/height ratio would present a constant surface as it dissolved, providing that the diameter remained relatively constant. The slow dissolution of a silver dollar, for example, might be expected to proceed with relatively constant surface since the area would remain constant at $2\pi r^2$ (neglecting the edge), whereas a sphere would undergo a vast change in surface since its area is $4\pi r^2$ and the radius would decrease with dissolution.

A typical example of a compressed tablet surrounding an erosion core is the Pyribenzamine Lontab (Ciba). The core contains carnauba wax and stearyl alcohol, which are melted together with Pyribenzamine, granulated, and compressed to form the core. The 100-mg Lontab is taken every 8-12 hr in place of two or three separate tablet or elixir doses.

Donnatal Extentab (Robins) has an outer colored pan coating containing the I dose. The core is enteric-coated and slowly dissolves in the intestines, releasing the equivalent of two additional doses. The total of three doses provides sustained effects for 10-12 hr.

Typical examples of laminated erosion-core tablets are Tedral SA and Peritrate SA (Warner-Chilcott). The 80-mg Peritrate SA contains 20 mg in the I layer and 60 mg in the S core. The core releases drug over an 8-hr period, and the overall duration is given as 12 hr since therapeutic blood levels are maintained for 4 hr after the core is expended. Tedral SA contains 90 mg of theophylline in each of the I and S, ephedrine HCl (16 mg in I, 32 mg in S) and 25 mg of phenobarbital in I only.

A number of manufacturers produce sustained-release tablets based on the erosion-core mechanism coupled with an initial dose. Some of these are listed in the summary given in Table 5.

Table 5

Partial Listing of Marketed Long-acting Oral Dosage Forms and Their Probable Categories[a]

Designation	Manufacturer	Typical Product
(a) Slow-erosion Core with Initial Dose		
Chronotab	Schering	Disophrol Chronotab
(Note: Chronotab is also used to designate repeat action in "Disomer Chronotab")		
Enduret	Boehringer Ingelheim	Preludin Enduret
Extentab	Robins	Donnatal Extentab
LA	Beecham-Massengill	Obedrin-LA
Lontab	Ciba	Pyribenzamine Lontab
LP	Dow	Novahistine LP
Singlet	Dow	Novahistine Singlet
SA	Warner-Chilcott	Peritrate SA Tedral SA
Sustained-Action	Schering	Drixoral
(b) Erosion Core Only		
Dospan	Merrell	Tenuate Dospan
Tempotrol	Philips Roxane	Geroniazol TT
Ten-Tab	Riker	Tepanil Ten-Tab
Timespan	Roche	Mestinon Timespan Roniacol Timespan
(c) Repeat-action Tablets		
Chronotab	Schering	Disomer Chronotab
(Note: Chronotab is also used to designate sustained-action in "Disophrol Chronotab")		
R–A	McNeil	Butisol R–A Clistin R–A
Repeat Action	Merrell	Bentyl Repeat Action Tablets
Repetab	Schering	Chlortrimeton Repetab Demazin Repetab Polaramine Repetab

[a]Estimated from product descriptions in *Physicians' Desk Reference*, 27th ed., Medical Economics, Oradell, N. J., 1973.

Table 5 (Continued)

Designation	Manufacturer	Typical Product
Timed-Release	Dorsey	Triaminic Tablets Triaminic Juvelets Tussaminic
(d) Pellets in Capsules		
Continuous Action	Menley James	Contac
Sequels	Lederle	Diamox Sequels Bamadex Sequels Pathilon Sequels
Spansules	Smith, Kline and French	Dexamyl Spansules Ornade Spansules Teldrin Spansules (many others)
=span	Wallace	Meprospan
Tembids	Ives	Isordil Tembids Capsules
Tempules	Armour	Nicobid
TD	Geigy	DBI-TD
(e) Enteric-coated Pellets in Capsules		
Medules	Upjohn	Medrol Medules
(f) Pellets in Tablets		
P.A.	Searle	Pro-Banthine P.A.
Spacetabs	Sandoz	Bellergal Spacetabs
Sustained Action	Key	Nitroglyn
Tembids	Ives	Isordil Tembids Tablets
(g) Leaching		
Gradumets	Abbott	Desbutal Gradumet Desoxyn Gradumet Fero-Gradumet
Sustained	Pfizer	Metamine Sustained
(h) Ion-exchange		
Strasionic	Pennwalt	Biphetamine Ionamin Omni-Tuss (liquid) Tussionex (liquid)

Table 5 (Continued)

Designation	Manufacturer	Typical Product
(i) Complexation		
Durabond	Mallinckrodt	Nalertan Obotan Rynatan (tablets and liquid)
(j) Microencapsulation		
Plateau Caps	Marion	Duotrate Pavabid
–Span	USV	Cerespan Histaspan Nitrospan
	Breon	Measurin

b. Erosion Core Only. Many drugs may not require an initial dose. That is, the onset may not be important if the patient is primarily interested in maintaining blood levels. In such cases a prolonged-action dosage form may be more appropriate than a sustained-release form. Typical examples are erosion-core tablets of an anorexic agent such as Tenuate Dospan (Merrell) and Tepanil Tentabs (Riker). The equivalent of three normal doses of the drug are contained within a uniform-release erosion core. Table 5 lists additional examples of prolonged-action tablets that are of the erosion-core type.

Another aspect of prolonged-action medication involves the fact that an initial dose may be required only when the patient first begins therapy and not accompanying every dose. One method previously used to deal with this problem was an erosion core without an initial-dose compartment. The dosage regimen was adjusted to include several tablets to initiate therapy followed by a maintenance dose every 12 hr.

c. Repeat-action Tablets. As previously defined, repeat-action tablets are not forms of continuous therapy but represent intermittent dosing by the administration of a single dosage form. They are discussed here primarily to avoid the possibility of confusing them with sustained-release tablets. When a repeat-action tablet is cut in two, the cross-sectional appearance will often be similar to that of the tablet in a tablet shown in Eq. (28). However, the labeling (Timed-Release, Repetabs, R-A, Repeat Action) and the description of the release pattern should indicate the difference. Several examples of such products and the manufacturers are given in Table 5.

d. Pellets in Capsules. The original sustained-release product was introduced on the market in October 1952 by Smith, Kline and French Laboratories. The

Spansule (SKF) consists of medicated pellets in a hard gelatin capsule. An average Spansule contains two to four times the normal single dose. The drug is contained within small pellets. There may be three to four different groups, each containing 100 pellets per group. One group of pellets is left uncoated to act as the initial dose. A slowly permeable lipid membrane is used to coat the remaining groups, and the rate of permeability is controlled by the thickness of this layer along with its composition. The second group of pellets may be thinly coated, the third coated medium, and the fourth coated to a thickness sufficient to last about 9 hr.

If each pellet in a group behaved exactly alike, then the spansule would release its drug like a repeat-action tablet; but this is not the case. The drug-release pattern approaches a normal type of distribution within each group. For example, the mean value for a group may be 3 hr, but the pellets may be distributed over a range of, say, ±30%. It is this distribution pattern that results in a sustained-release effect. As the pellets in subsequent groups begin to overlap somewhat, the sum total of the release patterns approaches a constant. Thus release of drug is nearly continuous and dependent only on the rate of permeation of the pellets by moisture from the g.i. fluids. See Table 5 for examples.

e. Enteric-coated Pellets in Capsules. Earlier we discussed the "all-or-none" effect of enteric-coated tablets. It was also pointed out that the average stomach emptying time might be statistically meaningful for a large group of people, but that a given individual could be at either end of the time range when swallowing one tablet. Now what if that individual were to swallow several hundred tablets? The predictability of the event would again be placed on a statistical basis. This is the principle of the Medule (Upjohn). The drug is incorporated into pellets of uniform size and uniform coating of a styrene–maleic acid copolymer which does not dissolve in the stomach. The release rate is dependent upon the stomach emptying rate for the pellets. Since there are a large number of pellets, their stomach emptying will be randomized, with an overall pattern approaching a normal distribution. By appropriate spacing of the dosage regimen some overlap can be achieved, resulting in a total release pattern that approaches a constant value.

It should be noted here that the Spansule and Medule do not really fit our model. One might picture the mechanism involved in these capsules by imagining a rubber stamp which will print a curve similar to those commonly seen for a normal distribution. If the stamp is used to print a series of such curves along the x axis of a piece of graph paper, it is possible to choose a constant time interval between the starting points so that the sum of the curves is a constant. Let us examine this analogy in the case of a spansule. If there are four groups of pellets, we will need to stamp four times. Since the total blood level will be the sum of the effects of all the pellets, all of the overlapped lines must be added. Thus with proper spacing of the individual curves, the overall sum can be made to approach a constant value as function of time. Table 5 lists additional products using this principle.

f. Pellets in Tablets. The same principle used in the Spansules can be employed in tablets. Pellets are prepared in the manner previously described, mixed with appropriate tabletting agents, and compressed into tablets. Bellergal Spacetabs (Sandoz) may be considered as one example of this approach. See Table 5.

g. Leaching. Leaching is rather unusual in that the tablet shell excreted in the feces differs very little in appearance from the original tablet ingested by the patient. The shell is actually a plastic matrix that passes through the entire body intact. It may be thought of as a plastic sponge which contains drug within the pores. As the tablet passes through the g.i. tract the drug is leached out by the g.i. fluids at a rate that is relatively independent of pH, g.i. motility, and enzymes. Thus the shell that is excreted intact has been depleted of its drug content.

Gradumets (Abbott) represent one application of this principle. The initial dose is controlled by the geometry of the tablet. Since the channels open to the surface of the tablet, there is a certain amount of drug that comes into immediate contact with g.i. fluids. This drug dissolves at once and supplies an initial dose. The amount in this dose is thus dependent on surface area, which is controlled by the geometry of the tablet.

The design of a Gradumet is obviously tailored to the specific drug to be used. The size of the channels, the ratio of drug to soluble and insoluble ingredients, the tablet geometry, and so on, must all be made compatible with the physical-chemical properties of the drug as well as its pharmacokinetic properties. This means that combining two drugs into a Gradumet presents a technological problem. One interesting solution to this problem can be found in the example Desbutal Gradumet (Abbott). Barbiturates and amphetamines are commonly employed in combinations. Pentobarbital and methamphetamine hydrochloride have been combined into a laminated Gradumet which is actually two independent Gradumets with a common interface. (Eq. 28). Thus the pair of agents can be administered in combination, yet the release mechanism can be tailored to the individual drugs.

h. Ion-exchange Resins. The Strasionic (Pennwalt) principle involves administration of capsules containing salts of drugs with a polystyrene sulfonic acid resin. This resin salt exchanges drug for ions as it passes through the g.i. tract. For example, an amine drug might be exchanged as

$$\underset{\text{Amine drug resinate}}{[RSO_3^- \ldots {}^+H_3N{-}R']} \overset{X^+}{\rightleftharpoons} RSO_3^- X^+ + R'NH_3^+ \tag{29}$$

where $X^+ = H^+, Na^+, K^+$, and so on, or

$$[RSO_3^- \ldots {}^+H_3N{-}R'] \overset{Y^-}{\rightleftharpoons} RSO_3^- + RNH_2 + HY \tag{30}$$

Amine drug resinate

where $Y^- = OH^-$, Cl^-, and so on. The rate of release is thus proportional to the concentration of the ions present in the g.i. tract. The contributions by H^+ and OH^- are negligible in g.i. fluids. We can estimate the total concentrations of Na^+, K^+, and Cl^- from published data as given here in Table 6 [44]. Although some ions, such as bicarbonate, are not included in this table, it can be seen that the sums of the ions listed remain fairly constant throughout the g.i. tract. These concentrations would obviously vary with changes in volume of g.i. fluids due to liquid intake. However, the constant-release principle is based upon a relatively constant exchange rate.

Table 6

	Concentration (mg%)			
Ion	Gastric Juice	Small Intestine	Large Intestine	Bile
Na^+	115	322	347	340
K^+	40	17	34	28
Cl^-	500	313	310	338
Sum	655	652	691	706

i. Complexation. Pharmacists who still remember their dispensing lectures no doubt recall the warning regarding the preparation of solutions of alkaloids in vehicles such as wild cherry syrup. Syrups that are high in tannins (wild cherry syrup is made from the bark) can result in precipitation of the drug-tannin complex in the case of amine drugs. This principle is employed by Mallinckrodt to produce long-acting oral dosage forms. These tablets contain a complex of the amine drug with tannic acid, $RCOO^- \, {}^+H_3N{-}R$, and the method is referred to as the Durabond principle. The clinician will have no problem remembering these forms, since they are conveniently namedRyna*tan*, Obo*tan*, and Naler*tan*.

j. Microencapsulation. Microencapsulation is perhaps the most recent addition to oral prolonged-release mechanisms. Drug powders (or in some cases particles) are covered with a thin coating that behaves like a dialysis membrane. The drug is released by diffusion through the membrane rather than by disintegration and dissolution. Gastrointestinal fluids diffuse through the membrane to form a saturated solution of drug within the sac or cell. Then the drug undergoes passive diffusion from this highly concentrated solution within the cell through the membrane to the less concentrated g.i. fluids. The rate of release is thus governed by the diffusion properties of the drug with respect to the membrane. The microencapsulated drug can be incorporated into tablets or capsules. Release rate can be controlled by the size of the drug particles that are encapsulated, the surface area of the cells, and the permeability of porosity of the membrane coating. Several manufacturers employ this technique; examples are given in Table 5.

5. *Choice of Drugs for Sustained-release Products and Evaluation of the Dosage Form*

a. Candidates for Long-acting Dosage Forms. We might begin this discussion by giving eight reasons why a drug would not be a wise choice for a sustained-release type of product:

1. Very short half-life
2. Long half-life
3. Large dose
4. Very potent drug
5. Poorly absorbed drug
6. Poorly soluble drug
7. Blood levels do not mirror biological activity
8. Actively absorbed drug

This list is by no means complete, but it should serve to stimulate the reader's thoughts with regard to criteria. A drug with a very short half-life will require too much in the sustained-release pool relative to a normal dose. If a drug has a long half-life, say 12 hr, there is no need to have a sustained form. A large dose, 1-2 g, for example, becomes impossible. Imagine a drug with a 1-hr half-life and a 1-g dose. The initial dose, I, would be 1 g and the S portion could easily be 4 g for a grand total of 5 g. "Now open wide, Johnny, and get ready for a big swallow!"

The question of a potent drug in a long-acting form may be more controversial. In my opinion it is not good practice to swallow five doses of a potent agent, especially if the margin of safety is relatively small. In spite of the fact that a well-designed, long-acting formulation should behave in a predictable manner, there is always that chance of an unexpected event in biological systems, and the potential for increased absorption is there. My reasoning behind eliminating poorly absorbed drugs as candidates is somewhat the same. Consider drugs such as hexamethonium or pentolinium, which are discussed in Practice Problem 5. These are fairly potent agents. They are extremely variable in their response upon oral administration, and this is easily understood when you consider that a patient is really swallowing 20 doses if a drug is only 5% absorbed. If, by some quirk of biological fate, the patient is able to absorb more on a given day, the potential for overdose is there. Now put such a drug in a sustained-release form. How much will be administered—80 doses? If the drug is poorly absorbed because it cannot pass the g.i. wall, then it must remain in the g.i. tract. That means a continuous-release dosage form is resulting in a pool of available but unabsorbed drug in solution in the g.i. tract.

What about the drug that is poorly absorbed because it is poorly soluble? Release from the dosage form must be the rate-limiting step. If the drug is poorly soluble and thus poorly absorbed, then it is likely that dissolution of the drug itself is rate-determining. The dosage form is therefore not governing the absorption pattern but may be superfluous, as undissolved drug particles in the g.i. tract would behave independently of the formulation.

If the therapeutic activity of a drug is independent of its concentration, it would seem to be irrational to expend time, effort, and money in an attempt to maintain constant blood levels. Reserpine has a 15-min half-life, yet its activity persists for as long as 48 hr [45]. Since reserpine may act by irreversibly inhibiting monamine oxidase, the duration may be related to the time of formation of new enzymes by the body. Thus the pharmacological activity occurs independently of the time course for drug in the blood, and pharmacokinetic parameters calculated from blood level data would not be therapeutically meaningful when applied to development of a prolonged-release product.

An actively absorbed drug generally exhibits a preferential area of the g.i. tract for its absorption. If this is an enzyme-transport process, that area will be located where the enzymes exist in greatest density. Producing a prolonged-release pattern before reaching that site makes little sense, since all of the drug that arrives in solution will behave in the same manner as it would in the case of a normal dosage form. Releasing drug after the formulation has passed by the site will give decreased absorption compared to the normal case. The overall problem makes the chances for success very slim for a drug that is primarily absorbed actively.

b. Evaluating Sustained-release Products. Naturally the clinical evaluation of sustained-release products should include all of the statistical parameters normally encountered in a good experimental design. It is not the intent here to review biomedical statistics and experimental design. However, it is considered appropriate to examine some of the components of a good clinical evaluation and to emphasize those aspects unique to long-acting products. This becomes especially apparent when one begins examining the literature in this area, since it is exceedingly easy to locate studies with conclusions that cannot be readily accepted in light of the experimental design.

Obviously, the study should be designed to remove bias. In spite of the fact that double-blind techniques are commonly employed, many such studies do not include a placebo or make any attempt to disguise the dosage forms. Sustained-release formulations are generally unique in appearance. The value of a double-blind study based on information collected by clinicians interviewing patients becomes rather questionable when the dosage forms have such distinguishing characteristics that a brief mention of it by the patient removes the blind. An interesting study was carried out to test the efficacy of the double-blind. One hundred patients were given a drug by a group of interns and the results were determined subjectively. Excellent results were obtained in 61% of the cases. A known placebo was introduced and 56% response obtained. When the same tests were carried out using a double-blind technique with unknown placebo, only 38% excellent results were reported. How common is the problem of experimental design affecting interpretation? An analysis of 100 consecutive articles in a group of medical journals revealed that 45 did not compare the treatment with a control and an additional 18 had inadequate control for a total of 63%.

It does not seem unreasonable that a manufacturer could produce a placebo which would appear like the real thing. Sometimes it is not possible to use a placebo, as patients should not go untreated. Comparison with standard forms or other sustained-release products then becomes the only alternative. While a Latin square design involving placebo, standard, and new product is ideal, the elimination of placebo should result in at least a crossover approach. Yet it is a common occurrence to find a group divided in two and treated with two drugs without any attempt at crossover. It goes without saying that the normal unbiased methods for random selection of patients should be employed in all tests.

A problem that is unique to sustained-release forms is proving that they are indeed sustained-release. This may not be as easy as it appears at first. Certainly the release pattern of a sustained-release preparation should be independent of pH, enzymes, agitation, and any other variables that might be encountered in the g.i. tract. This type of behavior can be tested in vitro, but negative results are more meaningful than postive ones. That is, if the dosage form is unpredictable in vitro, then the in vivo behavior will certainly not be more reliable. However, good results in vitro do not ensure success in the clinic. There is no substitute for clinical proof. At best, in vitro tests can be correlated with blood level data for use in quality control, but studies done in a beaker do not prove therapeutic utility. In fact, clinical proof that sustained-release dosage forms produce the desired release patterns within the g.i. tract itself does not demonstrate that they will provide sustained therapeutic responses. The release of drug in the g.i. tract is not the final test for a constant absorption rate. Absorption of a given drug may vary as the dosage form travels down the g.i. tract. Thus X-ray studies commonly employed to follow the behavior of an ingested long-acting formulation can document only the release pattern. While this is certainly important, the absorption pattern must be determined by other methods.

The most obvious criterion for sustained release is the appearance of the time course for the drug in the blood. The formulation is designed to produce steady-state blood levels, and the level of success can be determined directly from blood or urine assays as a function of time. While this seems simple enough, there are some problems associated with the choice of a reference standard in addition to the problems encountered in developing suitable analytical methods. It is common practice to compare the sustained-release form of the drug to the normal dosage regimen of the same drug. While this is a necessary part of a good study, it has been criticized as being incomplete. It does not prove that the sustained-release form works, because there is no comparison made with a single but equal dose of the same drug. Hollister [46] has suggested that a study should include a single normal dose, the normal dosage regimen, the sustained-release form, and a single dose of drug equal to the amount in the sustained-release form. In his commentary, "Measuring Measurin: Problems of Oral Prolonged-action Medications" [9], he demonstrated similar results from tablets and sustained-release tablets based on *salicylate* time course in blood following equal doses. The rank order for peak *acetylsalicylic acid* plasma levels (at 30 min) was roughly 7/4.5/3 (in μg/ml) for (buffered tablets/plain tablets/sustained-release tablets). The beta phase (which begins at approximately 1 hr) appeared similar for all three products with respect to acetylsalicylic acid. Furthermore, using this approach he demonstrated several cases where essentially equivalent blood level patterns were obtained with a single dose of drug equal to that contained in the "long-acting" form [46]. Obviously, it will not always be possible to administer such a large dose, but Hollister's point appears to be well conceived for those cases where it is possible.

Even if the sustained-release form does indeed work, it does not follow automatically that this results in a proven clinical advantage. The results must be compared to the current "standard" of therapy and the advantage demonstrated. This is best done by objective studies. Some real clinical manifestation of the disease should be measured quantitatively as a function of time. Such tests have been developed for adrenergics, cholinergics, sympathomimetics, parasympathomimetics, ganglionic blockers, vasodilators, antitussives, antacids, and countless others [47]. It is becoming increasingly difficult to accept the argument that no clinical test exists as a justification for a purely subjective study. However, when subjective tests are conducted, the credibility of the resultant data is completely dependent on the experimental design.

6. *Rational Clinical Use of Sustained-release Products*

The rational use of sustained-release products is based upon an understanding of their construction and the principle by which they are meant to function. Those employing the erosion-core principle, for example, contain several doses and depend on the geometry of the intact core for their continuous release pattern. Anything that would destroy this structure could result in an overdose. While this seems obvious enough, it cannot be taken for granted that this is common knowledge. In one report a markedly greater response was observed when tablets of the slow-release type were chewed by the patient before swallowing [48]. The workers concurred with other investigators who recommended chewing of the tablets as a routine procedure. In making use of sustained-release forms, it is good practice to avoid the introduction of new variables that may not have been present in the original evaluation studies. Thus beverages such as hot drinks that might soften fats or waxes, alcoholic beverages that might dissolve coatings, and so on, should be avoided. A worthwhile precaution would be to warn patients against the simultaneous ingestion of any foods or drugs that might affect the integrity of the dosage form with resultant increase in drug release rate.

It is not an uncommon practice to administer sustained-release preparations or fractions of them to children. There are several factors that would raise doubt regarding the wisdom of this procedure. Children are not little adults. The dosage regimen for a child should be one that is specifically developed for that purpose independently of the adult regimen and not calculated by applying some arbitrary equation to adjust the adult dose. It should be obvious that a given fraction arrived at by any formula cannot be considered optimum for every drug known to man when administered to a given child. However, this is a problem associated with pediatric posology in general, and there are some more specific problems with respect to the present subject of long-acting products.

We might first begin with the potential biological differences. The release pattern and the amount of drug in the slow-release compartment is directly related to the desired blood level and biological half-life in adults. Of course, these will be average values for an adult population. It is reasonable to expect that the distribution volume, biological half-life, and perhaps desired blood level would all be different for children. The Vd will be a function of the child's weight. The $t_{1/2}$ may be longer due to undeveloped enzyme systems with resultant decrease in metabolic rate. There may also be differences in urinary clearance values, protein binding, absorption, and so on. In short, it does not seem rational to administer either the whole or a part of long-acting adult dosage form to a child, especially since these forms will contain several doses.

There are additional problems associated with the administration of a fraction of a sustained-release dosage form. These are related to the physical make-up of the formulations themselves. For example, how can one take one-half the contents of a Spansule? Some physicians direct the parents to open the gelatin capsule and pour out one-half of the pellets. But which half do they obtain? Stratification of pellets in a mixture is a well-known "unmixing" problem to the pharmaceutical industry. A drum of granulation may have to be remixed before tabletting if it has been moved or stored long enough to result in different analyses at the top and bottom of the mixture. A Spansule may contain four groups of pellets. One cannot expect to pour one-half of each group out on a spoon and get one-half of the release pattern on ingestion.

Erosion-type products may be broken or cut in half, but this is not without its problems. Obviously, if an enteric coating is involved in the time-lapse mechanism it will be destroyed. Less obvious is the fact that one-half of the tablet has more than one-half the surface area. How much more will vary with the geometry of the original tablet. The surface will be greater than half, and thus the release rate will also be greater than half. The result would be blood levels that are greater than half and shorter duration than the original tablet. The relative blood levels and duration can be calculated rather simply.

Practice Problem 13

The relative dimensions as estimated with a ruler and the duration of action as stated in the manufacturer's product information are listed in Table 7 for several products. Choose from the list of categories the appropriate descriptive phrase that best describes each product. Then calculate what you would expect to be the relative blood level (%) and duration (hr) following administration of one-half of the dosage form. (Hint: Use the relative release rate and dosage form lifetime to estimate the answers.)

Table 7

Product	Duration (hr)	Relative Dimensions[a]
Mestinon Timespan	ca. 6	1 X 1 X 3
Pyribenzamine Lontab	8	core diameter = 2 thickness = 1
Tenuate Dospan	12	3 X 5 X 12
Triaminic Timed Release Tablets	8	core diameter = 4 thickness = 1
Rynatan	12	1 X 2 X 5

[a]Geometric formulae for areas: circle = πr^2; sphere = $4\pi r^2$; rectangle = length X width.

List of Types of Dosage Forms

1. Erosion core only
2. Pan-coated erosion core
3. Press-coated erosion core
4. Repeat action
5. Laminated tablet/core
6. Spansule pellets in capsule
7. Enteric pellets in capsule
8. Spansule pellets in tablet
9. Leaching from plastic matrix
10. Polystyrene sulfonic acid resin
11. Tannic acid complex
12. Microencapsulation

Practice Problem 14

(a) Why are Desbutal Gradumets (Desoxyn and Nembutal) formulated as 2-layer tablets? (Note: This combination tablet is no longer available in the United States.)

(b) A patient has complained to his physician that the undisintegrated tablets (Desbutal Gradumets) are appearing in his feces. The physician, in turn, asks the pharmacist if he is perhaps using "old stock." What should he answer?

(c) Would you object to the patient ingesting the following substance along with or immediately following the use of a Spansule and why: coffee or tea; saline cathartic; a Manhattan?

V. DOSAGE REGIMENS

The development of an optimum dosage regimen, which balances patient convenience with proper body content of drug, is an essential consideration for rational therapy with a drug product. Figure 6 introduced the concept of achieving a certain desirable blood level following administration of a single oral dose of the drug. But few drugs are used in a single dose. Some examples of single-dosage drugs are headache remedies, digestive aids, antinauseants, laxatives, anthelmintics, antacids, or others which you may call to mind that are used in one or two doses as the occasion arises. The large majority of drugs are administered repetitively on either a maintenance regimen (as in cardiovascular diseases) or to the end of prescribed course of therapy (as in treatment with an antibiotic). Figure 10 illustrates a typical blood level curve for an oral dose repeated every four hours.

For many drugs a desirable minimum plasma concentration can be determined. Kruger-Thiemer [49] has stressed the clinical significance of maintaining constant minimum inhibitory blood concentrations for certain antimicrobial agents. For other agents, such as digoxin, theophylline, procainamide, and gentamycin, a rather narrow range of minimum and maximum blood concentration can be defined. A multiple-dosage regimen can be calculated for either type of drug, that is, those which simply require a minimum or those which have a narrow margin of safety. The only prerequisite is that the desired therapeutic response must be related to a corresponding concentration of drug in blood.

The complexity of the equations employed for dosage regimen calculations is related to the pharmacokinetic model describing the situation. For example, a dosage regimen for a one-compartment model drug, administered by repetitive equal rapid I.V. injections, is easily calculated. But a multicompartment model drug administered orally becomes quite complex, and accurate assessments may

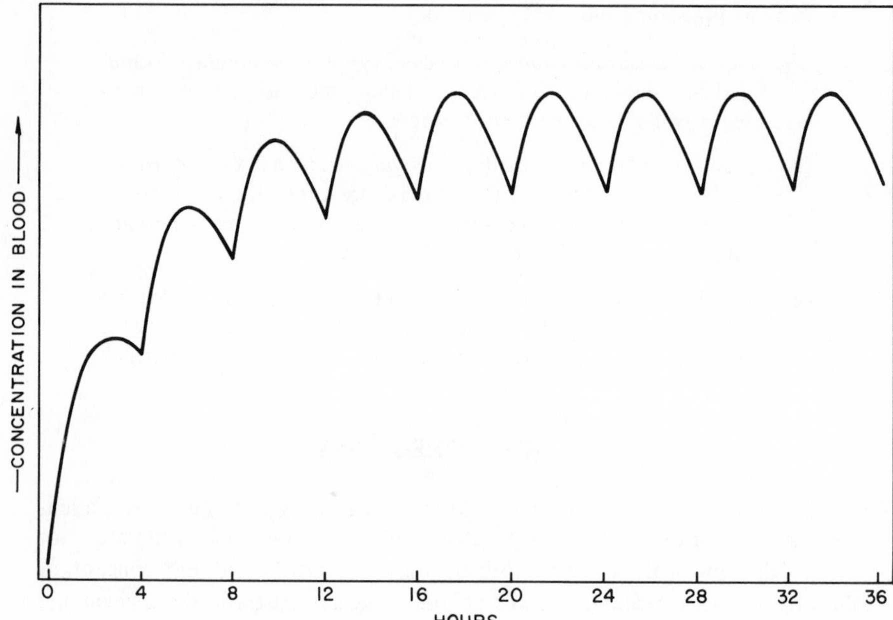

Fig. 10. An equal dose is administered orally every 4 hr.

require a value for the absorption rate constant, k_1. Since values for k_1 are often not readily obtainable, approximate methods have been devised for estimating reasonable dosage regimens. The present treatment will deal with the I.V. case of a one-compartment drug and the methods for making model-independent estimates for drugs administered by extravascular routes. Literature references for more complex treatments will be cited.

Regardless of the route of administration or the pharmacokinetic model, there are only two parameters which can be adjusted in developing a regimen for a given drug. These are the size of the dose and the frequency of administration. The amount of a drug in the body at any given time will be a function of how much drug is administered and how often it is administered. If we know the mathematical relationship between the body content and the dose and frequency, we can estimate a regimen to maintain any desired body level. Provided that a desirable therapeutic body content can be clinically defined, the optimum regimen can then be calculated to provide that level during repetitive multiple-dose therapy. The following sections are designed to illustrate this statement.

A. Accumulation During Repetitive Intravenous Dosing

Accumulation is most simply considered for rapid intravenous injections of a dose of drug described by a *one-compartment model* and administered at a fixed time interval, τ. An ordinary first-order equation will describe the loss from the body following a rapid intravenous injection:

$$\ln D = \ln D_0 - \beta t \tag{31}$$

D_0 is the dose and D is the total amount remaining in the body. The equation may be rearranged to define the natural logarithm of the fraction of the dose remaining, f, as

$$\ln f = \ln \frac{D}{D_0} = -\beta t \tag{32}$$

which can be rearranged to include the well-known half-life expression,

$$t_f = \frac{\ln f}{-\beta} \tag{33}$$

Thus, the time for the body content to reach any fraction of the administered dose is simply the natural logarithm of that fraction divided by the negative value for beta.

Consider the case where rapid equal intravenous doses of this drug are administered repetitively at a fixed time interval, τ. For example, let us say that the dose was administered every time a half-life had elapsed. Then $\tau = t_{1/2}$. Just prior to the second injection, one-half of the dose would remain in the body. Upon injection the body would contain 1.5 doses. Before the third dose, 0.75 doses remain. After the third dose, 1.75 doses are present. The drug is accumulating within the patient. What does accumulation mean? After each subsequent dose there is more drug within the patient than after the previous dose. Therefore the administered dose is greater than the dose eliminated. But there is a limit. Just as we observed in Sec. IV, a steady state will be achieved when the rate of drug supply becomes equal to its rate of loss. The difference between the present case and that of a constant-rate I.V. infusion is that the repetitive-dose steady state will fluctuate between a minimum and a maximum value as a function of time. This pattern (illustrated in Fig. 10) is shown quantitatively in Table 8 for the dosage intervals where $\tau = t_{0.5}$ and $\tau = t_{0.75}$. Once the body has reached the steady state, it is a necessary condition that the equivalent of a single dose is eliminated during each period of time equal to τ. This is implicit in the definition of steady state, which asserts simply that the dose administered is equal to that which has been eliminated. In Table 8 it is readily apparent that the difference between the body content before and after each dose approaches a constant value that is equal to a single dose. Thus during each dosage interval, τ, a single dose is eliminated and then replaced by the injection. The body content (or dose remaining in the body, D) before each subsequent dose will be called the minimum, so that

$$D_{min} = (P_{min})\, Vd \tag{34}$$

and the peak or maximum value

$$D_{max} = (P_{max})\, Vd \tag{35}$$

Table 8

The Fraction of the Dose in the Body Immediately Before and After Rapid I.V. Administration, Where $\tau = t_f$ for a One-compartment Drug

Number of Doses	f = 0.50		f = 0.75	
	Before Dose	After Dose	Before Dose	After Dose
1	0	1.00	0	1.00
2	0.50	1.50	0.75	1.75
3	0.75	1.75	1.313	2.313
4	0.875	1.875	1.734	2.734
5	0.938	1.938	2.050	3.050
6	0.969	1.969	2.288	3.288
7	0.984	1.984	2.466	3.466
8	0.992	1.992	2.600	3.600
9	0.996	1.996	2.700	3.700
10	0.998	1.998	2.775	3.775
∞	1.000	2.000	3.000	4.000

Practice Problem 15

(a) A drug that is distributed according to a one-compartment model has a $t_{1/2}$ value of 6 hr. A 210-mg dose is administered by rapid intravenous injection every 12 hr. If the Vd is 40 liters, what value will be achieved for P_{min} and P_{max}?
Answer: P_{min} = 1.75 mg/liter; P_{max} = 7 mg/liter

(b) Construct a single figure showing three accumulation plots for D vs t following rapid I.V. injections when f = 0.5, f = 0.75 (data in Table 8), and f = 0.25 (part a) and $\tau = t_f$.

Practice Problem 15 was designed to familiarize you with the kinetics of drug accumulation. The equations for quickly estimating D_{max} and D_{min} are quite simple and obvious once you have understood the time profile in your plot for part (b) of that problem. Keep in mind that the dosage interval, τ, is defined as the time to deplete the body content to the fraction f. Replacing t_f in Eq. (33), by τ provides the equation describing this:

$$\tau = \frac{\ln f}{-\beta} \tag{36}$$

We have observed that D_{max} is always *one dose* larger than D_{min}. Your figure in part (b) should show: $D_{max} = 4$, $D_{min} = 3$ (f = 0.75); $D_{max} = 2$, $D_{min} = 1$ (f= 0.5); $D_{max} = 1.33$, $D_{min} = 0.33$ (F = 0.25). The difference is always *one dose*, as you would expect for the steady state where each subsequent dose replaces the one that has been lost. You will have no problem remembering this equation.

$$D_0 = D_{max} - D_{min} \tag{37}$$

It is also a simple matter to calculate either D_{max} or D_{min} directly. The time of decrease from D_{max} to D_{min} is equal to the dosage interval, τ. Since we have defined $\tau = t_f$ (Eq. 36), then, by definition, $D_{min} = f(D_{max})$. We know that one dose was lost during this time interval (Eq. 37), so $D_0 = (1 - f)D_{max}$. This can also be derived by substituting $f(D_{max})$ for D_{min} in Eq. (37) and rearranging to obtain

$$D_{max} = \frac{D_0}{1 - f} \tag{38}$$

The previous examples (Table 8 and Practice Problem 15) set f = 0.75, 0.50, and 0.25, and $\tau = t_f$. Equations (37) and (38) will provide the same steady-state approximations. Try them. (A mathematical derivation for Eqs. (37) and (38) is provided in Appendix D.)

The estimation of P_{min} and P_{max} may be a practical problem in therapy or in a research problem. Equation (38) may be written in terms of the plasma concentration:

$$P_{max} = \frac{B}{1 - f} \tag{39}$$

and

$$P_{min} = \frac{B(f)}{1 - f} = f(P_{max}) \tag{40}$$

where B is the intercept value for β-phase plasma data as shown in Chap. 2, Fig. 10.

B. Average Steady-state Levels for Any Route and Model

The average amount in the body at steady state, during constant repetitive dosing at fixed time intervals, may be defined for *any route and model* (in which elimination occurs only from the central compartment) as

$$\bar{D}_{ss} = \frac{F(D_0)}{\beta\tau} = \frac{F(D_0)1.44t_{1/2}}{\tau} \tag{41}$$

where F is the fraction of the administered dose that is absorbed. For an intravenous injection, F = 1. This equation was originally derived for a one-compartment model [50] and later applied to multicompartmental models [51]. For a *one-compartment model*, the plasma concentration corresponding to the value $\overline{D}_{ss}$ would be calculated from

$$\overline{P}_{ss} = \frac{\overline{D}_{ss}}{Vd} \tag{42}$$

where Vd is calculated by any of the methods described in Chap. 3. As noted in that chapter, the calculated value for Vd may vary with the method used for a drug described by a model employing more than one compartment. Since the values $\overline{P}_{ss}$ and $\overline{D}_{ss}$ are steady-state values, one would expect the steady-state estimate for Vd to provide the best $\overline{P}_{ss}$ estimates in Eq. (42). See Chap. 3, Sec. II.B.2 and II.F (Eq. 65) for a discussion of the methods to calculate Vd_{inf}. If the Vd values are estimated following a single rapid intravenous dose (Eq. 10 or 12 in Chap. 3), the resulting estimates for $\overline{D}_{ss}$ obtained from the product of $(\overline{P}_{ss})(Vd)$ will overestimate the actual amount in the body [52]. The degree of error appears to increase as the values for k_{21}/k_2 and $t_{1/2}$ decrease. For example, it has been calculated that the percent error is 70% for penicillin G, 32% for lidocaine, 23% for ethchorvynol, but negligible for warfarin [52]. Thus, for a *two-compartment model*,

$$\overline{P}_{ss} = \frac{\overline{D}_{ss}}{Vd_{inf}}$$

Practice Problem 16

(a) If the desired average plasma level for a drug is 0.4 mg%, what dose should be given orally on a regimen of every 6 hr around the clock? The drug is 85% absorbed and the patient weighs 70 kg. The Vd value is 140 liters and $t_{1/2}$ is 3.5 hr.
Answer: 783 mg

(b) If identical average plasma levels are to be maintained with a 500-mg capsule, how often should it be administered?
Answer: 3.83 hr

C. Repetitive Oral Dosing for Minimum Effective Concentrations

If absorption is sufficiently fast relative to elimination, the equations developed for rapid intravenous injections (Eqs. 37 and 38) may be used for a first approximation of steady-state maxima and minima. More accurate estimates are obtained using equations which include values for the absorption rate constants [53-55]. However, these are rather complex, and the rate constant values for absorption are not readily available for most drugs. One approximation that has been employed to calculate the steady-state minimum in cases where $k_1 \gg \beta$ is

$$P_{min} = \frac{B_{app} f}{1 - f} \tag{43}$$

which is similar to Eq. (40) except that the apparent beta intercept, B_{app}, is determined from extrapolation of terminal data following a single oral dose [56]. This equation is based upon a one-compartment model, but Wagner and Metzler [54] have pointed out that fairly reasonable estimates result for many two-compartment cases. There are two variables which may be adjusted in developing a regimen with Eq. (43). These are B_{app} (which is proportional to dose) and f (which is related to τ by Eq. 36). Thus the size of the dose and the dosage interval can be altered to design a convenient regimen with any desired minimum steady-state plasma concentration. Although the values for D_0 and τ may be altered, there will be an ideal combination if plasma levels are to be maintained within a narrow range. If the size of the dose is fixed, for example, the ideal value for τ will then be fixed. This is illustrated in Fig. 11, where the dose size is constant for all three cases but the values for τ are altered. This can be illustrated with two examples taken from Schumacher [56]. In Practice Problem 17 the dose size is fixed and the interval must be calculated. In Practice Problem 18 the interval is fixed and the dose must therefore be adjusted.

Practice Problem 17: Calculation of the Dosage Interval to Maintain M.I.C. with 500-mg Capsules of Tetracycline

A single oral dose of tetracycline (500-mg capsule) is found to give a linear terminal semilog plot for total drug in blood vs time. The equation for this line is: $\ln(P_t) = \ln(3.9\ \mu g/ml) - (0.0729\ hr^{-1})(t)$. Calculate the dosage interval that will provide a M.I.C. of 0.8 μg/ml of free tetracycline if 50% of the drug in the blood is bound to serum protein.
Answer: 16.9 hr

Practice Problem 18: Calculation of the Oral Dose of Tetracycline to Maintain M.I.C. with a 12-hr Dosage Interval

In the previous problem 500-mg capsules were used to calculate a dosage interval. The regimen which resulted was one capsule every 16 or 17 hr. This is not a convenient interval. A regimen of morning and night (every 12 hr) would be more reasonable. Using the information in Practice Problem 17, calculate the dose to be administered every 12 hr.
Answer: 287 mg (Hint: Assuming that blood levels are proportional to dose, calculate the value for B_{app} when τ = 12 hr and therefore f

= 0.417. The value for B_{app} is 2.24, which is 57.4% of 3.90. Therefore the new dose is 57.4% of 500 mg.)

During the steady state a drug is administered on a fixed dose and dosage interval. The patient thereby maintains a relatively constant amount of drug in the body. The previous problem demonstrates the manner in which the dose or time interval may be altered and still maintain the steady state. When the 12-hr interval was employed, a maintenance dose of 287 mg was sufficient. However, 500 mg was needed when the 17-hr interval was used. In the steady state, a single dose of drug is eliminated during each τ interval and then replaced by the next dose. Therefore the difference between the minimum and maximum in the steady state is a single maintenance dose. This was illustrated in Table 8. The shorter the interval chosen for τ, the smaller the maintenance dose. This was just observed in the previous two problems, where 287 mg replaced 500 mg. Thus the shorter the τ interval, the smoother the blood-time profile during steady state and the less the difference between P_{min} and P_{max}. This may be an important consideration in developing a regimen for a drug with a narrow margin of safety.

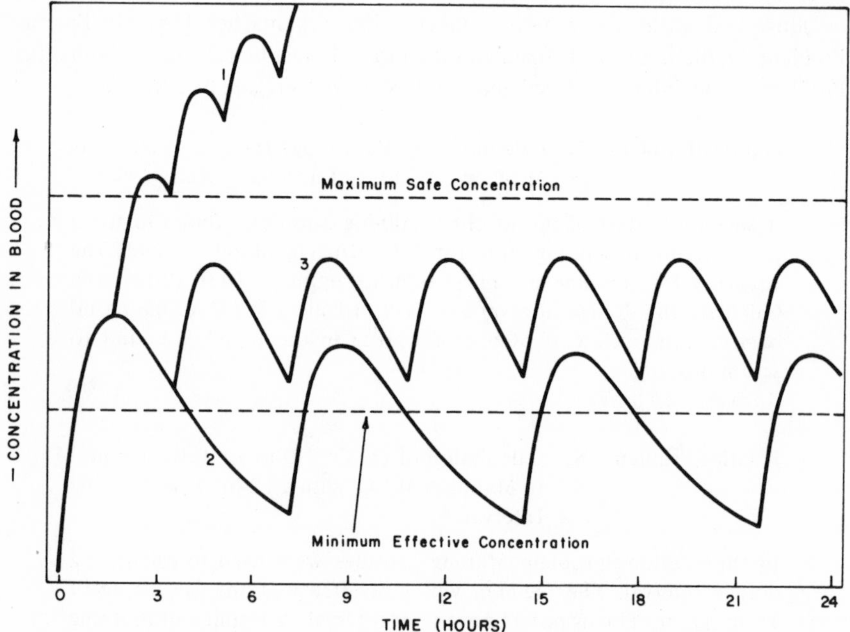

Fig. 11. The objective of the multiple-dosage regimen is to maintain the patient's blood level within the maximum and minimum concentrations shown in the figure. The dosage interval, τ, is too short in curve 1, too long in curve 2, and ideal in curve 3. The initial dose used for this simulation is 33% more than the maintenance dose, and k_1 is three times larger than k_2.

D. Calculation of Loading Dose

In Fig. 10 a fixed dose is administered every 4 hr and roughly 16 hr is required to achieve the steady state. Contrast that to the time course of curve 3 in Fig. 11, where the steady state is practically attained with the first dose. The difference is the fact that in curve 3 of Fig. 11 a loading dose equal to 33% more than the maintenance dose was used. Kruger-Thiemer [57] has pointed out that a nearly optimum regimen with little or no accumulation results when the loading dose is twice that of the maintenance dose and $\tau = t_{1/2}$ (provided that $k_1 \gg \beta$). Thus, for drugs which do accumulate, a loading dose can provide the shortest onset.

If a drug has a short half-life, a dosage regimen may not be designed to result in accumulation. The various penicillins, for example, have $t_{1/2}$ values of 0.5 to 1.0 hr (see Chap. 5). Oral penicillin tablets are generally administered every 4-6 hr. Assuming that absorption is relatively rapid and elimination is first order, one would estimate that 94% of a dose is eliminated in four half-lives or 2-4 hr. Thus administration of tablets every 4-6 hr will not result in accumulation, since each dose is administered to an empty patient. The time course of drug in blood after each dose would therefore appear like a single-dose treatment.

For those drugs which do accumulate during a multiple-dose regimen, an onset period representing the time to reach the steady state can be observed. As seen for the case of constant intravenous infusion, this onset is related to the $t_{1/2}$ of the drug. In other words, a drug with a long $t_{1/2}$ will have a longer onset than one with a shorter $t_{1/2}$ (all other parameters being equal). The amount of drug in the body at the steady state is dependent upon the bioavailable dose, the dosage interval, and the $t_{1/2}$. The ratio of drug in the body to bioavailable dose is defined by the equation

$$\frac{D_{ss}}{FD_0} = \frac{(1.44t_{1/2})}{\tau} \tag{44}$$

which is obtained by rearranging Eq. (41). Thus a drug that is completely absorbed (F = 1) will accumulate 1.44 times the dose if administered every half-life. If it is administered at intervals that are one-half of the value for the half-life, then 2.88 times the dose will accumulate. Thus we see that the number of doses which accumulate is directly proportional to the $t_{1/2}$ and inversely proportional to the dosage interval.

The onset is due largely to the $t_{1/2}$. For a one-compartment drug 90% of the steady-state content is achieved in roughly three to four half-lives [53,58]. A two-compartment drug may require even longer [59]. If one estimates (for example) that five half-lives are required for accumulation, it follows that a drug with a 12-hr half-life will not reach steady state for 2.5 days. Thus, a loading dose may be indicated for improved therapy. For example, a 4-day regimen of a drug with a 20-hr half-life would not achieve the steady state level during the course of therapy if the onset time for that drug were five half-lives. The use of a sufficiently large initial dose will result in steady-state levels throughout the 4 days. How does one calculate the initial dose or the loading dose, D*? It is calculated from the maintenance dose, D_0, and the value for f using the equation

$$D^* = \frac{D_0}{1 - f} \tag{45}$$

Thus, the initial dose, D*, is calculated from the maintenance dose, D_0, and the fraction, f, which is calculated from the elimination constant, β and the dosage interval, τ by use of Eq. (36). Equation (45) may be used for either the oral or intravenous route of administration provided that the maintenance dose, D_0 has been determined for the same route. That is the reason why Eq. (45) is identical to Eq. (38) for calculating D_{max} by the I.V. route, where the bioavailability factor, F, is equal to one. Thus, for the intravenous case, the loading dose is equal to D_{max}. For an extravascular route, D* will generally be larger than D_{max}, since the bioavailability factor will be less than one. Equation (45) may be applied to either one- or two-compartment model drugs provided that absorption and distribution are complete before the administration of each consecutive maintenance dose.

Practice Problem 19: Calculating Loading Dose

Calculate a loading dose to be used for each of the maintenance regimens (doses and intervals) that you estimated in Practice Problems 16, 17, and 18.
Answer: (PP16a) 1.13 g; (PP16b) 940 mg; (PP17) 705 mg; (PP18) 492 mg

One final complication, that will be mentioned here but not solved, is the problem of calculating a dosage regimen when drugs are not administered at uniform time intervals "around the clock." If the indicated dosage regimen for a drug is four times a day, it is unlikely that it will be taken once every 6 hr. The most common definition found in hospital formularies for q.i.d. is either 10-2-6-10 or 9-1-5-9 [60]. Thus a 12-hr period follows the last dose each night. Figure 12 illustrates drug plasma-time profiles for this type of dosage regimen at two different doses. Methods have been devised for computerized calculations of plasma level-time courses for such cases [60].

E. Adjustment of Dosage Regimen in Renal Failure

There are many specific examples of recommendations for adjustment of the dosage regimen for a drug administered to a patient during renal failure. This consideration is of paramount importance in cases where the drug has a narrow

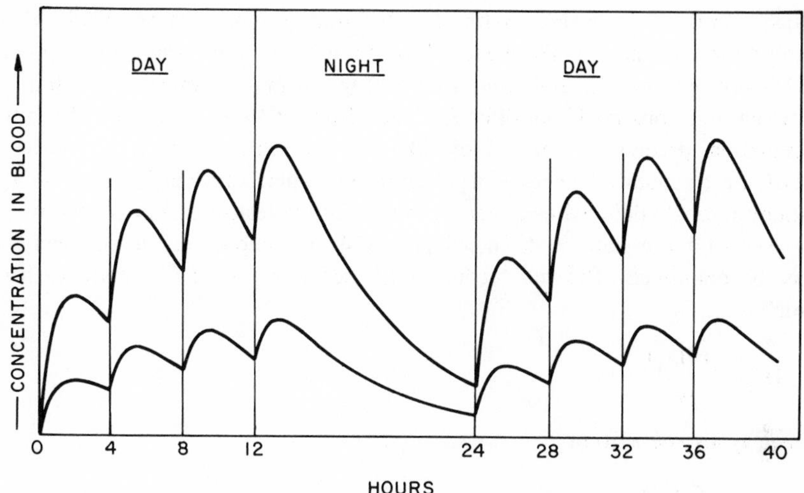

Fig. 12. A typical regimen of one tablet four times a day on a schedule of 10-2-6-10 or 9-1-5-9. Two different doses are illustrated over the first and second day of the regimen.

margin of safety. Administration of such a drug on a normal or average basis can result in much higher levels of drug accumulation during the steady state, causing side effects to the patients. One summary, containing more than 60 drugs, lists the probable side effects in patients with renal failure and the recommended maintenance-dosage intervals to avoid toxicities [61]. It contains a brief discussion of the use of creatinine clearance values in dosage adjustment and an excellent bibliography containing 78 references complete with titles. A number of investigators have recommended dosage adjustment based upon renal clearance values as an indicator of renal function. Notable among these examples are cephalosporins, digoxin, digitoxin, gentamicin, kanamycin, and procainamide [62].

The approach generally used is a very simple one. It is based on the assumption that

$$\beta = \beta_m + \beta_e \tag{46}$$

where the total elimination rate constant, β, is the sum of the first-order rate constants for metabolism, β_m and excretion, β_e. (This equation is discussed in Chap. 3, Secs. II.D.2 and II.D.3.) Thus the assumptions are that β remains first-order during renal failure and that metabolism remains constant but not saturated so that β_m remains constant. The change in β (or $t_{1/2}$) for the patient in renal failure is thus ascribed to the equation

$$C_R = (\beta_e)\,Vd \tag{47}$$

which assumes a constant value for Vd during renal failure. While these assumptions are commonly made, they do not represent the only approach which may be used. Several studies have simply found an empirical relationship between the observed half-life for the drug (which represents the total elimination process as defined by β) and the value for renal clearance of creatinine or inulin. The resulting "calibration" plot can then be used for the patient in renal failure whose clearance value for the test substance is known.

Any of the equations discussed previously for developing dosage regimens may be employed. The most commonly used is Eq. (41) (discussed earlier), which is

$$\bar{D}_{ss} = \frac{F(D_0)}{\beta\tau}$$

This may also be written

$$\bar{P}_{ss} = \frac{F(D_0)}{(Vd)\beta\tau} \tag{48}$$

Adjustment of dosage using these equations is obvious on inspection. Suppose the $t_{1/2}$ during renal failure is twice the normal value, so that β is reduced to one-half of its normal value. The patient would develop a steady-state plasma level, $\bar{P}_{ss}$ twice that of the normal patient. The adjustable parameters, D_0 and τ, may be altered in order to maintain a $\bar{P}_{ss}$ value equal to that in the patient with normal kidney function. Therefore, one could maintain the dosage interval constant and administer one-half the dose. Alternatively, the dose may be kept constant and the dosage interval made twice as long. Any combination in which (D_0/τ) results in one-half the initial value will work. In choosing τ one must consider convenience, whereas D_0 will be limited by available dosage strengths. It is also well to keep in mind that D_{max} is one maintenance dose larger than D_{min}. Thus smaller maintenance doses result in less fluctuation of body content during steady state. This could be a critical factor in choosing a convenient (D_0/τ) ratio for a drug which has a low therapeutic index.

An excellent example of adjustment of dose during renal failure by altering only the dosage interval, τ can be found in the product information for gentamicin sulfate injection. For example, the recommended τ values (in hr) as a function of C_R of creatinine (in ml/min) are 8 (>70); 12 (35-70); 18 (24-34); 24 (16-34); 36 (10-15); and 48 (5-9). Thus in extreme renal failure, where creatinine clearance is only 5-9 ml/min, the drug is administered only once every 2 days rather than once every 8 hr as is the case for the patient with normal kidney function.

The following problem, adapted from a reported request for drug information [63], illustrates how to adjust the dosage regimen based upon a fixed value for τ and a smaller maintenance dose.

Practice Problem 20: Adjusting the Maintenance Dose During Renal Failure

A 60-kg patient who has been taking 1.5 g of ethambutol in a single oral daily dose has undergone a kidney transplant and has a creatinine clearance value of 40 ml/min. Should the daily dosage of ethambutol be altered in order to maintain a steady-state body content which is similar to that before the operation? Assume the half-life for this drug in this patient was 6.5 hr before the transplant and that 80% of the drug was excreted intact by the kidneys (normally).

Answer: The dose should be reduced to 698 mg (or approx. 700 mg)

Solution: The value for β (normal) is 0.107, of which $\beta_e = 0.0853$ and $\beta_m = 0.0214$ (all in hr^{-1}). Using Eq. (47) which states that β_e is proportional to C_R, and assuming Vd constant allows calculation of β_e (renal failure) = (40/120) β_e (normal) = (0.333)(0.0853) = 0.0284 hr^{-1}. Thus, assuming β_{met} constant gives β (renal failure) = $\beta_m + \beta_e$ (renal failure) = 0.0214 + 0.0284 = 0.0498 hr^{-1}. Rearranging Eq. (41) yields D_0 (renal) = D_0 (normal) [β(renal)/β(normal)] = (1.5 g)(0.465) = 0.698 g. Since the value for β in renal failure is 46.5% of the normal value, the maintenance dose is reduced to 46.5% that of the normal dose.

Practice Problem 21

Recalculate the dose for this patient if the schedule is changed so that a dose is administered every 12 hr.

Answer: 350 mg.

There are several review articles on methods for adjusting doses during renal failure. A few are listed here for the interested reader [64–69].

REFERENCES

1. D. D. Breimer, On the Biological Availability of Drugs, *Pharmaceutisch Weekblad, 108*, 309 (1973).
2. P. A. Shore, B. B. Brodie, and C. A. M. Hogben, The Gastric Secretion of Drugs, *J. Pharmacol. Exp. Therap., 119*, 361 (1957).
3. C. A. M. Hogben, L. S. Schanker, D. J. Tocco, and B. B. Brodie, Absorption of Drugs from the Stomach, II, The Human, *J. Pharmacol. Exp. Therap,. 120*, 540 (1957).
4. L. S. Schanker, Absorption of Drugs from the Rat Colon, *J. Pharmacol. Exp. Therap., 126*, 283 (1959) and leading references.
5. E. Overton, *Arch. Ges. Physiol., 92*, 115 (1902).
6. J. Travell, Influence of Hydrogen Ion Concentration on Absorption of Alkaloids from Stomach, *J. Pharmacol. Exp. Therap., 69*, 21 (1940).

7. T. D. Sokoloski,, Solutions and Phase Equilibria, in *Remington's Pharmaceutical Sciences*, 15th ed,. Mack Publishing Co,. Easton, Pa,. 1975.
8. J. R. Leonards, The Influence of Solubility on the Rate of Gastrointestinal Absorption of Aspirin, *Clin. Pharmacol. Ther,. 4*, 476 (1963) and references therein.
9. L. E. Hollister, Measuring Measurin: Problems of Oral Prolonged-action Medications, *Clin. Pharmacol. Ther., 9*, 345 (1968). (Note: See Fig. 4 for previously unpublished data.)
10. E. B. Truitt and A. M. Morgan, Gastrointestinal Factors in Aspirin Absorption, *J. Pharm. Sci., 53*, 129 (1964), and Evaluation of Acetylsalicylic Acid Esterase in Aspirin Metabolism, *J. Pharm. Sci., 54*, 1640 (1965).
11. Examples of sodium or potassium salts of weak acid drugs showing increased absorption rates may be found in H. Juncher and F. Raaschou, *Antibiotic Med. Clin. Ther., 4*, 497 (1957); C. C. Lee, R. C. Anderson, F. G. Henderson, H. M. Worth, and P. N. Harris, *Antibiotic Chemother., 8*, 354 (1958); and E. Nelson, *J. Pharm. Sci., 47*, 297 (1958).
12. Examples of salts of weakly basic drugs showing increased absorption rates may be found in B. B. Brodies and C. A. M. Hogben, *J. Pharm. Pharmacol., 9*, 345 (1957); E. Nelson, *J. Pharm. Sci., 48*, 96 (1959); and W. Morozowich, T. Chulski, W. E. Hamlin, P. M. Jones, J. I. Northram, A. Purmalis, and J. G. Wagner, *J. Pharm. Sci., 51*, 993 (1962).
13. E. Nelson, E. L. Knoechel, W. E. Hamlin, and J. G. Wagner, Influence of the Absorption Rate of Tolbutamide on the Rate of Decline of Blood Sugar Levels in Normal Humans, *J. Pharm. Sci., 51*, 509 (1961).
14. J. Haleblian and W. McCrone, Pharmaceutical Applications of Polymorphism, *J. Pharm. Sci., 58*, 911 (1969).
15. J. W. Poole, G. Owen, J. Silverio, J. N. Freyhof, and S. B. Rosenman, Physicochimical Factors Influencing the Absorption of the Anhydrous and Trihydrate Forms of Ampicillin, *Current Therap. Res., 10*, 292 (1968).
16. J. R. Marvel, D. A. Schichting, and C. Denten, The Effect of a Surfactant and Particle Size on Griseofulvin Plasma Levels, *J. Invest. Dermat., 42*, 197 (1964).
17. M. Kraml, J. Dubuc, R. Gaudry, and D. Beall, Gastrointestinal Absorption of Griseofulvin, II, *Antibiot. Chemother., 12*, 239 (1962), and Gastrointestinal Absorption of Griseofulvin, I, *Arch Dermat., 87*, 179 (1963).
18. R. G. Crounse, Effect of Use of Griseofulvin, *Arch. Dermat., 87,* 176 (1963).
19. H. Blank, Antifungal and Other Effects of Griseofulvin, *Am. J. Med., 39*, 831 (1965).
20. H. E. Paul, K. J. Hayes, M. F. Paul, and A. R. Borgmann, Laboratory Studies with Nitrofurantoin, *J. Pharm. Sci., 56*, 882 (1967).
21. J. D. Conklin and F. J. Hailey, Urinary Drug Exctetion in Man During Oral Dosage of Different Nitrofurantoin Formulations,*Clin. Pharmacol. Ther., 10*, 534 (1969).
22. F. J. Hailey and H. W. Glascock, Gastrointestinal Tolerance to a New

Macrocystalline Form of Nitrofurantoin: A Collaborative Study, *Current Therap. Res., 9,* 600 (1967).

23. M. A. Schwartz and F. H. Buckwalter, Pharmaceutics of Penicillin, *J. Pharm. Sci., 51,* 1119 (1962).
24. J. P. Hou and J. W. Poole, β-Lactam Antibiotics: Their Physicochemical Properties and Biological Activities in Relation to Structure, *J. Pharm. Sci., 60,* 503 (1971).
25. J. G. Wagner, W. Veldkamp,and S. Long, Enteric Coatings, IV, *J. Pharm. Sci., 49,* 128 (1960).
26. J. G. Wagner, Biopharmaceutics: Absorption Aspects, *J. Pharm. Sci., 50,* 359 (1961).
27. V. C. Stephens, J. W. Conine, and H. W. Murphy, Esters of Erythromycin, IV, *J. Pharm. Sci., 48,* 620 (1959).
28. R. S. Griffith and H. R. Black, A Comparison of Blood Levels After Oral Administration of Erythromycin and Erythromycin Estolate, *Antibiotic Chemother., 12,* 398 (1962).
29. P. H. Tardrew, J. C. H. Mao, and D. Kenny, Antibacterial Activity of 2′-Esters of Erythromycin, *Appl. Microbiol., 18,* 159 (1969).
30. V. C. Stephens, C. T. Pugh, and N. E. Davis, A Study of the Behavior of Propionyl Erythromycin in Blood by a New Chromatographic Method, *J. Antibiot. (Tokyo), 22,* 551 (1969).
31. W. E. Wick and G. E. Mallitt, New Analysis for the Therapeutic Efficacy of Propionyl Erythromycin and Erythromycin Base, *Antimicrob. Ag. and Chemother.,* p. 410 (1968).
32. R. S. Griffith and H. R. Black, Comparison of the Blood Levels Obtained After Single and Multiple Doses of Erythromycin Estolate and Erythromycin Stearate, *Am. J. Med. Sci., 247,* 69 (1964).
33. J. A. Gronroos, H. A. Saarimaa, and J. L. Kalliomaki, A Study of Liver Function During Erythromycin Estolate Treatment, *Current Therap. Res., 9,* 589 (1967) and leading references.
34. L. S. Goodman and A. Gilman, *The Pharmacological Basis of Therapeutics,* 4th ed., The Macmillan Co., New York, 1970, p. 1040.
35. R. G. Remmers, G. M. Sieger, N. Anagnostakos, J. C. Corbett, and A. P. Doerschuk, Metal-acid Complexes with Members of the Tetracycline Family, III, *J. Pharm. Sci., 54,* 49 (1965) and references therein.
36. J. Scheiner and W. A. Altemeier, Experimental Study of Factors Inhibiting Absorption and Effective Therapeutic Levels of Declomycin, *Surgery, 114,* 9 (1962).
37. The following reviews have summarized observed differences in bioavailability of products: (a) J. G. Wagner, Generic Equivalence and Inequivalence of Oral Products, *Drug Intell. and Clin. Pharmacol., 5,* 115 (1971); (b) Symposium on Formulation Factors Affecting Therapeutic Performance of Drug Products, *Drug Information Bull., 3,* No. 1, Jan.-June (1969); (c) *Bioavailability of Drugs (B. B. Brodie and W. M. Heller, eds.),* S. Karger, New York, 1972; and (d) (Anon.), Biological Availability, A Statement by the Pharmaceutical Society of Great Britain, *Drug Intell. and Clin. Pharm., 7,* 117 (1973).

7, 117 (1973).

38. (a) A. J. Aguiar, L. M. Wheeler, S. Fusari, and J. E. Zelmer, Evaluation of Physical and Pharmaceutical Factors Involved in Drug Release and Availability from chloramphenicol Capsules, *J. Pharm. Sci., 57,* 1844 (1968); (b) A. J. Glazko, A. W. Kinkel, W. C. Alegnani, and E. L. Holmes, An Evaluation of the Absorption Characteristics of Different Chloramphenicol Preparations in Normal Human Subjects, *Clin. Pharmacol. Therap., 9*, 472 (1968).
39. H. Bell, H. Johansen, P. K. M. Lunde, H. A. Andersgaard, P. Sinholt, T. Midtvedt, E. Hollum,Absorption and Dissolution Characteristics of 14 Different Oral Chloramphenicol Preparations Tested in Healthy Human Male Subjects, *Pharmacology, 5*, 108 (1971).
40. W. H. Barr, J. Adir, and L. Garrettson, Decrease of Tetracycline Absorption in Man by Sodium Bicarbonate, *Clin. Pharmacol. Therap., 12*, 779 (1971).
41. J. G. Wagner, P. K. Wilkinson, H. J. Sedman, and R. G. Stoll, Failure of USP Tablet Disintegration Test to Predict Performance in Man, *J. Pharm. Sci., 62*, 859 (1973).
42. J. G. Wagner, Estimation of Defect Rate, *J. Pharm. Sci., 62*, Open Forum Page VI, (1973).
43. H.C. Standiford, M.C. Jordan, and W.M. Kirby, Clinical Pharmacology of Carbenicillin Compared with Other Penicillins, *J. Infect. Dis., 122,* 9 (Sup.), 1970.
44. G. J. Martin, *Ion Exchange and Adsorptive Agents*, Little, Brown & Co., 1955.
45. For a discussion of this and other subjects related to this chapter, see Chap. 2, by G. Levy, in *Prescription Pharmacy,* (J. B. Sprouls, Jr., ed.), J. B. Lippincott Co., Philadelphia, 1963.
46. L. E. Hollister, Studies of Delayed-action Medications, *New Eng. J. Med., 266*, 281 (1962); *Current Therap. Res., 4*, 471 (1962); *Clin. Pharmacol. Therap., 4*, 612 (1963).
47. *Animal and Clinical Pharmacologic Techniques in Drug Evaluation*, Vol. I (1964) (J. H. Nodine and P. E. Siegler, eds.), and Vol. II (1967) (P. E. Siegler and J. H. Moyer, eds.), Year Book Medical Publishers, Chicago.
48. J. C. King, Clinical Experience with a New Long-acting Antacid-Anticholinergic Preparation, *Am. J. Gastroenterol., 32*, 509 (1959).
49. E. Kruger-Thiemer, Formal Theory of Drug Dosage Regimens, *J. Theor. Biol., 13*, 212 (1966).
50. J. G. Wagner, J. I. Northram, C. D. Alway, and O. S. Carpenter, Blood Levels of Drug at the Equilibrium State After Multiple Dosing, *Nature, 207*, 1301 (1965).
51. M. Gibaldi and H. Weintraub, Some Considerations as to the Determination and Significance of Biological Half-life, *J. Pharm. Sci., 60*, 624 (1971).
52. D. Perrier and M. Gibaldi, Relationship Between Plasma or Serum Drug Concentration and Amount of Drug in the Body at Steady State Upon Multiple Dosing, *J. Pharmacokin. and Biopharm., 1*, 17 (1973).
53. J. M. Van Rossum, Pharmacokinetics, in *Drug Design*, Vol.I (E. J. Ariens, ed.), Academic Press, New York, 1971, p. 507.
54. J. G. Wagner and C. M. Metzler, Prediction of Blood Levels After Multiple Doses from Single-dose Blood Level Data: Generated with Two-compart-

ment Open Model Analyzed According to the One-compartment Open Model, *J. Pharm. Sci., 58*, 87 (1969).
55. R. G. Wiegand, J. D. Buddenhagen, and C. J. Endicott, Multiple Dose Excretion Kinetics, *J. Pharm. Sci., 52*, 268 (1963).
56. G. E. Schumacher, Practical Pharmacokinetic Techniques for Drug Consultation and Evaluation, I, Use of Dosage Regimen Calculations, *Am. J. Hosp. Pharm., 29*, 474 (1972).
57. E. Kruger-Thiemer,Dosage Schedule and Pharmacokinetics in Chemotherapy, *J. Pharm. Sci., 49*, 311 (1960).
58. J. M. Van Rossum, Pharmacokinetics of Accumulation, *J. Pharm. Sci., 57*, 2162 (1968).
59. J. G. Wagner, *Pharmacokinetics*, J. M. Richards Laboratory, Grosse Pointe Park, Mich., 1969, p. 139.
60. P. J. Niebergall, E. T. Sugita, and R. L. Schnaare, Calculation of Plasma Versus Time Profiles for Variable Dosing Regimens, *J. Pharm. Sci., 63*, 100 (1974).
61. W. M. Bennett, I. Singer, and C. H. Coggins, A Practical Guide to Drug Usage in Adult Patients with Impaired Tenal Function, *J. A. M. A., 214*, 1468 (1970). See also Ref. 67.
62. For these drugs and others, see references in R. H. Reuning and J. A. Visconti, A New Function-oriented Course: Individual Adjustment of Drug Dosage, *Amer. J. Pharm. Educ., 38* (May 1974).
63. Dias Rounds, Request Number 4, *Drug Intell. and Clin. Pharm., 5*, 251 (1971).
64. L. Dettli, Drug Dosage in Patients with Impaired Renal Function, *Post Grad. Med. J., 46*, 32 (Suppl.), (1970).
65. M. Mayersohn, Dosage Regimen Calculations in Patients with Renal Insufficiency, *Can. J. Hosp. Pharm., 24*, 215 (1971).
66. J. G. Wagner, *Biopharmaceutics and Relevant Pharmacokinetics*, Drug Intell. Publications, Hamilton, Ill., 1971, Chap. 28.
67. W. M. Bennett, I. Singer, and C. H. Coggins, Guide to Drug Usage in Adult Patients with Impaired Renal Function. A Supplement, *J.A.M.A., 223*, 991 (1973). See also Ref. 61.
68. R. H. Levy and G. H. Smith, Dosage Regimens of Antiarrhythmics, I and II, *Am. J. Hosp. Pharm., 30*, 398 and 494 (1973).
69. D. L. Guisti, Clinical Use of Penicillins in Patients with Renal and Hepatic Insufficiency. I. The Penicillins, II. The Cephalosporins., *Drug Intell. and Clin. Pharmacy, 7*, 62 and 252 (1973).

Chapter 5

PHARMACOKINETIC ASPECTS OF STRUCTURAL MODIFICATIONS IN DRUG DESIGN AND THERAPY*

*Adapted with permission of the copyright owner from a review by R. E. N. in *J. Pharm. Sci.*, *62*, 865 (1973).

I. INTRODUCTION

The clinical implications of variations in bioavailability from various dosage forms has received widespread attention [1-3]. It is well recognized that dosage-form design plays a major role in determining both the rate and extent of the release of active ingredients following administration of the product to the patient. The significance of pharmacokinetics in the design, evaluation, and rational use of drug products has been stressed in the previous chapters. Consideration has been given to the routes and rates of drug administration and to the effects of prolonged-action products, dissolution rate, particle size, inert ingredients, pH, and so on, upon the absorption of drugs following oral administration. Indeed, absorption aspects (in fact, formulation factors) comprise the primary impact of biopharmaceutics in clinical practice. Most of what has been reported applies primarily to gastrointestinal absorption and may be described as attempts to:

1. Maximize absorption rate by increasing the dissolution rate (as in micronization, salts of acids or bases, buffers, amorphous or metastable polymorphs, etc.)
2. Extend duration by decreasing release rate from the dosage form

(sustained release, repository injections of slowly soluble salts, macrocrystals, free acid or base instead of salt, etc.)

3. Decrease loss of degradation in the stomach (acid insoluble esters or salts, chemically stable derivatives, enteric coating, etc.)

Relatively few studies have been reported in which the goal has been to define substituent-group effects on the total drug–organism interaction including not only biological responses but also correlations among drug absorption, distribution, and excretion with pharmacological effects. Examples illustrating such effects can be found by examining classes of drugs where both pharmacokinetic studies and biological responses have been reported and then deducing, where possible, the connection between them. The results disclose three important facts:

1. Pharmacokinetic parameters do influence biological response, and they are indeed critical in drug design.
2. They can be modified by rather subtle structural changes.
3. There is a great need for basic studies in this field.

The ultimate goal is to design a drug molecule having a desired pharmacologic effect resulting from the proper balance of absorption, distribution, intrinsic activity, metabolism, and excretion without resorting to the costly and time-consuming process of screening large numbers of analogs.

It is common practice to consider the effects of substituent groups in a series of molecules upon the "drug–receptor" interaction (Fig. 1). Typically some assumptions are made regarding the interaction between the parent compound and the "receptor." Molecular modifications are made, and the basic assumptions are tested. Generally, abnormalities (unexpected results) are explained by modifying the concept of the "receptor" and occasionally even by modifying the concept of the drug structure, as in the case where the observed activity is explained by arguing for a particular conformation being the preferred one for that molecule *only* when it is in the vicinty of *that* receptor. In many cases the conclusions are based upon dose-response curves, and the dose is assumed to be

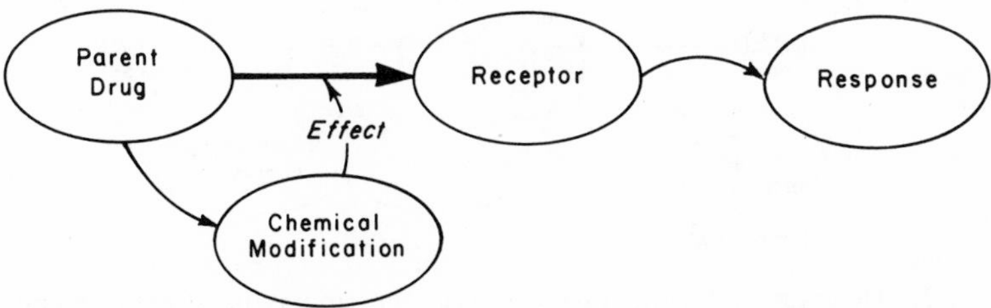

Fig. 1. Simplified model for considering the effect of various substituent groups on the drug-receptor interaction.

responsible for the magnitude of the response. However, it is well recognized (albeit seldom evaluated) that the time course for a drug at the "receptor" must also be considered. The onset, duration, and intensity of effect may be considered as a function of at least two factors:

1. Transport processes effecting the time course at the "receptor site"; delivery and removal from the site
2. Interaction between drug and receptor after arrival at the site

Figure 2 is a schematic representation used to illustrate how modification of a parent structure can influence the drug available to the receptor site. The following processes can be altered by changing a substituent group on a drug (D):

1. Supply and loss
   a. Release from dosage form–rate and/or amount
   b. Stability in depot
   c. Binding in depot (DB)
   d. Transfer from depot to central compartment (rate and/or amount)
   e. Elimination rate from central compartment
2. Distribution
   a. Binding in central compartment (DB)
   b. Binding in peripheral compartment (DB)
   c. Rate and volume of distribution
   d. Transfer to receptor site
3. Drug-receptor interaction

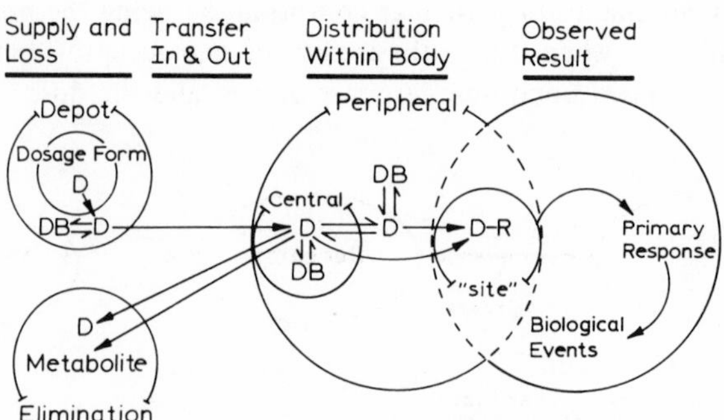

Fig. 2. Diagram of various rate processes which may be altered by chemical modification of a drug, thereby affecting the time course for drug at its site of action. The symbols and interactions are explained in the text.

Consider the case where two "equipotent" drugs are administered but one results in a decreased biological response due to failure to reach the site. How many potential explanations for this can you identify in Fig. 2? (There are more than ten.)

An obvious challenge for any attempt to "optimize" all of the above factors is physically locating the receptor site and defining an ideal time course for the drug-receptor interaction—for example, "hit and run," sustained effect, and so on. Although quite arbitrary, it may be stated that an *ideal drug* should:

1. Reach the site of action
2. Arrive rapidly in sufficient quantity
3. Remain for a sufficient duration
4. Be excluded from other sites
5. Be removed from the site when appropriate

Although the use of compartmental analysis of drugs in the body is quite common and well publicized, relatively little use has been made of a priori considerations of pharmacokinetic parameters in drug design and modification. The most significant question ultimately is "Does this alteration in pharmacokinetic behavior improve the course of therapy with this drug?" It is difficult to envision a model system that will lend itself to simple assessments of such questions. Indeed, this is the challenge of future development.

This chapter will be limited to pharmacokinetic parameters associated with compartmental analysis as described in Chap. 3. The therapeutic implications of the effects of molecular modification on pharmacokinetic parameters will be emphasized.

II. ANTIMICROBIAL AGENTS

A. Systemic Antibiotics

1. Goals for Derivative Formation

In order to optimize the clinical effectiveness of known systemic antibiotic agents, several goals are generally pursued. These will be discussed in detail in later sections, but briefly they may be summarized as follows:

1. Increase amount and/or rate of oral absorption of the drug from the dosage form
2. Increase distribution of the drug to the tissues
3. Increase biological half-life
4. Decrease binding to food and/or plasma proteins
5. Decrease minimum inhibitory concentration

Many successful attempts at achieving one or more of these goals can be cited.

For example, increased rates of oral absorption have been obtained by using salt forms of the parent drug such as potassium salts of penicillins or sodium salts of sulfonamides. The amount of penicillin absorbed orally has been improved by increasing gastric stability through molecular modification. Optimizing the oil/water partition coefficient through ester formation has resulted in improved oral absorption of erythromycin and lincomycin. Molecular modification of tetracyclines resulting in increased tissue distribution has been the object of much research.

The emphasis on improved tissue distribution of antimicrobial agents has increased in the past several years. Spitzy and Hitzenberger [4] have stated that "bacteria germinate more frequently in the tissues than in blood," while Pratt [5] states that "bacteria are more common in other tissues than blood." Several other authors stress the importance of tissue concentrations [6-8]. Fabre et al. [9] have stated that antibiotic effectiveness depends upon penetration into tissues and particularly inflammed tissues. Thus, if binding values were equal, an antibiotic with greater tissue distribution would appear to be reaching the site of action with better efficiency.

The development β-lactamase-resistant pencillins has resulted in increased biological half-life and higher postdistribution body levels. Both penicillin and tetracyclines serve as examples of types of drugs where attempts to increase half-life and to reduce binding to food and/or plasma proteins have been attempted. These examples are discussed more completely in later sections dealing with absorption, prodrug formation, and effects of molecular modification on given classes of agents.

2. *Penicillins*

a. Structural Requirements and Ideal Properties. Penicillins contain two major parts, the 6-aminopenicillanic acid moiety and various side chains (R) attached to the nucleus through an amide linkage (Table 1). The antimicrobial activity of the antibiotic is associated with the intact β-lactam ring, since rupture of the ring at any point results in loss of activity [10,11]. The presence of the free carboxyl group and sulfur atom are necessary, since removal of the sulfur or derivative formation through the carboxyl group results in marked reduction or loss of activity [10-12]. The structure of the side chain can vary widely and appears to control the relative potency of various derivatives. Small changes in the structure of the side chain can also result in large changes in the pharmacokinetic parameters, as will be shown later. In general, it can be stated that the goal of molecular modification of penicillins is to produce and ideal penicillin which will be stable toward acids and β-lactamases, well absorbed and distributed, less bound to plasma proteins, have a broad spectrum and high antibacterial activity. In terms of pharmacokinetic parameters, it should possess a long $t_{1/2}$ and large Vd.

Table 1

Structures of Some Common Penicillins

Penicillin nucleus: RCONH–(β-lactam/thiazolidine ring system with S, N, C=O, gem-dimethyl)–CO_2H

Name	R
Penicillin G	C_6H_5–CH_2–
Penicillin V	C_6H_5–O–CH_2–
Methicillin	2,6-(OMe)$_2$$C_6H_3$–
Oxacillin	3-phenyl-5-methylisoxazol-4-yl (Ph, N, O, Me)
Cloxacillin	3-(2-Cl-phenyl)-5-methylisoxazol-4-yl (Cl, N, O, Me)
Dicloxacillin	3-(2,6-Cl$_2$-phenyl)-5-methylisoxazol-4-yl (Cl, Cl, N, O, Me)
Nafcillin	2-ethoxynaphth-1-yl (OEt)
Ampicillin	C_6H_5–CH(NH_2)–
Carbenicillin	C_6H_5–CH(CO_2H)–

b. Effect of Molecular Modification on Gastric Stability and Dissolution Rate. Schwartz and Buckwalter [13] have discussed the relative gastric stability of penicillins as the primary factor in determining bioavailability. Penicillin G and methicillin are very unstable in acid, having half-lives of 3.5 and 2.3 min respectively, at pH 1.3, 35°C. On the other hand, ampicillin has a half-life of 660 min under the same conditions. The dramatic change in $t_{1/2}$ appears to be due to electronic effects of the protonated amine in acidic solution. In general, an electron-withdrawing group attached to the α-carbon inhibits the electronic displacements necessary for cleavage of the β-lactam ring. The inhibition diminishes when the electron-withdrawing group is present elsewhere in the side chain.

The dissolution rate and rate of oral absorption of penicillins has been increased by forming the potassium salt of the carboxylic acid such as potassium penicillin G and V. Highly insoluble salts are formed with amines such as procaine and N,N′-dibenzylethylenediamine, which dissolve very slowly. These salts are injected intramuscularly, where they form a slowly released depot of the drug—thus extending the duration of plasma levels.

c. Pharmacokinetic Analysis of the Results of Side-chain Modifications. The effect of molecular modification of the side chain can be illustrated by considering the isoxazolyl penicillins, which are a group of closely related derivatives with varied pharmacokinetic behavior (Table 2). They differ in

Table 2

Isoxazolyl Penicillins

Penicillin[a]	Pss (mg/liter)[b]	C_R(ml/min)[c]	Vd(liter)[c]
Oxacillin	9.7	226	14
Cloxacillin	15	162	10
Dicloxacillin	25	113	10

[a] For structures, see Table 1.
[b] Taken from Ref. 17.
[c] Calculated from Ref. 17.

structure only in the number of chlorine atoms present on the benzene ring in the side chain. Early studies attributed higher dicloxacillin serum levels to increased oral absorption. The ratios of serum levels following oral administration in one study were roughly 2/1 for dicloxacillin/cloxacillin [14]. In another study similar ratios of 2.3/1.4/1 for dicloxacillin/cloxacillin/oxacillin were obtained for both the oral and intravenous route of administration [15]. This precludes absorption being the sole factor responsible for different plasma profiles.

The percent absorption was calculated from

$$\% \text{ absorption} = 100\% \, (\text{Area}_{\text{oral}}/\text{Area}_{\text{I.V.}}) \tag{1}$$

using the areas under the curves. Some improvement in absorption with increasing chlorine substitution was noted; dicloxacillin was absorbed 80%, cloxacillin 77%, and oxacillin 67%. However, this is not a sufficient difference to explain the dramatic contrast in plasma levels following oral administration. Such curves cannot be compared directly in spite of the seemingly minor structural differences, and each derivative must be considered pharmacokinetically as a new drug. The values of all four rate constants (k_1, k_{12}, k_{21}, and k_2) may change with the addition of chlorine atoms, and their contributions to the time course must be considered.

Dittert et al. [16] demonstrated that penicillins are distributed according to a two-compartment model. Therefore, before we consider the effect of chlorine substitution on pharmacokinetic parameters, we should note a basic problem in evaluating the Vd of such drugs. As was pointed out in Chap. 3, the calculated value for Vd is independent of the method used to determine it only if a drug is truly distributed according to a one-compartment open model. However, if the drug is distributed according to a multicompartment open model, the value of Vd is dependent upon the rate constants. The value obtained by the extrapolation method may not agree with that obtained by the steady-state method. By using constant intravenous infusion to obtain a steady-state plasma level, the T′/P′ ratio will be the equilibrium ratio and the Vd will be independent of k_2. This offers one approach to comparing distribution of analogs using a method that should produce more controlled results than one that is influenced by elimination. With this in mind we can now proceed to do Sample Problem 1, which will demonstrate how to explain the observed differences in plasma concentrations of the three isoxazolyl penicillins.

Sample Problem 1

Oxacillin, cloxacillin, and dicloxacillin were administered to a group of subjects in a study by Rosenblatt et al. [17]. Using constant intravenous infusions of 250 mg/hr, they obtained the steady-state plasma levels given in Table 2. Clearance values and apparent volumes of distribution are also given. Using additional data for the fraction excreted in the urine, it can be shown that 44%, 38%, and 26.5% of oxacillin, cloxacillin, and dicloxacillin, respectively, are eliminated by nonrenal mechanisms.

(a) Calculate β for each penicillin.
Solution: The value for β can be calculated using the equation,

$$\beta = \frac{k_0}{\mathrm{Vd}\ P_{ss}} \tag{2}$$

which is taken from Eq. (65) in Chap. 3. Thus, for oxacillin

$$\beta = \frac{(250\ \mathrm{mg/hr})}{(14\ \mathrm{liters})(9.7\ \mathrm{mg/liter})}$$

$$\beta = 1.83\ \mathrm{hr}^{-1}$$

Similarly, β for cloxacillin and dicloxacillin are calculated to be 1.65 hr^{-1} and 1.00 hr^{-1}, respectively.

(b) Calculate β_e and β_m (nonrenal) for each penicillin.
Solution: Assuming that no metabolic or excretion mechanisms have become saturated at the plasma levels employed in these studies, β is the sum of β_e and β_m. Therefore, urinary excretion data for oxacillin indicate that

$$\beta_m = 0.44\beta$$

$$\beta_m = 0.81\ \mathrm{hr}^{-1}$$

and

$$\beta_e = \beta - \beta_m = 1.02\ \mathrm{hr}^{-1}$$

Similarly, β_m is found to be 0.63 hr^{-1} and 0.26 hr^{-1} for cloxacillin and dicloxacillin, respectively. The values of β_e for cloxacillin and dicloxacillin are 1.02 hr^{-1} and 0.74 hr^{-1}, respectively.

(c) Explain the differences in the observed steady-state plasma levels.
Solution: The values calculated in parts (a) and (b) have been entered in Table 3 together with the values of Vd and P_{ss} from Table 2. The dicloxacillin/cloxacillin/oxacillin plasma steady-state concentration ratio is 2.6/1.7/1, which is very similar to the oral and I.V. ratios.

Table 3

Penicillin	P_{ss} (mg/liter)	Vd(liters)	$\beta(\mathrm{hr}^{-1})$	$\beta_e(\mathrm{hr}^{-1})$	$\beta_m(\mathrm{hr}^{-1})$
Oxacillin	9.7	14	1.84	1.03	0.81
Cloxacillin	15	10	1.67	1.03	0.63
Dicloxacillin	25	10	1.00	0.74	0.26

From the values of Vd given in Table 3, it can be concluded that the difference between the steady-state plasma levels of dicloxacillin and cloxacillin cannot be due to a difference in distribution, since Vd is the same for each. However, when consideration is also given to β, it becomes clear that the plasma levels may be explained as follows: Dicloxacillin levels are higher than those of cloxacillin due to decreased elimination; cloxacillin levels are higher than oxacillin levels primarily due to decreased Vd; dicloxacillin levels are higher than oxacillin levels due to both decreased elimination and Vd.

(d) What is the effect of increasing chlorine substitution on β_e and β_m?
Solution: From the data in Table 3 it can be seen that addition of chlorine to oxacillin results in a decrease in β_m. The addition of one chlorine to oxacillin apparently does not affect β_e, but addition of the second chlorine decreases β_e. The same general trend can be seen in the clearance values, where increasing chlorine substitution results in decreased clearance.

Sample Problem 1 contains several features which merit further discussion. Dicloxacillin has the longest half-life (smallest β) of the isoxazolyl penicillins shown in Table 1. The addition of two chlorine atoms to oxacillin has thus increased its duration. It is generally agreed that extending the duration of penicillins in the blood is a clinical advantage, since they have such short $t_{1/2}$ values [18]. Some speculation exists regarding the reason why this change in half-life has occurred. Increasing the number of chlorine atoms on oxacillin decreases its hydrophilicity. Thus for the isoxazolyl penicillins in Table 2, renal and nonrenal elimination decreases with increasing lipophilicity. The major pathways for the elimination of penicillins are the active transport systems of the kidney tubules and liver. It has been suggested by Nayler [19] that since tubular secretion and inactivation involve passage across lipid membranes, there probably exists an optimum partition coefficient for these transfers. Since the isoxazolyl penicillins are the most hydrophobic penicillins in clinical use, they probably have partition coefficients in excess of the optimum so that any increase in lipophilicity would result in a lower tendency for the necessary transfer to occur. These observations are somewhat supported by the fact that penicillin G has a renal clearance of 400 ml/min, which approaches the renal plasma flow rate of 650 ml/min, while addition of chlorine to the already hydrophobic oxacillin decreases the clearance from 226 to 113 ml/min, which is roughly the value for glomerular filtration (Chap. 3).

Another interesting feature of Sample Problem 1 is that the $t_{1/2}$ values for oxacillin and cloxacillin (calculated using β) would be approximately the same. Thus, the difference in metabolism between oxacillin and cloxacillin could have been overlooked if only a comparison of β or half-life had been made. The half-life parameter indicates the time required to eliminate half the drug from the body. Yet clearance values in Table 2 indicate that oxacillin is cleared 1.4 times faster than cloxacillin. This may be explained by noting that the apparent volume of distribution of oxacillin is 1.4 times larger than cloxacillin. Thus, the difference in renal clearance between the drugs is exactly offset by the increase in volume of distribution.

Similar analyses can be extended to other penicillins. Differences in steady-state plasma levels are frequently (and erroneously) attributed solely to differences in elimination. The next problem will further demonstrate the need to consider parameters other than β.

Sample Problem 2

The observed steady-state plasma levels for various penicillins following I.V. infusions of 500 mg/hr and half-life values are given in Table 4.

Table 4

Observed Steady-state Plasma Concentrations for Various Penicillins Following I.V. Infusion of 500 mg/hr

Penicillin	P_{ss} (mg/liter)	$t_{1/2}$ (hr)
Carbenicillin	73	1.00
Dicloxacillin	51	0.71
Cloxacillin	30	0.42
Ampicillin	29	0.98
Oxacillin	19	0.39
Nafcillin	18	0.55
Penicillin G	16	0.61

(a) What rank order would be predicted solely on the basis of elimination?
Solution: Based solely on elimination, the penicillin with the longest half-life would be predicted to have the highest plasma concentration. Therefore, the rank order would be carbenicillin > ampicillin > dicloxacillin > penicillin G > nafcillin > cloxacillin > oxacillin.

(b) Another parameter must be considered in order to predict the observed steady-state plasma levels correctly. Calculate the value of this parameter for each penicillin.
Solution: The value of Vd must also be considered when predicting the observed steady-state plasma concentrations. The value of Vd for each penicillin can be calculated using the equation

$$Vd = \frac{k_0}{\beta P_{ss}} \qquad (3)$$

The value for β may be calculated from the half-life values given in Table 4 using the equation

$$\beta = \frac{0.693}{t_{1/2}} \tag{4}$$

For example, the Vd of carbenicillin is

$$Vd = \frac{(500 \text{ mg/hr})(1.00 \text{ hr})}{(0.693)(73 \text{ mg/liter})}$$

$$Vd = 10 \text{ liter}$$

In a similar fashion the remaining Vd values were found to be dicloxacillin, 10 liters; cloxacillin, 10 liters; ampicillin, 24 liters; oxacillin, 15 liters; nafcillin, 22 liters; and penicillin G, 28 liters.

Sample Problem 2 shows that both elimination and volume of distribution are determining factors of the steady-state plasma concentrations. Neither of the parameters, Vd or β when considered alone will enable correct prediction of the steady-state plasma levels. However, a few single parameter comparisons can be made from the data in Table 4. Differences in plasma levels among carbenicillin, cloxacillin, and dicloxacillin are due solely to elimination differences, since the Vd of each is similar. Conversely, carbenicillin levels are higher than ampicillin levels entirely due to a difference in Vd.

Table 5

Values for Selected Pharmacokinetic Parameters[a] for Several Penicillins

Penicillin	$t_{1/2}$ (hr)	Vd (liters)	C_R (ml/min)[b]
Carbenicillin	1.0	10	86
Dicloxacillin	0.88, 0.71, 0.7	13, 10, 9.4, 16	88, 162, 130
Cloxacillin	0.42, 0.6	10, 11, 23	162, 287
Ampicillin	1.0, 0.8	22, 20, 25, 30	283, 210,[c] 312
Oxacillin	0.7, 0.38, 0.40	27, 14, 13, 15, 26	190,[c] 402
Nafcillin	0.55	21	160[c]
Methicillin	0.43	22	350
Penicillin V	0.53, 0.43, 0.52	51, 54	393
Penicillin G	0.70, 0.5, 0.84–0.93,[d] 0.6–0.99[e], 0.54, 0.65, 0.78	26, 22, 37–47,[d] 35	433, 386,[c] 340–480,[d] 393

[a]The values were taken from Refs. 14–19 or calculated from data contained in them.

[b]Renal clearance values.

[c]Units are ml/min/1.72 m^2.

[d]Variation due to ambulatory vs bed rest.

[e]Variation attributed to size of dose.

The values of some selected pharmacokinetic parameters are given in Table 5. These parameters are the ones which are used most often to make comparisons between analogs. These parameters also can be used to calculate other parameters of interest, as outlined above.

3. Tetracyclines

a. Structural Requirements and Ideal Properties. Since the isolation in 1947 of the first known member of the tetracycline family, many semisynthetic derivatives have been prepared and their properties extensively studied. Tetracyclines are tetrahydronaphthacene derivatives composed of four rings. Some of the more common tetracyclines are shown in Table 6. The antimicrobial activity of the tetracyclines is associated with the tricarbonylmethane (C_1, C_2, and C_3), the dimethylamino (C_4), and phenolic diketone (C_{10}, C_{11}, and C_{12}) moieties. The phenolic diketone appears to be essential, since molecular modification of that system results in complete loss of activity. Modification of the tricarbonylmethane or dimethylamino moieties drastically reduces the activity. Substitution of various groups on positions 5-9 results in differences in antimicrobial activity, distribution of the drug to tissues, and binding to plasma proteins, but does not affect activity as greatly as do the other three moieties. The tetracyclines are bacteriostatic agents and appear to produce this effect by inhibiting bacterial protein synthesis through alternation of the RNA-ribosome complex [20-24].

Table 6

Structures of Various Tetracyclines

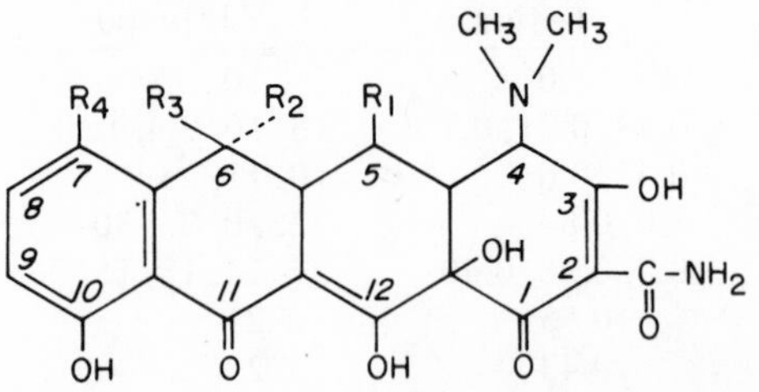

Name	R_1	R_2	R_3	R_4
Tetracycline	H	OH	CH_3	H
Chlortetracycline	H	OH	CH_3	Cl
Demethylchlortetracycline	H	OH	H	Cl
Oxytetracycline	OH	OH	CH_3	H
Methacycline	OH	$=CH_2$	–	H
Minocycline	H	H	H	$-N(CH_3)_2$
Doxycycline	OH	H	CH_3	H

In general, molecular modifications of the basic tetracycline structure have reflected attempts to improve absorption, decrease binding to plasma proteins, improve distribution to the tissues, and decrease minimum inhibitory concentrations. These attempts are examples of research directed toward preparation of an ideal tetracycline. The ideal tetracycline is one which would be rapidly and completely absorbed, only slightly bound to plasma protein, distributed throughout the proper tissues, of long duration, and possess high intrinsic antimicrobial activity. In terms of pharmacokinetic parameters, an ideal tetracycline might therefore have a large Vd and long $t_{1/2}$.

b. Absorption and Distribution. The basic tetracycline molecule has three pK_a values of 3.3, 7.7, and 9.5 [25] associated with the tricarbonylmethane, phenyl diketone, and dimethylamino groups, and thus will be ionized over the entire pH range which a molecule would encounter after oral administration. This fact, coupled with the tendency of tetracyclines to form complexes with substances in the stomach, implies that their oral absorption might be slow and incomplete. Oral administration of tetracycline HCl with 200 ml of water containing 2.0 g of $NaHCO_3$ resulted in a 50% decrease in absorption relative to absence of $NaHCO_3$ [26]. When the tetracycline was dissolved prior to administration, no differences were observed.

Although much has been done regarding factors that decrease tetracycline absorption, relatively little has been reported on the effect of molecular modification upon the absorption process per se. Considerable effort has been made to examine distribution of various tetracyclines into body tissues. Although the value of Vd is a valuable tool in calculating infusion rates and dosage regimens, predicting multiple dose plasma levels, as an indicator of protein binding, and so in, it does not indicate *where* the drug has been distributed once it has left the plasma. This has been discussed in some detail in Chap. 3. Specific organ levels can be determined by surgically removing various tissues and analyzing for the drug. For example, using this approach the ratio of total tetracycline in muscle tissue to the concentration in canine serum has been correlated with chloroform/water partition coefficients [27,28]. The tetracycline with the highest partition coefficient had the highest muscle concentration. The observed order of the tetracyclines studied was 6-demethyl-6-deoxytetracycline $\gg$ doxycycline $\gg$ tetracycline $\gg$ demethylchlortetracycline = methacycline $\gg$ oxytetracycline. In another study [29] concentrations of tetracycline, demethychlortetracycline, and chlortetracycline were determined in no less than 47 organs, tissues, or fluids using radiolabeled compounds. Results indicate that all nonfat tissues are penetrated by the antibiotics within 4.5 hr after I.V. injection and that tissue distribution of tetracycline is generally less than that of the other two.

Doxycycline content in 12 organs sampled operatively in 81 patients was compared with the serum levels at the time of tissue removal and the tissue-to-serum ratios calculated for each organ [9]. These ratios varied from approximately 2 for the kidney, lung, and bladder to less than 0.7 for the appendix and adipose tissue. When the serum concentrations were corrected for binding, the ratios became 13.4 for the kidney, 12.2 for the lungs, 6.3 for muscle, and 3.9 for lymph node. The concentration in all organs usually fell in the range 2-4 μg/g of tissue and always was above 1 μg/g which was considered to be amply bacteriostatic.

There is some indication that lipid solubility plays a major role in the distribution of tetracyclines and that serum protein binding may be less of a factor. Tetracyclines permeate both extra and intracellular fluid, and calculated values of Vd in man [4,30] exceed the volume of total body water—thus indicating that some form of binding must occur.

c. *Binding to Dairy Products and Various Divalent or Trivalent Cations.* It became apparent soon after the introduction of chlortetracycline in 1948 that concomitant administration of aluminum hydroxide gel resulted in decreased biological activity for the antibiotic [31]. Decreased gastrointestinal absorption due to complexation with divalent and trivalent cations, such as calcium, magnesium, aluminum, and so on, indicates that the co-administration of milk or antacids to diminish the potential side effects of anorexia, nausea, and vomiting (often observed with tetracycline therapy) must be avoided. In Chap. 4 the data of Scheiner and Altemeir [32] were used to demonstrate the dramatic sensitivity of demethylchlortetracycline to complexation with heavy metals. Relative to equal doses in the fasting state, only 13% oral absorption takes place when the antibiotic is administered with 8 oz of milk and 22% with 20 ml of aluminum hydroxide gel. Thus development of tetracyclines with a lesser tendency toward complexation became a clinically significant research goal. However, since the sites considered most likely to be the site of complexation [33-35] are also necessary for antimicrobial activity, any direct molecular modification of these sites in order to reduce complexation is precluded. Modifications can be made only in positions such as 5-9, where the substituents will exert either electronic or steric effects upon binding.

Some measure of success has been obtained with newer tetracyclines. Doxycycline oral absorption is markedly less sensitive to food and homogenized milk. This is illustrated in the following problem.

Sample Problem 3

Rosenblatt et al. [36] studied the effect of diet on oral bioavailability of doxycycline and demethylchlortetracycline. Some of the results are illustrated in Fig. 3. The reported maximum plasma value (or peak height) and the time at which it occurred (t_{max}) for each of these eight curves is given in Table 7.

Table 7

Literature Values (Ref. 36) for Peak Plasma Levels (P_{max}, μg/ml) and Their Time of Occurrence (t_{max}, hr) Following Single Oral Doses of 300 mg of Demethylchlortetracycline or 100 mg of Doxycycline to Healthy Volunteers in a Crossover Study

Drug	Fasting		Nondairy Food		Skim Milk		Whole Milk and Food	
	P_{max}	t_{max}	P_{max}	t_{max}	P_{max}	t_{max}	P_{max}	t_{max}
Doxycycline	1.79	2	1.75	4	1.45	2	1.18	4
Demethylchlor-tetracycline	1.98	4	1.08	4	0.59	4	0.71	4

(a) Summarize the effect of (1) food, (2) skim milk, and (3) whole milk and food on the bioavailability of these two antibiotics and include a rough estimate of the percent reduction of oral absorption in each case.

Solution: The peak height may be used for a rough estimate provided that k_1 is relatively constant as indicated by the constancy of the t_{max} values (see Chap. 3). The t_{max} values for demethylchlortetracycline are constant at 4 hr. The estimates

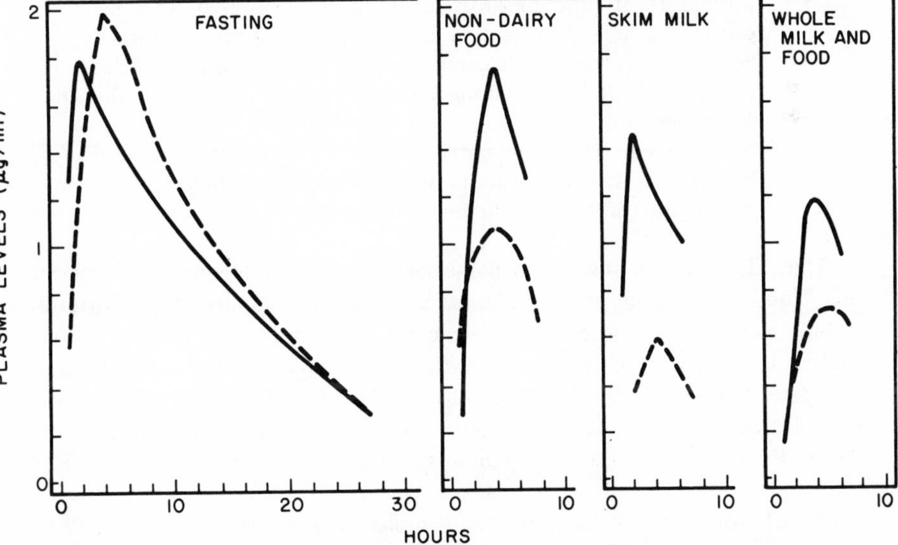

Fig. 3. The data of Rosenblatt et al. [36] have been used to construct these curves representing the time course in blood following single oral doses of 100 mg of doxycycline (solid line) or 300 mg of demethylchlortetracycline (dashed line).

are therefore: (1) food: (108/1.98) = 54% (or 46% reduction); (2) skim milk: (59/1.98) = 30% (70% reduction); (3) food and whole milk: (71/1.98) = 36% (64% reduction).

The t_{max} values for doxycycline are given as 2 hr and 4 hr. Therefore: (1) food appears to have delayed absorption but provided the same peak value; (2) skim milk: (145/1.79) = 81% (19% reduction); (3) food and whole milk: again absorption appears to be delayed. Since food and food with whole milk both have a t_{max} value of 4 hr, the effect of the whole milk can be estimated from (118/1.75) = 67% (33% reduction).

(b) How do these results compare with those calculated from Scheiner and Altemeir [32]?
Solution: See Sample Problem 1 in Chap. 4.

(c) Figure 3 shows fairly similar time profiles for the two tetracyclines in the fasting state for doses of 300 mg and 100 mg. What conclusions can be made regarding the oral absorption of demethylchlortetracycline relative to doxycycline?
Solution: None; additional information is required since these are two different chemical entities.

(d) Product information supplied with doxycycline hyclate for injection indicates that 40% of the dose is excreted by the kidney within 72 hr after administration to individuals with normal renal function. Rosenblatt et al. recovered 45.4 mg during 72 hr following oral ingestion of 100 mg by normal volunteers (creatinine clearance roughly 130 ml/min). What percent of the orally administered dose was absorbed in the Rosenblatt study?
Solution: It was apparently 100% absorbed, since urinary recovery of 45.4 mg exceeds the value calculated based on the 40% figure (or 40% of 100 mg = 40 mg).

Thus, doxycycline absorption has been shown to be less sensitive to skim milk, food, and homogenized milk when compared to demethylchlortetracycline. However, ingestion of antacids containing divalent or trivalent cations resulted in negligible absorption for both drugs. Similar results, although more pronounced, have been noted in another study [37]. When doxycycline was administered orally to humans together with aluminum hydroxide gel, the observed plasma concentrations (at an unspecified time) were reduced to 10% of normal.

Schach von Wittenau [38,39] found similar plasma levels at 1, 3, and 12 hr on day 1, and 0 and 12 hr on day 5 when doxycycline was administered in 100-mg doses every 12 hr with food, on an empty stomach, or with milk in a three-group crossover study. This design would not, however, detect differences that occurred between 3 and 12 hr on day 1, which is the period that contains the peak level in previous studies (Sample Problem 3, Fig. 3). This is the period which would result in major differences in curve areas. Results of in vitro binding studies [38] with calcium ion showed 19% of doxycycline, 36% of oxytetracycline, 40% of methacycline, 40% of tetracycline, and 75% of demethylchlortetracycline was bound. Thus, it appears that in vitro binding studies of this sort qualitatively predict in vivo absorption differences between doxycycline and demethylchlortetracycline in the presence of whole milk.

d. Effect of Binding on Distribution, Elimination, and Half-life. Differences in protein binding continue to cause confusion whenever comparisons between various derivatives are made. The significance of tissue and protein binding in relation to therapeutic efficacy remains unclear for many antibiotics. Readily reversible binding by serum or tissues may serve as a pool of active drug to prolong therapeutic levels [7]. For example, the antibacterial activity of three long-acting sulfonamides may be independent of their protein binding, but this binding may determine their duration [40]. However, this is not unequivocal for all drugs, since some researchers indicate that penicillins bound to protein lose their activity. It has been stated [7] that absorption, distribution, and inactivation may be more important than binding in determining penicillin therapy, presumably because of reversibility. However, other data [41] emphasize the decrease in bioavailability observed with penicillins due to inactivation by protein binding. The M.I.C. of eight penicillins in human serum is the same as that in broth when corrected for the bound fraction. Methacillin was least active in broth where there was no binding. However, in serum where it was bound to a lesser extent than the others studied, it not only required the lowest total concentration of drug to kill 99% of the inoculum, but it also acted more rapidly than any other penicillin.

It would seem that the tissue distribution of a drug would decrease with increasing serum binding as a result of the inability of the protein-bound form to diffuse from the plasma. However, data exist [16,41] which do not support this hypothesis in the case of penicillins. Similar values of Vd were obtained for four penicillins whose percent binding in plasma varied from 22 to 94% [16]. The fraction of the dose in the peripheral compartment was considered by the authors to be similar for all five penicillins studied [16].

While the significance of protein binding of antibiotics is still in dispute, there seems to be some agreement that, in general, reversibility of bound drug is the key factor. It has been noted and documented by authors of seemingly opposing views that reversible binding can serve to prolong drug action [7,41], whereas only irreversible binding removes the drug from the biophase. It would appear from present evidence that the significance of drug binding is probably dependent upon the strength of binding, and it has been calculated that protein binding will affect drug distribution only if the binding constant exceeds 10^4 [42].

The renal clearance of tetracyclines decreases with increasing protein binding

[9]. Urinary clearance is greater for oxytetracycline (73% free) and least for doxycycline (18% free). Chlortetracycline and minocycline are exceptions since they are excreted mainly in the bile. The $t_{1/2}$ appears to be related to protein binding only for those drugs that are primarily cleared by glomerular filtration. A drug that is excreted by tubular secretion does not appear to be influenced by protein binding. Penicillins which have high clearance values (reflecting tubular secretion) have half-lives which are relatively insensitive to protein binding. Data suggest that tetracyclines are primarily excreted by glomerular filtration rather than by tubular secretion, although the lack of precise serum protein binding measurements makes it difficult to calculate the individual contributions. Tetracyclines tend to accumulate during renal insufficiency, with chloretetracycline and doxycycline being notable exceptions. Chlortetracycline is excreted primarily in the bile, as previously mentioned. However, the reason why doxycycline does not accumulate remains unclear. Fabre et al. [9] reported that doxycycline clearance decreased during renal insufficiency without a concurrent increase in hepatic excretion despite a relatively constant $t_{1/2}$ in normal and anuric patients. More recent studies [37] into the extent of enzymatic or metabolic degradation of doxycycline in man and dog indicates that more than 90% of the intact drug was recovered from the urine and feces in both species. Thus excretion of intact doxycycline in feces appears to compensate for decreased renal clearance in uremic patients.

e. Tetracycline Half-lives. The extension of biological half-life to increase duration and decrease the frequency of administration has been a major research goal. Chlortetracycline first appeared in 1948 with a reported $t_{1/2}$ of 5.6 hr and a recommended dosage interval of 6 hr. Oxytetracycline and tetracycline were introduced soon after with reported half-lives of 8.2 and 9.2 hr respectively. In 1958, demethylchlortetracycline ($t_{1/2}$ of 11.8 hr) and methacycline were introduced as useful on a 12-hr regimen. Doxycycline ($t_{1/2}$ of 18–22 hr) marked a new stage in this evolution with the advent of once-a-day therapy.

However, the above half-lives do not appear to be unequivocal. Doluisio and Dittert [43] have redetermined the $t_{1/2}$ values for several tetracyclines and compared their results with those previously published. A summary of the data is contained in Table 8. In comparing the half-lives following a single oral dose to those determined after plateau steady-levels had been reached, they indicated that the $t_{1/2}$ of each of the four antibiotics increased significantly during the 6-day study. It is also apparent that the $t_{1/2}$ values do not vary as much as earlier data would indicate [44], and the range of the four $t_{1/2}$ values in the steady state appears to be 14 ± 3 hr. Antibiotic therapy usually involves the administration of more than a single dose. Therefore the values obtained during multiple dosing would appear to be of more significance in clinical use. The half-life values from single-dose studies failed to predict correctly the steady-state plasma levels obtained following multiple doses, whereas the steady-state $t_{1/2}$ values could be used to predict the observed levels [43]. Based on the fact that multiple dosing of antibiotics is the normal regimen has led Schach von Wittenau and Twomey [37] to refer to the $t_{1/2}$ observed for doxycycline after multiple dosing as the "practical" half-life. They estimate this value to be approximately 22 hr but warn that first-order kinetics are not appropriate for doxycycline elimination following multiple dosing for several days. This behavior is speculated to be due to slow release of drug stored in tissues [38].

Table 8

Apparent Biological $t_{1/2}$ Values for Four Tetracyclines[a]

Antibiotic	Single Dose	Multiple Doses	Steady State
Tetracycline	6.3, 5.6–9.3, 8.2, 8.0, 7.2, 7.3	10,[b] 9.5, 11	10.8
Demethylchlortetracycline	9.0, 6.3–13.3, 12.6, 10, 11, 12.7	14.7,[b] 14.7, 15	13.6
Methacycline	7.0, 14.3, 8.5, 9.6, 7.7	11.0,[b] 10.5, 11.5	14.3
Doxycycline	8.3, 11.7, 15, 15.1	14.5,[b] 22	16.6

[a]From Ref. 43.
[b]Values determined on days 4 and 5 of a multiple-dose regimen.

The biological half-life of a drug may be altered by such factors as the size of the dose, the age of the patient, whether the patient is ambulatory or confined to bed, variation in urinary excretion, co-administration of other drugs, protein binding, or disease. These variables must be controlled or accounted for through proper experimental design. Once this has been done, pharmacokinetic evaluation of $t_{1/2}$ and β become more meaningful.

It has been suggested that the increased $t_{1/2}$ values following multiple dosing might be due to a failure to obtain an accurate assessment of the terminal (or β) slope following a single oral dose [45]. Inclusion of part of the distribution phase could tend to make the $t_{1/2}$ appear smaller with a single dose, whereas this problem is eliminated during the steady state. This behavior has been illustrated using a hypothetical three-compartment model [45]. However, it would also apply to a two-compartment case, which may be appropriate for assessing tetracyclines [46].

A significant observation from the work of Doluisio and Dittert [43] is that all four tetracyclines have reasonably similar steady-state half-lives. It was also observed that they all produced comparable serum levels when administered every 12 hr at appropriate dosage levels. This can be easily understood in terms of what now may be considered classical approaches to dosage-regimen development. These approaches were considered in Chap. 4.

From the discussion presented in this section on tetracyclines, it can be concluded that significant factors to be considered in determining the effects of molecular modification upon the antibiotic activity of a series of derivatives are serum levels, Vd, and $t_{1/2}$. The meaning of these values must be interpreted in terms of the known effects of protein binding and other variables. The ultimate criteria for comparing serum levels of derivatives always must be based on how much is required to treat the disease in question. A derivative which produces a plasma level twice as high as the original drug is not an improved agent when ten times the original level is required.

4. *Miscellaneous Systemic Antimicrobial Agents*

a. Cephalosporins. The cephalosporins are a group of compounds having structures quite similar to penicillins. The more common cephalosporins are shown in Table 9. These compounds contain a β-lactam ring fused to a dihydrothiazine ring which composes the basic 7-aminocephalosporanic acid nucleus. Various groups are attached to this nucleus and are responsible for the observed differences in chemical and biological properties. The structural requirements for antimicrobial activity are quite similar to those of penicillins. An intact β-lactam ring is essential [10,11], and derivative formation through the free carboxyl group results in drastic reduction or complete loss of activity [10-12]. The goals of molecular modification of cephalosporins are to produce a drug which is stable toward acids and β-lactamases, is well absorbed and distributed, and is broad in spectrum and high in antibacterial activity.

The success obtained in pursuing these goals has been remarkable. Cephalosporins in general are more acid-stable than penicillins and are resistant to penicillin β-lactamase [10,47]. However, cephalosporin β-lactamases are known to exist and are very effective in inactivating the cephalosporins [48-51]. Cephalothin and cephaloridine (as well as the naturally occurring compounds cephalosporin C, N, and P not shown in Table 9) are not well absorbed. However, molecular modifications have resulted in the production of cephaloglycin and cephalexin, which are well absorbed orally and resistant to decomposition due to gastric acidity. Peak serum levels are obtained within 1 hr after oral administration of cephalogylcin and cephalexin in their free acid forms [52,53].

Cephalosporins are effective against many gram-positive and gram-negative organisms and are several times more active than the penicillins against gram-negative bacteria [54-56]. Cephalothin is effective against a wide variety of bacteria, particularly the β-lactamase producing *S aureus*, while it is notably ineffective against *Pseudomonas* and indole-positive *Proteus* [57-60]. Cephalori-

Table 9

Name and Structure of Some Common Cephalosporins

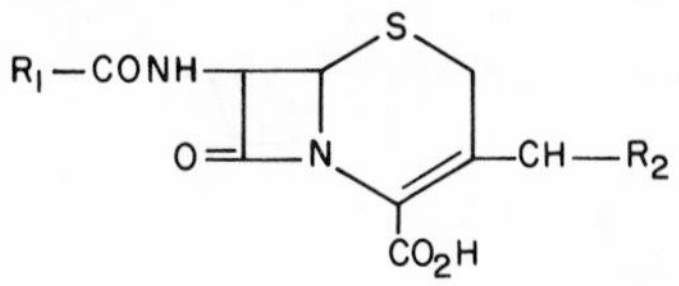

R_1—CONH— [cephem nucleus: β-lactam (C=O, N) fused to dihydrothiazine ring containing S; —CH—R_2; CO_2H]

Name	R_1	R_2
Cephalothin	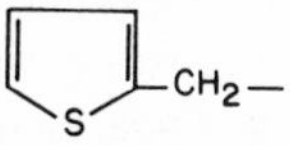 2-thienyl—CH_2—	—$OCOCH_3$
Cephaloridine	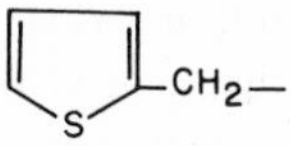 2-thienyl—CH_2—	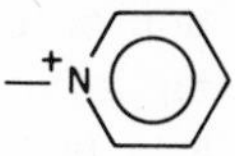 —^+N (pyridinium)
Cephaloglycin	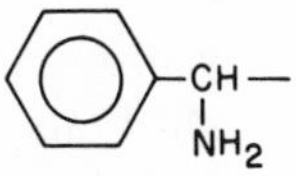 phenyl—CH(NH_2)—	—$OCOCH_3$
Cephalexin	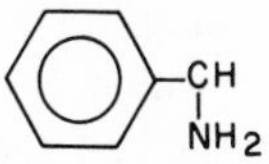 phenyl—CH(NH_2)	—H

dine and cephalexin are similar in that they do not have the acetoxy side chain on the dihydrothiazine ring. Of all the *desacetoxy* derivatives, cephaloridine is the most active, especially toward gram-negative organisms [61-63,55]. However, when cephaloridine, cephalothin, and cephaloglycin are compared, cephaloridine is the most effective against gram-positive organisms and cephaloglycin is the most effective against gram-negative bacteria [64-66].

Cephaloridine has several drawbacks to its clinical use when compared to the other cephalosporins. It is not well absorbed orally and has the potential of causing nephrotoxicity. Cephalosporins, in general, should be used only with extreme caution in those individuals sensitive to penicillins, since cross-allergenicity appears to occur [67].

b. Lincomycin and Clindamycin. Lincomycin is a naturally occurring substance produced by *Streptomyces lincolnensis.* Clindamycin is a semisynthetic compound differing from lincomycin only substitution of a chlorine for a hydroxyl at the 7-position.

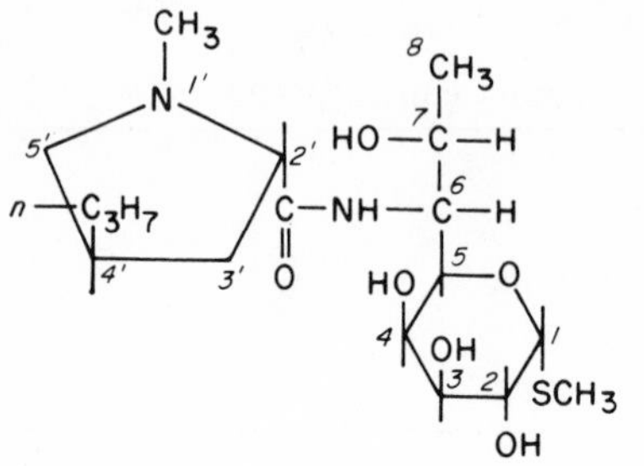

Lincomycin 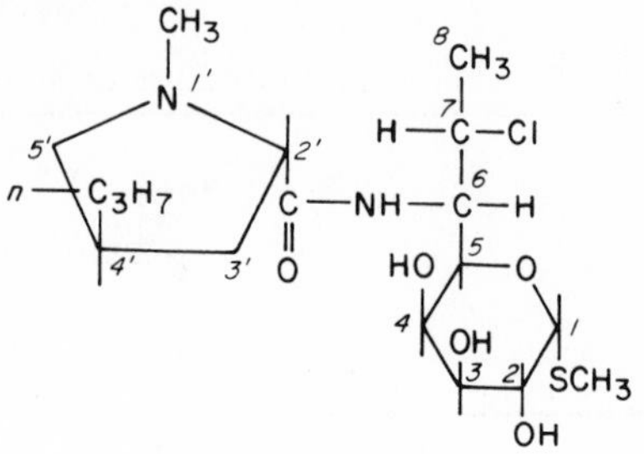 Clindamycin

Stereochemistry plays an important role in the activity of clindamycin. Replacement of the 7R-hydroxyl group of lincomycin with a 7R-chloro group increased biological activity by a factor of 1.6, while a 7S-chloro substituent increased activity by a factor of 4 [68]. Increasing the size of the R group at the C-4′ position on the pyrrolidine ring also increased activity, with a maximum effect being achieved with n-pentyl or n-hexyl chains [68,69]. However, the increase in activity over lincomycin was not as great in vivo (1.6X) as was observed in in vitro tests (10X).

Lincomycin and clindamycin are effective for the treatment of gram-positive organisms, especially those which are resistant to penicillins. Depending upon the concentration employed and the particular sensitivity of the organism, these drugs can be either bacteriostatic or bacteriocidal. Lincomycin has one serious drawback to its clinical use which is not manifested to as great an extent by clindamycin. Cases of severe and persistant diarrhea have been reported, and at times it has resulted in an acute colitis.

It has been shown that lincomycin is not quantitatively absorbed in the rat [70], but studies of tritium-labeled clindamycin in rats and dogs indicated that its absorption in these species was more nearly quantitative, since the area under plasma total radioactivity vs time curves following oral and parenteral administration were idential [71]. Lincomycin reaches peak serum levels in humans in 2–4 hr following oral administration and has a biological half-life of 5.4 hr whereas clindamycin reaches peak levels in about 45 min and has a biological half-life of 2.4 hr. The difference in oral absorption may be due to a large difference in lipid solubility between the two compounds. Lincomycin has an n-octanol/water partition coefficient of 3.6, while that for clindamycin is 145 [72]. Esterification of the C-2, C-3, C-4, and C-7 hydroxyls has resulted in prodrugs with improved oral absorption. This subject will be considered in detail in a later section.

c. Sulfonamides. Since the discovery in 1935 of this antibacterial activity, thousands of sulfonamide derivatives have been synthesized. The therapeutically useful agents are all derivatives of sulfanilamide, and some of these are shown in Table 10.

Table 10

Structure, Half-life, and Dosing Interval of Some Common Sulfonamides[a]

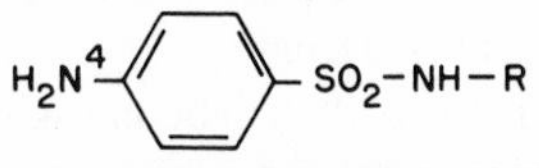

H_2N^4–⟨benzene ring⟩–SO_2–NH–R

Name	R	$t_{1/2}$ (hr)	τ (hr)
Sulfanilamide	H	9	8
Sulfathiazole	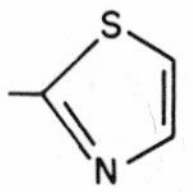 S, N	4	4
Sulfisoxazole	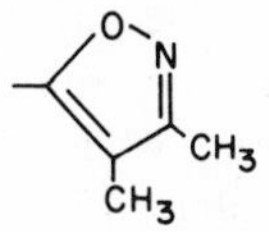 O, N, CH_3, CH_3	6	6
Sulfamethoxazole	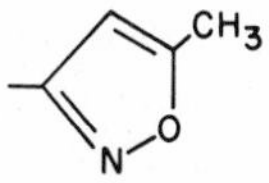 CH_3, N, O	11	12
Sulfadiazine	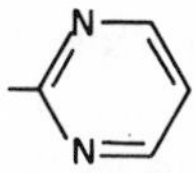 N, N	17	12
Sulfadimethoxine	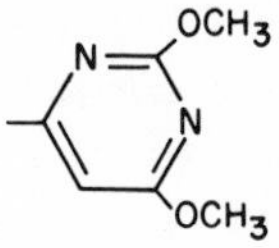 OCH_3, N, N, OCH_3	41	24
Sulfamethoxypyridazine	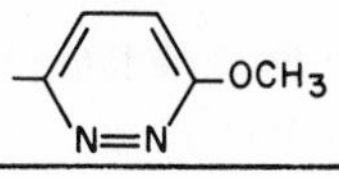 OCH_3, N=N	35	24

[a]From Ref. 73.

Notice should be taken of the wide range of half-lives shown in Table 10. The clinical utility of the various sulfonamides will depend in part upon their half-lives. For example, sulfisoxazole, with a relatively short half-life of 6 hr, is excreted as the free drug into the urine and rapidly reaches bacteriostatic levels. Sulfadimethoxine, on the other hand, has a $t_{1/2}$ of 41 hr, accumulates slowly in the urinary tract, and is used primarily for upper respiratory tract infections or other systemic soft tissue infections. Thus, $t_{1/2}$ serves as a qualitative guide as to whether a sulfonamide would have more potential in urinary tract or systemic infections.

Sulfonamides with long half-lives have been implicated in the development of Stevens-Johnson syndrome in children. Sulfas such as sulfadimethoxine (Madribon), sulfamethoxypyridine (Kynex and Midicel), and sulfameter (Sulla) all contain a warning statement in their labeling which points out the possible occurrence of this sometimes fatal side effect. Sulfonamides with short or intermediate half-lives are not required to bear the cautionary statement. Since the sulfas with shorter half-lives are generally effective for the same conditions, they should be employed whenever possible and the long half-life sulfas used only as a last resort.

Differences in the half-lives of sulfonamides can be attributed to differences in metabolism and urinary excretion. Sulfonamides are excreted in the urine as the free drug, N^4-acetylated metabolites, N^4-glucinonidates, or other soluble metabolites. Analysis of an 8-hr urine sample of human subjects following a 2-g oral dose revealed that sulfisonidine, sulfamethazole, and sulfisoxazole were excreted primarily as the free drug, while sulfaphenazole and sulfadimethoxine were excreted as the N^4-glucinonidates [74].

Urinary excretion of sulfonamides is affected by protein binding and the pK_a of the drug. Protein binding may increase the duration of the drugs, since only the unbound form will be subject to glomerular filtration, as was pointed out earlier. In general, sulfonamides are highly protein bound. For example, sulfamethoxazole and sulfisoxazole are 70 and 85% bound in blood, respectively [75]. Both ionic and hydrophobic forces are involved in protein binding [76-78]. The ionic binding is a function of the pK_a of the sulfonamide, while the hydrophobic binding is related to its lipophilicity. It has been shown for a series of 2-sulfapyridine derivatives having similar pK_a values around 6.4 that increasing *n*-octanol/water partition coefficients are accompanied by increasing protein binding [73]. Steric factors were also shown to play a role in protein binding, since the percent free of various sulfonamides with ortho-substituted heterocycles at the N′-position of the basic sulfonamide nucleus was always higher than that for the para-substituted derivatives [73].

The pK_a of the sulfonamide affects urinary excretion through another mechanism in addition to its effect on protein binding. Once the sulfonamide has passed through the glomerulus into the tubule, it may be passively reabsorbed via the un-ionized form, which passes across the membrane more readily than the ionized form. Thus, the biological half-life is increased by factors which favor this passive resorption process. The amount resorbed will depend upon the pK_a of the sulfonamide and the urinary pH, which in turn determines how much of the un-ionized species will be present. The $t_{1/2}$ of sulfaethidole, which has a pK_a of 5.1, was markedly increased from 4.2 to 11.4 hr when the urinary pH was changed from 8 to 5 [73]. It would also be expected that the more lipophilic the un-ionized species, the greater would be the resorption.

From the above discussion it may be concluded that pK_a and partition coefficient are important parameters in determining observed differences in sulfonamide therapy due to protein binding and urinary excretion.

B. Urinary Tract Antimicrobial Agents

The goals of molecular modification of agents used in the treatment of urinary tract infections are often contrary to some of those stated previously for systemic antimicrobial drugs. Although the following list of characteristics for an idealized urinary tract antimicrobial agent may seem somewhat arbitrary, examples from the current literature indicate that the goals of research in this area generally reflect these characteristics. The ideal urinary tract antimicrobial agent should possess the following properties:

1. High intrinsic antimicrobial activity
2. High urinary concentrations of intact drug or active metabolite
3. Short biological half-life
4. Low volume of distribution
5. Poor or rapidly reversible serum protein binding

Molecular modifications aimed at changing one of the above characteristics of a particular agent may affect the others, since urinary concentration, volume of distribution, biological half-life, and protein binding are often interdependent. As a consequence, it seems appropriate to discuss these characteristics both individually and collectively.

1. Intrinsic Activity

High intrinsic antimicrobial activity is a goal common to both systemic and urinary tract antibacterials. The organisms more frequently responsible for urinary tract infections are gram-negative bacilli such as *E. coli, Enterobacter (aerobacter) aeorgenes, Pseudomonas aeruginosa, Proteus vulgaris,* and various salmonellae and gram-positive streptococci and staphlococci [79]. In patients developing symptoms of urinary tract infections for the first time (and who have not been prevoiously catheterized or examined with the use of instruments), it would be reasonable to assume that the infection is due to either *E. coli* or one of the *Proteus* species and to initiate drug therapy on that basis [80]. The choice of the drug to be used may be altered if necessary after the results of sensitivity tests performed on a urinary specimen have been obtained and assessment of the clinical response has been made. The importance of sensitivity tests in those cases where a high level of activity is desired against a particular organism cannot be overemphasized. In one study comparing the activity of four tetracyclines against various common systemic and urinary tract pathogens, the conclusion was drawn that none of the tetracyclines tested exhibited a clear advantage over the others when the pathogens were considered as a group [81].

Urinary pH may also play an important role in limiting the activity of anti-infective agents. The minimum inhibitory concentrations of several sulfonamides have been correlated with their pK_a values [82], and the ionized species appear to possess greater activity than the un-ionized species [83]. Gentamycin activity against *Klebsiella, Pseudomonas aerugenosa,* and *Proteus mirabilis* has been shown to increase with increasing pH [84]. Figure 4 is taken from Ref. 84 to illustrate the type of results obtained. This behavior implies that alkalinization of urine might be a useful adjunct in gentamycin therapy. Streptomycin and kanamycin also have greater activity in alkaline urine [80]. Conversely, drugs such as penicillin G, tetracycline, nitrofurantoin, and methenamine are more active in acidic urine [80]. The necessity of an acidic urine for the activity of methamine will be discussed later in the section on prodrugs. Kunin [85] has discussed the management of pH during the treatment of urinary tract infections. He points out that daily use of pH-sensitive paper (Nitrazine ribbons) is necessary because of the varying response to agents used to alter urinary pH. Agents used orally to acidify the urine (and their total daily doses) are ammonium chloride (8–12 g), methionine (8–12 g), ascorbic acid (2 g), NaH_2SO_4 (2 g); and those to alkalize are Na_2HPO_4 (2 g), $NaHCO_3$ (12–24 g), acetazolamide (0.5–1.5 g) according to Kunin [85]. Table 11 summarizes the optimum urinary pH for agents considered useful in various urinary tract infections.

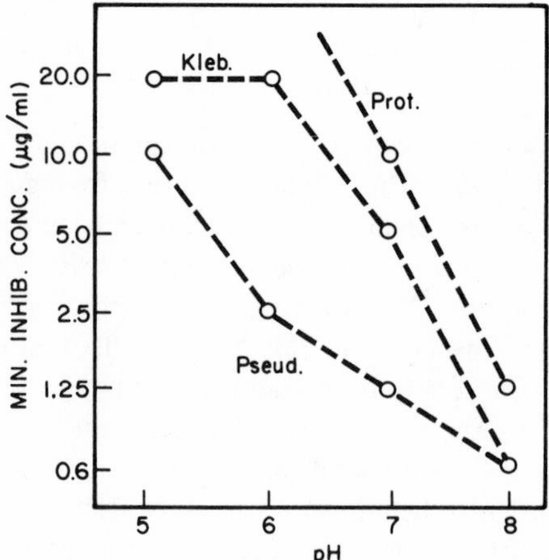

Fig. 4. Data taken from Ref. 84 showing the role of pH in gentamycin activity against *Klebsiella, Pseudomonas aerugenosa,* and *Proteus mirabilis.* As the pH increases, the M.I.C. decreases, illustrating an apparent *increase* in gentamycin activity.

Table 11

Optimum pH for Urinary Tract Anti-infective Agents[a]

Acid	Alkaline	Other
Tetracyclines	Erythromycin	Sufonamides (close to the pK_a)
Nitrofurantoin	Streptomycin	Penicillins (literature is contradictory)
Mandelamine	Kanamycin	Nalidixic acid (no pH adjustment needed)
Carbenicillin	Gentamicin	Chloramphenicol (not affected)
	Polymyxin B and E	Cephaloridine, Cephalexin, Cephalothin (pH 6-8)

[a]Recommendations by Kunin [85].

2. *Urinary Concentration, Half-life, and Protein Binding*

The ability to produce high concentrations of the drug or its active metabolite at the site of action is a desirable trait shared by both systemic and urinary tract antimicrobial agents. It is preferred that systemic agents possess a long half-life in order to maintain tissue levels at minimum inhibitory concentrations for a sufficient duration of treatment. However, for urinary tract antibacterials the $t_{1/2}$ should be relatively short so that the drug will reach the site of action rapidly and in sufficient quantity. Implicit in this statement is that urinary clearance is primarily responsible for the short half-life and not metabolism to inactive forms or other clearance processes.

The urinary clearance of these agents is a function of the mechanism of clearance, protein binding, and urinary pH. Since only the unbound form of a drug will undergo glomerular filtration, the extent and strength of protein binding will affect this type of urinary clearance. As previously stated, increased protein binding has been indicated as a possible cause of extended duration of several sulfonamides [40]. In this respect the mechanism of urinary clearance becomes important, since drugs which are actively secreted appear to be eliminated in a manner which is independent of protein binding [86]. Passive resorption of the drug can occur from the tubules, which results in lowering of the observed clearance. Maintenance of the urinary pH at a value where the drug exists primarily in the ionized form will inhibit this process. Thus, for weak acids such as the sulfonamides, an alkaline urine would result in minimal resorption.

3. *Volume of Distribution*

In general, urinary tract antimicrobial agents should have a low volume of distribution, which increases their selectivity for the urinary tract. The degree of tissue penetration desired will depend upon the site of infection. Infections of the lower urinary tract (bladder and urethra) such as cystitis are best treated with those agents which have low volumes of distribution and short half-lives. In cases where infection involves the upper urinary tract (kidney and ureters), tissue penetration becomes important and agents with a low Vd such as nitrofurantoin are ineffective. For this reason, pyelonephritis, which requires high, steady bacteriostatic levels in the parenchymal cells [9], is often treated using one of the tetracycline derivatives.

4. *Potential Toxicity Due to Renal Insufficiency*

Although cephaloridine, chloramphenicol, the colistins, neomycin, polymyxin, kanamycin, streptomycin, and gentamycin are effective against many of the organisms responsible for urinary tract infections, their use should be reserved for those cases which are resistant to other commonly used agents because of their potential for causing severe side effects. Ototoxicity has occurred with the use of gentamycin, kanamycin, and neomycin. Gentamycin and cephaloridine may result in nephrotoxicity, while blood dyscrasias are well-known side effects of chloramphenicol. The probability of the occurrence of these side effects is increased in those cases involving renal insufficiency due to higher and prolonged levels of these drugs and the increased difficulty in controlling their plasma levels.

III. OPTIMIZING ORAL ABSORPTION

Although the molecular requirements for oral absorption of drugs cannot be quantitatively defined at the present time, it is generally agreed that several factors are of primary importance. These factors are the drug's partition coefficient, its aqueous solubility, and its resistance to loss from the absorption site due to enzymatic or chemical degradation. Attempts to quantify the effects of molecular modification on these factors have been made and models proposed to explain the observed effects based on passive diffusion of drugs to, into, and through simulated membranes. Often a set of rules or constants derived from this type of research enable predictions to be made concerning the absorption and physicochemical properties of a new compound. Thus, a priori design of molecules having the desired absorption behavior and physicochemical properties may become possible. While this is not yet a reality, considerable progress has been made in the form of linear relationships that are predictive within a given series. The effect of molecular modification on the above factors and the relationships derived from research in this area will be discussed in the following sections.

A. Partition Coefficient

The pH-partition hypothesis for gastrointestinal drug absorption was discussed in Chap. 4. A few early reviews summarize the pertinent data [87-89]. Essentially the theory states that only the un-ionized form of the drug passes through a biological membrane. The membrane is regarded as lipoidal in nature, and the ease with which the drug passes through it increases with increasing lipophilicity of the drug. While there are undoubtedly many compounds whose absorption behavior follows this theory, a growing list of exceptions has necessitated refinement of the theory. For example, the absorption-rate constants for both ionized and un-ionized species of sulfaethidole and barbital have been determined in situ using rat stomach and intestine [90]. The ratios of the first-order constants for the neutral species to that of the ionized form was roughly 5 for sulfaethidole and 3 for barbital. At pH 6.1, approximately 42% of the sulfonamide is absorbed in the ionized form.

Other studies have been made concerning the absorption of compounds which are ionized over the entire pH range of the gastrointestinal tract either due to fixed ionic charges in compounds such as the quaternary ammonium drugs [91,92] or due to the pK_a of the compound such as in the case of methylene blue [93] and the tetracyclines [94]. Tetracyclines exist in the cationic form at acidic pH values, as anions at alkaline pH, and in zwitterionic form at relatively neutral pH values. They are too polar to partition into a nonpolar solvent, but will partition into *n*-octanol from pH 5.2 and 7.4 buffered aqueous solutions [95]. Thus, tetracyclines may have sufficient lipid solubility to be passively absorbed in vivo even though ionized. The partitioning of tetracycline into *n*-octanol as a function of the pH of the aqueous solution and its ionic form has been examined [94]; it was found that partitioning was greatest at those pH values where the concentration of the zwitterion species was highest. This is also the pH range where tetracyclines exhibit their greatest antibiotic effect [96]. In general, minocycline, doxycycline, and methacycline have the same pH-partition profile as tetracycline, but all are much more lipid-soluble—having zwitterions whose partition coefficients are 20-30 times that of tetracycline. These large differences in partition coefficients may also explain the large differences in tissue penetration and distribution discussed in earlier sections.

In some cases, what appears to be evidence contradicting the pH-partition hypothesis is really data showing dominance of other factors. For example, phenobarbital and pentobarbital are weak acids having pK_a values of 7.2 and 8.1, respectively. Therefore, it would be predicted that these drugs would be more rapidly absorbed from the acidic environment of the stomach than from the intestine. Instead, two to three times as much is absorbed from the intestine during a 10-min period as is abosrbed from the stomach in 1 hr [97]. This large difference is not due to preferential absorption of the ionized species but is due primarily to the much larger surface area of the intestine, which more than compensates for the decreased absorption of drug per unit area. Thus, the results of absorption experiments must be interpreted carefully and variables such as surface area controlled.

1. Partition Coefficient Adjustment Through Molecular Modification

In 1964, Fujita, Iwasa, and Hansch derived a substituent constant, π, which can be used to predict partition coefficients by summing the π values of the component parts of the molecule [98]. The π constant was defined by the Hammett-like relationship,

$$\pi x = \log \frac{Px}{Ph} = \log Px - \log Ph \qquad (5)$$

where Px is the partition coefficient of the molecule bearing the substituent x and Ph is the partition coefficient of the unsubstituted compound. The *n*-octanol/water system was chosen as the standard for determination of these constants, since it was felt that *n*-octanol possesses several properties which allow it to serve as a model for the hydrophobic and H-bonding effects that might be encountered in biological membranes [99]. This method for predicting partition coefficients has been demonstrated for many compounds with widely varying structures, such as diphenhydramine, diethylstilbesterol, and 6 α-fluroprednisolone [100-102]. A library of partition coefficients for the basic structures of various classes of chemotherapeutic agents, such as penicillins [103], phenothiazines [104], barbiturates [105], and so on, have been compiled and serve as a data base for a priori calculation of the partition coefficients of various derivatives. However, caution should be used when calculating π values, since various interactions may cause deviations from the π-value additivity rules [98,102,106-109].

2. Model Systems for Absorption Studies

The buccal absorption of drugs has been suggested as an in vivo method for studying the passage of drugs across biological membranes [110] and lends itself well toward studying the effects of the lipid solubility and pK_a of various compounds. This method has been used to examine the absorption of amines, alkyl-substituted acids, substituted phenylacetic acids, and various other carboxylic acids [111-116]. Several important relationships were derived from these studies. Absorption across the buccal membrane was shown to occur by passive diffusion. For a series of unbranched aliphatic acids ranging in chain length from butyric to dodecanoic, absorption was shown to increase with decreasing pH and increasing chain length. Rate constants, expressed as clearance values, for the absorption of ten carboxylic acids at pH 4 increased linearly with increasing partition coefficients (*n*-heptane/1 N HCl). A linear relationship was also found between the absorption of a series of amines and acids and log partition coefficient when the drugs were either 1 or 10% ionized. This linear relationship also held for amphetamines and ten fluramines. It had been previously calculated that the log transfer rate through a lipoidal barrier would be expected to increase linearly with log partition coefficient until a maximum constant value was approached [117].

Other investigators have developed an in vitro diffusion model for absorption studies [118]. This physical model consisted of a bulk aqueous diffusion layer and a lipid phase and has been used to interpret quantitatively and mechanistically the above in vivo buccal absorption data. For the alkanoic acids, a factor of 2.3 per methylene group for the buccal membrane–aqueous phase incremental partition coefficient was determined. This same model was satisfactorily tested on data for buccal absorption of various acids, and a value of 2.2 was obtained for the *p*-alkyl phenylacetic acid series [119]. This provided further evidence for the applicability of the diffusional model and the significance of the diffusion layer in buccal transport. The theory was extended to a multicompartment diffusion model, and data for the gastric, intestinal, and rectal absorption of sulfonamides and barbituarates was shown to fit the mdoel [120,121].

Studies on the intestinal absorption rate of more than 50 compounds were conducted in rats [122,123]. From extrathermodynamic considerations, an additivity rule was proposed to predict the effect of substituents on the absorption rate constant.

The effect of alkyl chain length of a series of *p*aminobenzoate esters on their physiochemical properties and ability to penetrate biological barriers has also been examined [124]. This diffusional model predicts a parabolic dependence of the maximum steady-state flux on chain length as the homologous series is ascended. Other studies also point to a parabolic relationship between biological activity and lipophilic character [125–128]. The parabolic nature of these relationships suggest that an optimum partition coefficient should exist for a given system. For example, optimum log partition coefficients for the absorption of various acids and bases from rat stomach and intestine have been estimates to be 1.97 and 1.39, respectively [129].

3. *Partition Coefficient Effects in Absorption Data*

Both in vivo and in vitro absorption studies indicate that the absorption of compounds with very small partition coefficients may be improved by increasing their lipophilicity. For example, clindamycin is much better absorbed than is lincomycin and has a much larger log partition coefficient value (2.16 vs 0.55, respectively) [72].

Esterification is a common method of increasing the partition coefficients of molecules. Applying the π-additivity principle, calculations indicate that the acetate ester of an alcohol will have a log partition coefficient value which is 0.89 units larger than that of the alcohol. Increasing the chain length of the ester will increase the log partition coefficient by 0.5 for each additional methylene group in the chain. Thus, the butyrate ester would have a value which is 1.89 units more than the parent alcohol. The C-2 propionate ester of lincomycin is more extensively absorbed than the parent compound [72], and the C-2 and C-7 butyrates are better absorbed from rat intestinal loops [130]. The oral absorption of a series of erythromycin esters has been examined and, based on areas under the plasma curves, the acetate and propionate esters appear to be better absorbed than the parent drug while the butyrate was absorbed markedly less [131]. However, these curves may not be indicative of absorption differences alone, since intact ester was present in significant amounts. If the blood level curves represent total erythromycin due to hydrolysis of the ester prior to assay, the differences cannot be attributed solely to absorption without further data.

This scheme illustrates the different rate processes which may affect the time

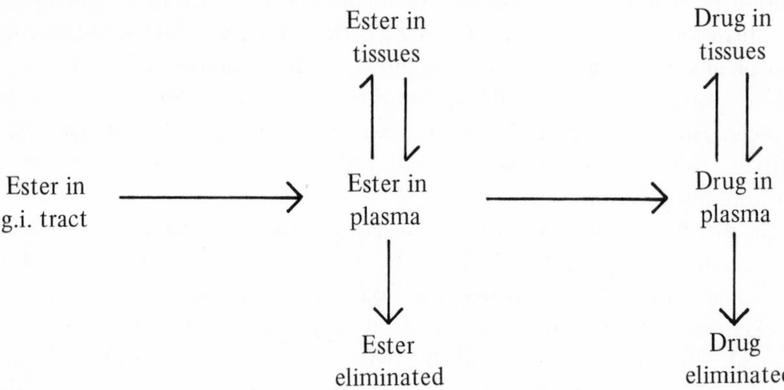

course of a drug and its ester in plasma. Due to differences in partition coefficients, the distribution and elimination of the intact ester may be greatly different than that of the drug itself. Thus, interpretation of blood level curves must be made carefully in order to avoid making erroneous conclusions as mentioned above regarding erythromycin esters. This will be discussed later in more detail.

B. Aqueous Solubility

The fastest rate of absorption by the oral route can generally be achieved by administering a solution of the drug. Thus, if one is concerned primarily with onset of action, the drug would best be administered in the form of an elixir, syrup, or aqueous solution. The rate-determining step for absorption would be the passive diffusion of the drug from the g.i. fluid through the membrane into the systemic circulation. However, when the drug is administered as a solid, there are certain conditions under which the dissolution step may be rate determining. A modified form of the Noyes-Whitney dissolution rate was previously discussed and is again given here:

$$\frac{dC}{dt} = \frac{kDS}{Vh}(C_s - C) \quad (6)$$

dC/dt is the rate of increase in concentration of the drug in the bulk solution in which the dissolution is taking place, k is a proportionality constant, D is the diffusion coefficient of the drug in the solvent, S is the surface area of undissolved solid, V is the volume of the bulk solution, h is the diffusion layer thickness around a particle, and C_s is the total solubility of the drug in the solvent. Among other things, it can be seen that increasing the total solubility of the drug would result in an increase in dissolution rate. The total solubility of weak acids as a function of the pH of the solvent was previously expressed as

$$S_T = S_0(1 + 10^{pH-pK_a}) \quad (7)$$

and for weak bases as

$$S_T = S_0(1 + 10^{pK_a-pH}) \quad (8)$$

where S_0 is the intrinsic solubility of the uncharged acid or base (see Chap. 4). Thus, molecular modification may alter the total solubility of a compound by altering its pK_a or intrinsic solubility.

The effects of molecular modifications on pK_a can often be predicted using the well-known Hammett equation and the appropriate σ and ρ values. Methods of predicting the effect on intrinsic solubility are not as well developed. Linear plots of log solubility vs π value have been obtained for a series of testosterone esters [132], substituted phenothiazines [133], and *p*hydroxybenzoate esters [134]. The slopes of the lines for these solids varied from approximately 2.4 to 3.1 per methylene group. A linear relationship has also been developed for solubility of many drug and druglike substances in binary aqueous solvents [135]. These methods should be used with caution when predicting aqueous solubility of solids, since unusual behavior may occur due to various factors such as entropic effects within a crystal.

C. Loss from Absorption Sites

It is reasonable to assume that if all other factors remain constant, decreasing the loss of a drug from the absorption site due to various degradation pathways will results in improved oral absorption of the compound. Indeed, much research has been aimed at increasing the gastrointestinal stability of various chemotherapeutic agents.

The penicillins have been extensively studied in this regard. As was pointed out earlier, the gastric stability of penicillins may be the primary factor in determining bioavailability [13]. Penicillin G and methicillin are rapidly hydrolyzed in the stomach to an inactive penicilloic acid, while ampicillin is relatively stable. An electron-withdrawing group on the α-carbon of the side chain confers a degree of gastric stability which depends upon the nature of this group. However, there is no group which can be said to stabilize the β-lactam ring completely [8].

Erythromycin is another compound which suffers from gastric instability. Erythromycin undergoes acid-catalyzed intramolecular cyclic ketal formation to an inactive form. Ester formation, which was previously discussed as one method for improving oral absorption (by increasing the partition coefficient) will also improve oral absorption by protecting the groups involved in the intramolecular reaction. Tetracyclines are yet another example. Complexation of tetracyclines with food or other gastric contents can drastically reduce their oral absorption.

IV. PRODRUGS

Prodrugs are compounds resulting from chemical modification of a biologically active compound which will liberate the active compound in vivo due to enzymatic or chemical attack. Stella [136] has reviewed some of the reasons for formation of prodrugs. The prodrug approach is widely used as a method of improving oral absorption of poorly absorbed drugs. Pharmacokinetic evaluations of prodrugs must be conducted carefully to avoid drawing conclusions about the time course of the active drug in the body, which are really based on data reflecting the absorption, distribution, and elimination of the intact prodrug. The ideal prodrug is one which is nontoxic, does not produce toxic fragments upon liberation of the active drug, releases the active drug at the desired rate, and is at least as stable as the parent compound toward degradative pathways which limit availability.

A. Nucleosides

The first examples of a nucleoside prodrug which improved oral absorption in humans appeared in 1961 [137]. Psicofuranine is not significantly absorbed from the gastrointestinal tract of humans. Prodrugs were prepared by esterification of the sugar hydroxyls, and the tetracetate was chosen for human trials on the basis of observed equivalent activity to the parent when compared subcutaneously in mice. Although no detectable levels could be determined after oral administration of psicofuranine in humans, its tetracetate is well absorbed. Assays with and without preliminary hydrolysis indicated that the prodrug was rapidly converted to free psicofuranine in the blood. The major difference in physicochemical properties between the drug and its prodrug appears to be enhanced lipid solubility of the tetracetate. The π-additivity principle indicates that the n-octanol/water log partition coefficient value should increase by 0.89 for each acetate ester or by 3.56 for the tetracetate. That a large increase in lipid solubility has occurred is evidenced by the water/chlororform partition coefficient of 992 for psicofuranine and 0.041 for the prodrug.

It is quite common to associate the term bioavailability with absorbability from an oral dosage form as a natural result of the immense research activity in that area. However, tissue binding or elimination may also be involved in limiting bioavailability, since the degree of success of a drug is dependent upon its ability to reach the site of action and its time course at that site.

The bioavailability of arabinosylcytosine (Ara-C) may be said to be limited by elimination due to metabolism which, therefore, limits its effectiveness. Pharmacokinetic studies were used to define the nature of the problem, and improved therapy was made possible by appropriate dosage regimens and also by the development of prodrugs. The details of this research are summarized as an illustration of the power of pharmacokinetics in drug design.

Ara-C is a cytotoxic agent which exerts antitumor and antiviral activity in a variety of animal neoplasms. It is effective for the treatment of acute myelogenous leukemia in man [138]. The greatest response in a single disease was observed in acute granulocytic leukemia, where 35 of 144 adequately treated patients (or 24%) achieved complete or partial remissions [139] and, more recently, 21 of 49 patients (43%) attained complete remissions through rapid drug injection followed by continuous drug infusion to maintain steady-state therapy for 4 hr per day [140].

This somewhat encouraging remission rate is even more astonishing when one considers the brief duration of this drug. When given by I.V. injection to humans, the resulting blood level data show biphasic first-order curves which are characteristics of a two-compartment open model. The initial loss from the blood is quite fast, having a $t_{1/2}$ of approximately 12 min, and may be attributed to simultaneous distribution and elimination [141–143]. At the end of the initial phase (α phase), over 80% of the nucleoside remaining in the blood and urine is in the form of a single inactive metabolite, arabinosyluracil (Ara-U), indicating both rapid and extensive deamination during the distribution phase [141]. The elimination phase (β phase) has a $t_{1/2}$ of approximately 111 min, and

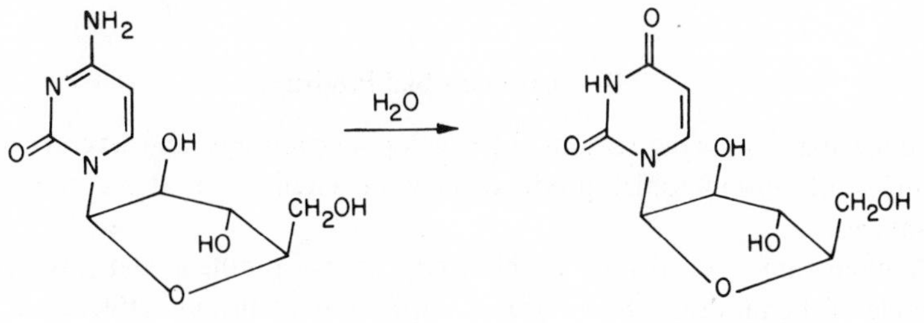

Ara - C Ara - U

nearly complete conversion to Ara-U by pyrimidine nucleoside deaminase occurs during this period. Uptake by red blood cells is rapid, and within 5 min cells attained 60% of the concentration found in plasma. However, the $t_{1/2}$ within the cell is only 2-3 min. Thus Ara-C exhibits a relatively short duration of bioavailability due to deamination to Ara-U, which apparently has no activity as an inhibitor of cell growth.

An increase in biological half-life may lead to increased remission rates, and evidence for this hypothesis can be found [144]. The plasma $t_{1/2}$ of Ara-C in leukemic patients following 30-min infusions in patients who experienced complete remissions was significantly longer than the $t_{1/2}$ values in those who did not respond to therapy. These results were presumably due to variations in deaminase activity among the subjects and suggest that deamination of Ara-C may cause failure of the drug to produce hematologic remissions in certain patients. Further support for this proposal may be taken from the demonstration that the dosage regimen markedly affects its therapeutic index. For example, superior results were obtained using either constant I.V. infusion or rapid injections every 8 hr rather than single daily injections [145,146]. The most effective schedule presently appears to be 200 mg/M^2/day given by continuous I.V. infusion [138], which yields steady-state plasma levels of about 0.15 μg/ml [141].

Another approach to increasing the duration of Ara-C is to develop a prodrug from which it would be slowly liberated. A single dose of arabinosylcytosine-5′-adamantoate was nearly as effective as an optimum schedule of Ara-C given every 3 hr parenterally to L1210 leukemic mice. The duration of cytotoxic plasma levels of Ara-C was greatly increased with the prodrug [147]. Several 5′-acylates had activity equal to or better than the 5′-adamantoate and appear to be more stable to pyrimidine nucleoside deaminase while still producing Ara-C via hydrolysis in plasma.

B. Antimicrobial Prodrugs

There are many possible reasons for developing prodrugs, and several successful examples of antimicrobial prodrugs may be cited to illustrate some of the advantages.

Methenamine constitutes a relatively simple problem and a well-known example of the prodrug which releases a urinary tract anti-infective. At acidic pH values methenamine is converted to formaldehyde, which is the active antimicrobial agent as shown here.

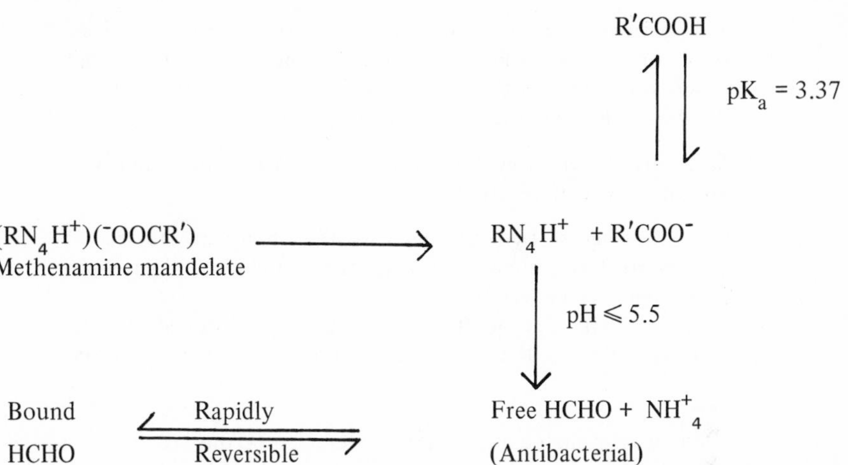

Methenamine is converted to formaldehyde if the pH of the medium is less than 5.5, and for this reason tablets of methenamine are often enteric-coated to prevent conversion in the stomach resulting in gastric upset and nausea. The enteric coating dissolves in the alkaline pH of the intestine where absorption occurs, allowing intact methenamine to enter the blood which is also too alkaline for conversion. It is cleared intact into the urine, where it becomes converted to formaldehyde if the pH is less than 5.5. The rate of conversion can be controlled by management of urinary pH. This is generally accomplished by administering methenamine as the mandelic or hippuric acid salt and supplementing with oral urinary acidifiers.

Sample Problem 4

The drugs listed in Table 12 were administered to a patient with gouty nephropathy who developed a urinary tract infection.

Table 12

Excerpts from a Patient Medication Record[a]

Drug	Days: 1–2	3–14	15–18	19–23	24	25–26	27–33
Sodium bicarbonate (I.V.)	X						
Allopurinol (300 mg/day)	X	X	X	X	X	X	X
Sodium bicarbonate (P.O. 6 g/day)			X	X	X	X	X
Mandelamine (2 g/day)				X	X		
Furadantin (400 mg/day)					X	X	
Macrodantin (400 mg/day)							X

[a]The authors are indebted to Dr. James Visconti for suggesting this sample problem and for supplying the necessary information.

(a) This patient received allopurinol to decrease uric acid levels. Based on your knowledge of renal clearance of uric acid, what other compound on this chart would cause excretion and how?
Solution: Review urinary clearance in Chap. 3.

(b) What drugs were used for his urinary tract infection, and why was the change necessary?

(c) Can you suggest two reasons why the choice of the second urinary tract anti-infective was not the best choice? What might have been used instead?
Solution: The pH of the urine will be controlled by the $NaHCO_3$. Review the Sec. II.B. for the pertinent information.

Carbenicillin was available only in parenteral form due to its poor oral bioavailability, which was presumably due to its low lipid solubility (it is a dicarboxylic acid) or its acid instability or both. At pH 2.0 it has a half-life of less than 30 min [148]. Once again esterification has been used to prepare a prodrug which would be more lipophilic and acid-stable, thereby decreasing loss at the site of absorption due to degradation. The prodrug carbenicillin indanyl sodium has been synthesized. It is the indanol ester of carbenicillin. The ester was quite stable when incubated in simulated gastric juice at pH 2.0 and 37°C for 1 hr, while under these same conditions carbenicillin was almost totally destroyed [148]. The prodrug is rapidly hydrolyzed in vivo after absorption so that it produces the same biological response as carbenicillin. The 5-indanol moiety is excreted in various conjugated forms, and differential assays have shown that only trace amounts of intact ester are present in the serum and urine [148]. In experimental urinary tract infections in one study, the effectiveness of the oral prodrug was generally as good or better than that of parenteral carbenicillin. The oral prodrug is useful only in urinary tract infections, since it has been shown that serum levels of carbenicillin from the oral prodrug are suboptimal [149].

Hetacillin is a prodrug of ampicillin which may be considered as a condensation product of acetone and ampicillin. Ampicillin and hetacillin are available in oral dosage forms as well as in dry powder form for reconstitution before injection. Concentrated solutions of hetacillin have been shown to be more stable [150]. Six hours were required for 10% loss of activity at room temperature for hetacillin, while ampicillin exhibited 10% loss under the same conditions in only 1 hr. This is an advantage to the user of reconstituted hetacillin. The oral absorption of hetacillin may be somewhat greater than that of ampicillin based on urinary recovery data [151,152], although one study reports decreased urinary recovery of ampicillin with the prodrug [153]. There have been a number of comparisons based on the plasma concentration-time profiles, but the meaning of these results is equivocal since assays failed to differentiate between drug and prodrug [154]. This problem will be discussed later in the section dealing with potential pitfalls in data interpretation.

The propionate and butyrate esters of erythromycin, which have been discussed earlier, can be considered to be prodrugs used to improve oral absorption by increasing partition coefficient and decreasing loss at the absorption site due to acid instability. Erythromycin base has a pK_a of 8.9 and thus would be ionized throughout the entire gastrointestinal tract. Intestinal absorption would be expected to be better than absorption from the stomach, and this has been shown to be the case in rats where it was most rapidly absorbed in the upper small intestine [131]. Two other forms, which are designed to bypass the stomach (where erythromycin is inactivated through cyclic ketal formation) are in common use. Erythromycin stearate resists dissolution in the stomach but dissociates rapidly in the intestines to give free erythromycin. Erythromycin estolate, by contrast, is probably absorbed largely as the intact ester and hydrolyzed in the blood to yield free erythromycin. The $t_{1/2}$ for erythromycin estolate hydrolysis in human serum has been reported to be 93 min [155]. However, the advantages of high serum levels of the propionate ester prodrug have been a matter of controversy. In a four-way crossover study (fasting and nonfasting) blood levels obtained after single and multiple doses of erythromycin estolate and erythromycin stearate were compared [156]. The estolate achieved higher blood levels at a faster rate both with and without food. However, the assay used was probably capable of hydrolyzing estolate esters, since the in vitro hydrolysis has been reported to vary from 0.5 hr at pH 8 to 5.0 hr at pH 5 [157]. Another study reported 20–35% free base and 65–80% ester present after the fifth dose of ester to humans, so that the average free base level was higher from the ester than that obtained by administration of the salt [158].

The use of esterification to increase partition coefficient as a means of increasing oral absorption is limited by the solubility of the resultant ester. The partition coefficient of a compound can be greatly increased by forming long-chain esters, but the oral absorption of these esters may be reduced due to their low water solubility. However, the relative insolubility of the long-chain esters can be an advantage in the development of pediatric oral formations, since the bad taste of some drugs when administered orally in solution can be more easily concealed by administering them as suspensions with suitable flavor additives. A balance must be found between increasing insolubility, which decreases oral absorption, and increasing partition coefficient, which increases absorption, by using an ester of the appropriate chain length.

Esters of lincomycin and clindamycin have been prepared in an effort to mask undesirable taste and maintain (or improve) oral absorption [159]. Lincomycin esters have been compared for activity by subcutaneous and oral routes in mice. The 2-hexanoate, 2-laurate, and 2-palmitate esters appear to be absorbed as well or better than clindamycin itself when all are administered as the hydrochloride salts at doses of 25 mg/kg equivalent to clindamycin base. In contrast to the erythromycin estolate, these esters apparently hydrolyze prior to absorption or very rapidly thereafter, so that the presence of intact ester does not complicate comparisons of plasma level-time profiles. In a pharmacokinetic study of clindamycin HCl and its palmitate ester in 52 children, it was found that mean serum levels of clindamycin following single doses of the palmitate were lower than those from the parent drug [160]. However, if the dosage was not adjusted for the difference in molecular weight between the base and the palmitate ester, this difference in dose is sufficient to explain the observed difference in serum levels.

In an excellent review of prodrugs and their properties, Sinkula has outlined some of the pharmaceutical reasons for drug modification [161]. Some of the properties which may be altered through derivative formation are as follows:

1. Mask the taste or odor of bitter or obnoxious drugs
2. Alter aqueous solubility
3. Improve ease of formulation of drugs difficult to formulate
4. Increase stability
5. Decrease gastric or intestinal irritation
6. Decrease pain on injection
7. Improve depot action
8. Improve absorption
9. Facilitate transport of the drug to the site of action

Except for those cases where derivatives revert back to parent drug before or immediately after absorption, the modification must be considered as potentially capable of affecting the absorption, distribution, and elimination kinetics in addition to performing the desired function.

V. PITFALLS IN DATA INTERPRETATION

A. Meaning of Parameters

Although it is important that the field of drug design and evaluation involve consideration of pharmacokinetic effects, it is equally imperative that the meaning and limitation of each parameter under comparison be understood. Earlier the values for Vd were compared at the steady state for three isoxazolyl penicillins. The steady state was chosen to avoid the effect of k_2 upon those values.

The calculation of Vd for a two-compartment model has been the subject of considerable confusion in the literature. The methods derived for use in the one-compartment model have been applied to the two-compartment model. However, unlike the one-compartment model case, the Vd values calculated by the various methods are not equal. This observation and the reasons behind it were discussed in Chap. 3.

The apparent volume of distribution of a drug, Vd, is not a volume at all. That is, it should not be considered as a particular physiological space within the body. It might be hypothetically defined as the volume of body water which would be required to contain the amount of drug in the body if it were uniformly present in the same concentration as it is in the blood. However, all compartments which contain the drug may not have equal concentration. Thus, any volume calculated utilizing the drug concentration in only one compartment can be only an *apparent* volume. It appears most useful to avoid all analogies to volumes and consider Vd simply as a proportionality factor which when multiplied by the concentration of drug in the blood gives the amount of drug present in the body.

Understanding the conditions which affect the Vd allows explanation of some clinical findings which might otherwise appear anomalous. A number of drugs, such as cephalexin, colistimethate, lincomycin, methicillin, and insulin, show decreased apparent volumes of distribution in patients with renal failure as compared to normal patients. Also, administration of probenecid, an inhibitor of renal tubular secretion of organic acids, reduces the volume of distribution of penicillin derivatives. These observations are not surprising in view of certain facts. Since the Vd does not necessarily represent a real volume, observed changes may not reflect any change in the tissues through which the drugs are distributed. The values obtained may depend upon the size of k_2 for a two (or more) compartment drug. Thus, comparisons of Vd for derivatives should either be interpreted in terms of the effects of k_2 on the distribution value or carried out at steady-state plasma levels.

When the latter method is used, the researcher must be certain that the steady-state has, in fact, been achieved before the data are used to calculate pharmacokinetic parameters such as Vd. In this regard the time required to approach steady-state levels becomes an important consideration. This time can be evaluated by considering the following equation for the plasma concentration as a function of time during constant intravenous infusion of a one-compartment model drug [162].

$$P = \frac{k_0}{Vd \cdot \beta}(1 - e^{-\beta t}) \tag{9}$$

The value of the plasma concentration at the steady state is

$$P_{ss} = \frac{k_0}{Vd \cdot \beta} \tag{10}$$

Inspection of these equations indicates that the steady state is achieved when $e^{-\beta t}$ approaches zero, which occurs when $t = \infty$. In a practical sense, however, the data become useful when the plasma level is sufficiently close to the theoretical steady-state value. For any fixed rate of infusion, k_0, the time to achieve a "practical" steady state is determined by β and thus by the $t_{1/2}$ of the drug. Table 13 summarizes the approach to P_{ss} after constant infusion is maintained for four to seven half-lives. Thus, the often-stated general rule of thumb that four to five half-lives are required to reach the steady state during constant intravenous infusion for one-compartment model drugs is based on achieving 94–97% of P_{ss}. For clinical purposes the patient may be assumed to be steady-stated after four half-lives, but for research purposes five or more half-lives might be more appropriate before data are used to calculate pharmacokinetic parameters. The time required to approach P_{ss} for two-compartment model drugs is more difficult to calculate. The equation for plasma concentration as a function of time can be written

$$P = \frac{k_0}{V_p k_2}\left[1 - \left(\frac{k_2 - \alpha}{\beta - \alpha}\right)e^{-\beta t} - \left(\frac{k_2 - \alpha}{\alpha - \beta}\right)e^{-\alpha t}\right] \tag{11}$$

Table 13

Percent of Steady-state Plasma Level Achieved at Various Time Intervals

Number of Half-lives	$e^{-\beta t}$	$(1 - e^{-\beta t})$	Percent P_{ss}
$4t_{1/2}$	$e^{-2.77}$	0.94	94
$5t_{1/2}$	$e^{-3.46}$	0.97	97
$6t_{1/2}$	$e^{-4.15}$	0.984	98
$7t_{1/2}$	$e^{-4.85}$	0.992	99

The interpretation of Vd values is complicated for many drugs, such as erythromycin, sulfonylureas, salicylates, and coumarin anticoagulants, which are bound to plasma proteins. The apparent volume of distribution should be calculated on the basis of freely diffusing drug, and thus a correction must be made for the fraction bound. If this correction is not made, two types of error can occur. When the assay method determines only free drug, the bound drug will be counted with drug distributed to the tissues and the calculated Vd will appear large. On the other hand, if the assay is for total drug, the value for Vd will be too small. If corrections are not made for protein binding, Vd values

2. *The Bioavailability of Drug Products*, American Pharmaceutical Association, Washington, D.C., 1973.
3. B. B. Brodie and W. M. Heller, eds., *Bioavailability of Drugs*, S. Karger, New York, 1972.
4. K. H. Spitzy and G. Hitzenberger, The Distribution Volume of Some Antibiotics, *Antibiot. Annu.*, *1957–1958*, 996.
5. R. Pratt, Antibiotics 1956–1961, *J. Pharm. Sci.*, *51*, 1 (1964).
6. C. M. Kunin, Pharmacology of the Antimicrobials, *Mod. Treat.*, *1*, 829 (1964).
7. G. H. Warren, The Prognostic Significance of Penicillin Serum Levels and Protein Binding in Clinical Medicine, *Chemotherapia*, *10*, 339 (1966).
8. J. P. Hou and J. W. Poole, β-Lactam Antibiotics: Their Physicochemical Properties and Biological Activities in Relation to Structure, *J. Pharm. Sci.*, *60*, 503 (1971).
9. J. Fabre, E. Milek, P. Kalfopoulos, and G. Merier, *Schweig, Med. Wschr.*, *101*, 625 (1971).
10. E. P. Abraham, *Advances in Pharmaceutical Sciences*, Vol. I (D. Perlman, ed.), John Wiley and Sons, New York, 1967, pp. 1–31.
11. K. E. Price, A. Gourevitch, and L. C. Cheney, Biological Properties of Semisynthetic Penicillins: Structure–Activity Relationships, *Antimicrob. Ag. Chemother.*, 670 (1966).
12. E. Kaczka and K. Folkers, in *The Chemistry of Penicillin* (H. T. Clarke, J. R. Johnson, and B. Robinson, eds.), Princeton University Press, Princeton, N.J., 1949, pp. 243–268.
13. M. A. Schwartz and F. H. Buckwalter, Pharmaceutics of Penicillin, *J. Pharm. Sci.*, *51*, 1119 (1962).
14. C. F. Gravenkemper, J. V. Bennett, J. L. Brodie, and W. M. M. Kirby, Dicloxacillin. In Vitro and Pharmacologic Comparisons with Oxacillin and Cloxacillin, *Arch. Internal. Med.*, *116*, 340 (1965).
15. Z. Modr and K. Dvoracek, *Advances in Biosciences* (G. Raspe, ed.), Pergamon Press, Elmsford, N.Y., 1970, p. 219.
16. L. W. Dittert, W. O. Griffin, J. C. LaPiana, F. J. Shainfeld, and J. T. Doluisio, Pharmacokinetic Interpretation of Penicillin Levels in Serum and Urine After Intravenous Administration, *Antimicrob. Ag. Chemother.*, p. 42 (1969).
17. J. E. Rosenblatt, A. C. Kind, J. L. Brodie, and W. M. M. Kirby, Mechanisms Responsible for the Blood Level Differences of Isoxazolyl Penicillins, *Arch. Int. Med.*, *121*, 345 (1968).
18. H. C. Standiford, M. C. Jordan, and W. M. M. Kirby, Clinical Pharmacology of Carbenicillin Compared with Other Penicillins, *J. Infect. Dis.*, *122*, 9 (Suppl.), (1970).
19. J. H. C. Nayler, Structure Activity Relationships in Semi-synthetic Penicillins, *Proc. Royal Soc. Lond.*, *179*, 357 (1971).
20. R. H. Connamaker and H. G. Mandel, Studies on the Intracellular Location of Tetracycline in Bacteria, *Biochem. Biophys. Acta.*, *166*, 475 (1968).

21. E. F. Gale, Mechanisms of Antibiotic Action, *Pharmacol. Rev., 15*, 481 (1963).
22. T. J. Franklin, Mode of Action of the Tetracyclines, *Symp. Soc. Gen. Microbiol., 21*, 192 (1966).
23. B. Parthier, Wirking mechanismen und Wirkungespektren der Antibiotica im Protein- und Nucleinsaurenstoffwechsel, *Pharmagie, 20,* 465 (1965).
24. G. H. Miller, S. A. Kahlil, A. N. Martin, Structure–Activity Relationships of Tetracyclines I: Inhibition of Cell Division and Protein and Nucleic Acid Synthesis in *Escherichia coli* W, *J. Pharm. Sci., 60*, 33 (1971).
25. L. J. Leeson, J. E. Krueger, and R. A. Nash, Concerning the Structural Assignments of the Second and Third Acidity Constants of the Tetracycline Antibiotics, *Tet. Lett., 18*, 1155 (1963).
26. W. H. Barr, J. Adir, and L. Garrettson, Decrease in Tetracycline Absorption in Man by Sodium Bicarbonate, *Clin. Pharmacol. Ther., 12*, 779 (1971).
27. M. Schach von Wittenau and R. Yeary, The Excretion and Distribution in Body Fluids After Intravenous Administration to Dogs, *J. Pharmacol. and Exp. Ther., 140*, 258 (1963).
28. M. Schach von Wittenau and C. S. Delahunt, The Distribution of Tetracyclines in Tissues of Dogs After Repeated Oral Administration, *J. Pharmacol. and Exp. Ther., 152*, 164 (1966).
29. R. G. Kelly and L. A. Kanegis, Tissue Distribution of Tetracycline and Chlortetracycline in the Dog, *Toxicol. and App. Pharmacol., 11*, 114 (1967).
30. C. M. Kunin, A. C. Dornbush, and M. Finland, *J. Clin. Invest., 38*, 1950 (1959).
31. F. E. Digangi and C. H. Rogers, Absorption Studies of Aureomycin Hydrochloride on Aluminum Hydroxide Gel, *J. Pharm. Sci., 38*, 646 (1949).
32. J. Scheiner and W. A. Altemeir, Experimental Study of Factors Inhibiting Absorption and Effective Therapeutic Levels of Declomycin, *Surgery, 114*, 9 (1962).
33. L. A. Mitscher, A. C. Bonacci, and T. D. Sokoloski, Circular Dichroism and Solution Conformation of the Tetracycline Antibiotics, *Tet. Lett., 51*, 5361 (1968).
34. N. A. Baker and P. M. Brown, Metal Binding in Tetracyclines–Cobalt (II) and Nickel (II) Complexes, *J. Am. Chem. Soc., 88*, 1314 (1966).
35. L. Z. Benet and J. E. Goyan, Thermodynamics of Chelation by Tetracyclines, *J. Pharm. Sci., 55*, 1184 (1966).
36. J. E. Rosenblatt, J. E. Barrett, J. L. Brodie, and W. M. M. Kirby, Comparison of in Vitro Activity and Clinical Pharmacology of Doxycycline with Other Tetracyclines, *Antimicrob. Ag. Chemother.*, 134 (1966).
37. M. Schach von Wittenau and T. M. Twomey, The Disposition of Doxycycline by Man and Dog, *Chemother., 16*, 217 (1971).
38. M. Schach von Wittenau, Some Pharmacokinetic Aspects of Doxycycline Metabolism in Man, *Chemother., 13*, 41 (Suppl.), (1968).

39. J. R. Migliardi and M. Schach von Wittenau, Pharmacokinetic Properties of Doxycycline in Man, 5th International Congress of Chemother., Vienna, Austria, June 26-July 1, 1967, p. 165.
40. R. C. Batterman, L. F. Tauber, and M. E. Bell, Long-acting Sulfonamides: In Vivo Correlation in Man of Protein Binding, Serum Concentration and Antimicrobial Activity, *Curr. Ther. Res., 8*, 75 (1966).
41. C. M. Kunin, Clinical Pharmacology of the New Penicillins. 1. The Importance of Serum Protein Binding in Determining Antimicrobial Activity and Concentration in Serum, *Clin. Pharmacol. and Therap., 7*, 166 (1966).
42. M. C. Meyer and D. E. Guttman, The Binding of Drugs by Plasma Proteins, *J. Pharm. Sci., 57*, 895 (1968).
43. J. T. Doluisio and L. W. Dittert, Influence of Repetitive Dosing of Tetracyclines on Biologic Half-life in Serum, *Clin. Pharmacol. and Therap., 10*, 690 (1969).
44. J. Fabre, J. S. Pitton, C. Virieux, F. L. Laureniet, J. P. Barnhardt, and J. C. Godel, Doxycycline; Absorption Distribution and Excretion of a New Wide-spectrum Antibiotic in Man, *Schweiz. Medizinische Wochenshrift, 97*, 915 (1967). Translation by Carl Demrick Associates, Inc.
45. M. Gibaldi and H. Weintraub, Some Considerations as to the Determination and Significance of Biological Half-life, *J. Pharm. Sci., 60*, 624 (1971).
46. J. M. van Rossum, in *Drug Design*, Vol. I (E. J. Ariens, ed.), Academic Press, New York, 1972, p. 509.
47. B. Crompton, M. Jago, K. Crawford, G. G. F. Newton, E. P. Abraham, Behavior of Some Derivatives of 7-Aminocephalosporanic Acid and 6-Aminopenicillanic Acid as Substrates, Inhibitors and Inducers of Pennicillinases, *Biochem. J., 83*, 52 (1962).
48. E. P. Abraham, The Cephalosporin C. Group, *Quart. Rev. Chem. Soc., 21*, 231 (1967).
49. E. Van Heyningen, in *Advances in Drug Research*, Vol. I. (N. J. Harper and A. B. Simmonds, eds.), Academic Press, New York, 1967, pp. 1-70.
50. J. T. Smith, J. M. T. Hamilton-Miller, and R. Knox, Bacterial Resistance to Penicillins and Cephalosporins, *J. Pharm. Pharmacol., 21*, 337 (1969).
51. M. R. Pollock, Enzymes Destroying Penicillin and Cephalosporins, *Antimicrob. Ag. Chemother.*, p. 292 (1964).
52. A. C. Kind, D. G. Kestle, H. C. Standiford, and W. M. M. Kirby, Laboratory and Clinical Experience with Cephalexin, *Antimicrob. Ag. Chemother.*, p. 361 (1968).
53. J. Pitt, R. Siasoco, K. Kaplan, and Louis Weinstein, Antimicrobial Activity and Pharmacological Behavior of Cephaloglycine, *Antimicrob. Ag. Chemother.*, p. 630 (1967).
54. R. R. Chauvette, E. H. Flynn, B. G. Jackson, E. R. Lavagnino, R. B. Morin, R. A. Mueller, R. P. Pioch, R. W. Roeske, C. W. Ryan, J. L. Spencer, and E. Van Heyningen, Chemistry of Cephalosporin Antibiotics. II. Preparation of a New Class of Antibiotics and the Relation of Structure

to Activity, *J. Amer. Chem. Soc., 84*, 3401 (1962).

55. M. Barber and P. M. Waterworth, Penicillinase-resistant Penicillins and Cephalosporins, *Brit. Med. J., 2*, 344 (1964).
56. R. R. Chauvette, E. H. Flynn, B. G. Jackson, E. B. Lavagnino, R. B. Morin, R. A. Mueller, R. P. Pioch, R. W. Roeske, C. W. Ryan, J. L. Spencer, and E. Van Heyningen, Structure-Activity Relationship Among 7-Acylamidocephalosporanic Acids, *Antimicrob. Ag. Chemother.*, p. 687 (1962).
57. K. N. Anderson and R. G. Petersdorf, Cephalosporin C and Cephalothin in Gram-negative Infections, *Antimicrob. Ag. Chemother.*, p. 724 (1962).
58. E. H. Flynn, Biological and Chemical Studies of the Cephalosporins, *Antimicrob. Ag. Chemother.*, p. 715 (1967).
59. E. W. Walters, M. J. Romansky, and A. C. Johnson, Cephalothin, A New Semisynthetic Broad-spectrum Antibiotic, *Antimicrob. Ag. Chemother.*, p. 706 (1962).
60. R. S. Griffith and H. R. Black, Treatment of Infections in Man with Cephalothin, *J.A.M.A., 189*, 823 (1964).
61. E. Van Heyningen and C. N. Brown, The Chemistry of Cephalosporins. IV. Acetoxyl Replacements with Xanthates and Dithiocarbamates, *J. Med. Chem., 8*, 174 (1965).
62. J. L. Spencer, F. Y. Siu, E. H. Flynn, B. G. Jackson, M. V. Sigal, H. M. Higgins, R. R. Chauvette, S. L. Andrews, and D. E. Bloch, Chemistry of Cephalosporin Antibiotics VIII. Synthesis and Structure-Activity Relationships of Cephaloridine Analogs, *Antimicrob. Ag. Chemother.*, p. 573 (1966).
63. J. L. Spencer, F. Y. Siu, E. H. Flynn, B. G. Jackson, and H. M. Higgins, Chemistry of Cephalosporin Antibiotics IX. Synthesis of Cephaloridine, *J. Org. Chem., 32*, 500 (1967).
64. W. E. Wick and W. S. Boniece, In Vitro and In Vivo Laboratory Evaluation of Cephaloglycin and Cephaloridine, *Appl. Microbiol., 13*, 248 (1965).
65. J. M. Applestein, E. B. Crosby, W. D. Johnson, and D. Kaye, In Vitro Antimicrobial and Human Pharmacology of Cephaloglycin, *Appl. Microbiol., 16*, 1006 (1968).
66. L. B. Hogan, W. J. Holloway, and R. A. Jakubowitch, Clinical Experience with Cephaloglycin, *Antimicrob. Ag. Chemother.*, p. 624 (1967).
67. R. Thornburn, J. E. Johnson, and L. E. Cluff, Studies on the Epidemiology of Adverse Drug Reactions, *J. A. M. A., 198,* 345 (1966).
68. A. Burger, *Medicinal Chemistry*, 3rd ed., Part I, Wiley-Interscience, New York, 1970, p. 348.
69. B. J. Magerlein, R. D. Birkenmeyer, and F. Kagan, Chemical Modification of Lincomycin, *Antimicrob. Ag. Chemother.*, p. 727 (1966).
70. C. E. Meyer and C. Lewis, Absorption and Fate of Lincomycin in the Rat, *Antimicrob. Ag. Chemother.*, p. 169 (1963).
71. F. F. Sun, Disposition of Clindamycin in Rat and Dog, *Fed. Proc., 29*, 677 (1970).

72. W. Morozowich, The Design of Orally Absorbed Drugs, 13th Annual National Industrial Pharmaceutical Research Conference, June 24, 1971.
73. J. K. Seydel, in *Drug Design*, Vol. I, (E. J. Ariens, ed.), Academic Press, New York, 1971, p. 368.
74. G. Zbinden, *Advances in Chemistry, Series 45, Molecular Modification in Drug Design*, American Chemical Society, Washington, D.C., 1964, p. 32.
75. T. Struller, Long-acting and Short-acting Sulfonamides. Recent Developments, *Antibiot. Chemother, 14*, 179 (1968).
76. T. Fugita and C. Hansch, Analysis of the Structure-Activity Relationship of the Sulfonamide Drugs Using Substituent Constants, *J. Med. Chem., 10*, 991 (1967).
77. M. Nakagaki, N. Koga, and H. Terada, Studies on the Binding of Chemicals with Proteins. II. The Mechanism of Binding of Several Sulfonamides, *Yakugaku Zasshi, 84*, 516 (1964).
78. W. Scholtan, Die Bindung der Sulfonamide an Eiweisskorper, *Arzneim-Forsch., 14*, 348 (1964).
79. M. A. Krupp and M. J. Chatton, *Current Diagnosis and Treatment*, Lange Medical Publications, Los Altos, Calif., 1972, p. 491.
80. W. H. Hughes and H. C. Stewart, *Concise Antibiotic Treatment*, Appleton-Century-Crofts, New York, 1970, pp. 27-29.
81. D. N. Holvey, R. L. Iles, and J. C. LaPiana, Serum Concentrations and Recovery in Urine of Four Tetracycline Analogs, *Curr. Ther. Res., 12*, 536 (1970).
82. J. K. Seydel, Sulfonamides, Structure-Activity Relationship, and Mode of Action, *J. Pharm. Sci., 57*, 1455 (1968).
83. C. L. Fox and H. M. Rose, Ionization of Sulfonamides, *Proc. Soc. Exptl. Biol. Med., 50*, 142 (1942).
84. A. A. Lindberg, H. Bucht, and L. O. Kallings, Treatment of Chronic Urinary Tract Infections with Gentamycin, *Gentamycin First Innal. Symp., Paris,* January, 1967, pp. 75-83.
85. C. M. Kunin, *Detection, Prevention and Management of Urinary Tract Infections*, Lea & Febiger, Philadelphia, 1972, p. 183.
86. B. B. Brodie, Displacement of One Drug by Another from Carrier or Receptor Sites, *Proc. Roy. Soc. Med., 58*, 946 (1965).
87. L. S. Schanker, Mechanisms of Drug Absorption and Distribution, *Ann. Rev. Pharmacol., 1*, 29 (1961).
88. L. S. Schanker, Passage of Drugs Across Body Membranes, *Pharmacol. Rev., 14*, 501 (1962).
89. R. R. Levine and E. W. Pelikan, Mechanism of Drug Absorption and Excretion, *Ann. Rev. Pharmacol, 4*, 69 (1964).
90. W. G. Crouthamel, G. H. Tan, L. W. Dittert, and J. T. Doluisio, Drug Absorption IV: Influence of pH on Absorption Kinetics of Weakly Acidic Drugs, *J. Pharm. Sci., 60*, 1160 (1971).
91. R. R. Levine and E. W. Pelikan, The Influence of Experimental Procedures and Dose on the Intestinal Absorption of an Onium Compound, Benzomethamine, *J. Pharmacol. and Exp. Therap., 131*, 319 (1961).
92. R. H. Reuning, B. L. Ross, B. J. Shoemaker, and S. S. Watson, Positive

Influence of an Acidic Medium on the Intestinal Absorption of a Quaternary Ammonium Compound in the Rat, *Pharmacologist, 13*, 195 (1971).

93. A. R. DiSanto and J. G. Wagner, Pharmacokinetics of Highly Ionized Drugs II: Methylene Blue–Absorption, Metabolism and Excretion in Man and Dog after Oral Administration, *J. Pharm. Sci., 61*, 1086 (1971).
94. J. L. Colaizzi and P. R. Klink, pH-Partition Behavior of Tetracyclines, *J. Pharm. Sci., 58*, 1184 (1969).
95. J. T. Doluisio and J. V. Swintosky, Drug Partitioning II. In Vitro Model for Drug Absorption, *J. Pharm. Sci., 53*, 597 (1964).
96. C. M. Kunin and M. Finland, Clinical Pharmacology of the Tetracycline Antibiotics, *Clin. Pharmacol. Therap., 2*, 51 (1961).
97. R. R. Levine, Factors Affecting Gastrointestinal Absorption of Drugs, *Digestive Diseases, 15*, 171 (1970).
98. T. Fujita, J. Iwasa, and C. Hansch, A New Substituent Constant, π, Derived from Partition Coefficients, *J. Amer. Chem. Soc., 86*, 5175 (1964).
99. C. Hansch and W. J. Dunn, Linear Relationships Between Lipophilic Character and Biological Activity of Drugs, *J. Pharm. Sci., 61*, 1 (1972).
100. E. Miller and C. Hansch, Structure-Activity Analysis of Tetrahydrofolate Analogs Using Substituent Constants and Regression Analysis, *J. Pharm. Sci., 56*, 92 (1967).
101. Corwin Hansch, in *Drug Design*, Vol. I, (E. J. Ariens, ed.), Academic Press, New York, 1971, p. 289.
102. G. L. Flynn Structural Approach to Partitioning: Estimation of Steriod Partition Coefficients Based upon Molecular Constitution, *J. Pharm. Sci., 60*, 345 (1971).
103. A. E. Bird and A. C. Marshall, Correlation of Serum Binding of Penicillins with Partition Coefficients, *Biochem. Pharmacol., 16*, 2275 (1967).
104. E. J. Lien and C. Hansch, Correlation of Ratios of Drug Metabolism by Microsomal Subfractions with Partition Coefficients, *J. Pharm. Sci., 57*, 1027 (1968).
105. C. Hansch and S. M. Anderson, The Structure-Activity Relationship in Barbiturates and Its Similarity to That in Other Narcotics, *J. Med. Chem., 10*, 745 (1967).
106. D. J. Curie, C. E. Lough, R. F. Silver, and H. L. Holmes, Partition Coefficients of Some Conjugated Heteroenoid Compounds and 1,4-Napthoquinones, *Can. J. Chem., 44*, 1035 (1966).
107. W. P. Purcell, J. G. Bensley, R. P. Quintana, and J. A. Singer, Application of Partition Coefficients, Electrical Moments, Electronic Structures and Free-energy Relationships to the Interpretation of Cholinesterase Inhibition, *J. Med. Chem., 9*, 297 (1966).
108. J. Iwasa, T. Fujita, and C. Hansch, Substituent Constants for Aliphatic Functions Obtained from Partition Coefficients, *J. Med. Chem., 8*, 150 (1965).
109. C. Hansch and S. M. Anderson, The Effect of Intramolecular Hydrophobic

Bonding on Partition Coefficients, *J. Org. Chem., 32*, 2583 (1967).

110. A. H. Beckett, R. N. Boyes, and E. J. Triggs, Kinetics of Buccal Absorption of Amphetamines, *J. Pharm. Pharmacol., 20*, 92 (1968).
111. A. H. Beckett and E. J. Triggs, Buccal Absorption of Basic Drugs and Its Application as an In Vivo Model of Passive Drug Transfer Through Lipid Membranes, *J. Pharm. Pharmacol., 19*, 315 (1967).
112. A. H. Beckett and A. C. Moffat, The Influence of Alkyl Substitution in Acids on Their Performance in the Buccal Absorption Test, *J. Pharm. Pharmacol., 20*, 2395 (1968).
113. A. H. Beckett and A. C. Moffat, Correlation of Partition Coefficients in *n*-Heptane–Aqueous systems with Buccal Absorption Data for a Series of Amines and Acids, *J. Pharm. Pharmacol., 21*, 1445 (1969).
114. A. H. Beckett and A. C. Moffat, The Influence of Substitution in Phenylacetic Acids on Their Performance in the Buccal Absorption Test, *J. Pharm. Pharmacol., 21*, 1395 (1969).
115. A. H. Beckett and A. C. Moffat, Kinetics of Buccal Absorption of Some Carboxylic Acids and the Correlation of the Rate Constants and *n*-Heptane–Aqueous Phase Partition Coefficients, *J. Pharm. Pharmacol., 22*, 15 (1970).
116. M. J. Taraszka, Absorption of Clindamycin from the Buccal Cavity, *J. Pharm. Sci., 59*, 873 (1970).
117. R. G. Stehle, Diffusional Model for Transport Rate Studies Across Membranes, *J. Pharm. Sci., 56*, 1367 (1967).
118. N. F. H. Ho and W. I. Higuchi, Quantitative Interpretation of in Vivo Buccal Absorption of *n*-Alkanoic Acids by the Physical Model Approach, *J. Pharm. Sci., 60*, 537 (1971).
119. K. R. M. Vora, W. I. Higuchi, and N. F. H. Ho, Analysis of Human Buccal Absorption of Drugs by Physical Model Approach, *J. Pharm. Sci., 61*, 1785 (1972).
120. A. Suzuki, W. I. Higuchi, and N. F. H. Ho, Theoretical Model Studies of Drug Absorption and Transport in the Gastrointestinal Tract I, *J. Pharm. Sci., 59*, 644 (1970).
121. A. Suzuki, W. I. Higuchi, and N. F. H. Ho, Theoretical Model Studies of Drug Absorption and Transport in the Gastrointestinal Tract II, *J. Pharm. Sci., 59*, 651 (1970).
122. H. Nogami, M. Hanano and H. Yamada, Studies on Absorption and Excretion of Drugs. XI. Relation Between Chemical Structure and Absorption Rate, Intramolecular Interaction Constant, Additivity Rule and Prediction for Intestinal Absorption Rate Coefficient, *Chem. Pharm. Bull., 16*, 586 (1968).
123. H. Nogami, M. Hanano, and H. Yamada, Studies on Absorption and Excretion of Drugs. X. Relation Between Chemical Structure and Absorption Rate. Substituent Constant for Absorption Rate Coefficient of Foreign Organic Compounds, *Chem. Pharm. Bull., 16*, 580 (1968).
124. G. L. Flynn and S. H. Yalkowsky, Correlations and Predictions of Mass Transport Across Membranes I: Influence of Alkyl Chain Length on

Flux-determining Properties of Barrier Diffusant, *J. Pharm. Sci., 61*, 838 (1972).

125. J. T. Penniston, L. Beckett, D. L. Bentley, and C. Hansch, Passive Permeation of Organic Compounds Through Biological Tissue: A Non-steady-state Theory, *Mol. Pharmacol., 5*, 333 (1969).

126. T. Higuchi and S. S. Davis, Thermodynamic Analysis of Structure-Activity Relationships of Drugs: Prediction of Optimal Structure, *J. Pharm. Sci., 59*, 1376 (1970).

127. J. W. McFarland, On the Parabolic Relationship Between Drug Potency and Hydrophobicity, *J. Med. Chem., 13*, 1192 (1970).

128. C. Hansch and J. M. Clayton, Lipophilic Character and Biological Activity of Drugs II: The Parabolic Case, *J. Pharm. Sci., 62*, 1 (1973).

129. E. J. Lien, Physicochemical Properties and Gastrointestinal Absorption of Drugs, *Drug Intel., 4,* 7 (1970).

130. H. P. Fletcher, H. M. Murray, and T. E. Weddon, Absorption of Lincomycin and Lincomycin Esters from Rat Jejunum, *J. Pharm. Sci., 57*, 2101 (1968).

131. C. Lee, R. C. Anderson, F. G. Henderson, H. M. Worth, and P. N. Harris, Pharmacology and Toxicology of Erythromycin Propionate, *Antibiot. Ann.*, 1958-1959, p. 354.

132. K. C. James and M. Roberts, The Solubilities of the Lower Testosterone Esters, *J. Pharm. Pharmacol., 20*, 709 (1968).

133. A. L. Green, Ionization Constants and Water Solubilities of Some Aminoalkylphenothiazine Tranquillizers and Related Compounds, *J. Pharm. Pharmacol., 19*, 10 (1967).

134. F. Shihab, W. Sheffield, J. Spronts, and J. Nematholhahi, Solubility of Alkyl Benzoates I: Effect of Some Alkyl *p*-Hydroxybenzoates (Parabens) on the Solubility of Benzyl *p*-Hydroxybenzoate, *J. Pharm. Sci., 59*, 1574 (1970).

135. S. H. Yalkowsky, G. L. Flynn, and G. L. Amidon, Solubility of Nonelectrolytes in Polar Solvents, *J. Pharm. Sci., 61*, 983 (1972).

136. V. J. Stella, Chemical Modification of Drugs to Overcome Pharmaceutical Problems, *Austral. J. Pharm Sci., NS 2*, 57 (1973).

137. H. Hocksema, G. B. Whitfield, and L. E. Rhuland, Effect of Selective Acylation on the Oral Absorption of a Nucleoside by Humans, *Biochem. and Biophys. Res. Comm., 6*, 213 (1961).

138. G. P. Bodey, E. J. Freireich, R. W. Monto, and J. S. Hewlett, Cytosine Arabinoside (NSC-63878) Therapy for Acute Leukemia in Adults, *Cancer Chemother. Rep., 53*, 59 (1969).

139. J. S. Hewlett, J. Battle, R. Bishop, W. Fowler, S. Schwartz, P. Hagen, and J. Lewis, Phase II Study of A-8103 (NSC-25154) in Acute Leukemia in Adults, *Cancer Chemother. Rep., 42*, 25 (1964).

140. B. Goodell, B. Leventhal, and E. Hendersen, Cytosine Arabinoside in Acute Granulocytic Leukemia, *Clin. Pharmacol. and Therap., 12*, 599 (1971).

141. D. H. W. Ho and E. Frei, Clinical Pharmacology of 1-β-D-arabinofuranosyl Cytosine, *Clin. Pharmacol. Therap., 12*, 944 (1971).

142. R. L. Dedrich, D. D. Forrester, and D. H. W. Ho, In Vitro-in Vivo Correlation of Drug Metabolism—Deamination of 1-β-D-arabinofuranosylcytosine, *Biochem. Pharmacol., 21*, 1 (1972).

143. W. A. Creasy, Tumor Inhibitory Effects of Combinations of the Vinca Alkaloids with Actinomycin D, *Biochem. Pharmacol., 15*, 367 (1966).

144. B. C. Baguley and E. M. Falkenhaug, Plasma Half-life of Cytosine Arabinoside (NSC-63878) in Patients Treated for Acute Myeloblastic Leukemia, *Cancer Chemother. Rep., 55*, 791 (1971).

145. E. Frei, J. N. Bukers, and J. S. Hewlett, Dose Schedule and Antitumor Studies of Arabinosyl Cytosine (NS 63878), *Cancer Res., 29*, 1325 (1969).

146. J. J. Wang, O. S. Selawry, T. J. Vieltie, and G. P. Bodey, Prolonged Infusion of Arabinosyl Cytosine in Childhood Leukemia, *Cancer, 25*, 1 (1970).

147. G. L. Neil, H. H. Buskirk, T. E. Moxley, R. C. Manak, S. L. Kuentzel, and B. K. Bhuyan, Biochemical and Pharmacologic Studies with 1-β-D-Arabinofuranosycytosine 5′-Adamantoate, A Depot Form of Cytarabine, *Biochem. Pharmacol., 20,* 3295 (1971).

148. K. Butler, A. R. English, A. K. Knirsch, and J. J. Korst, Metabolism and Laboratory Studies with Indanyl Carbenicillin, *Del. Med. J., 43*, 366 (1971).

149. J. F. Wallace, E. Atalus, D. M. Bear, N. K. Brown, H. Clark, and M. Turck, Evaluation of an Indanyl Ester of Carbenicillin, *Antimicrob. Ag. Chemother.*, p. 223 (1970).

150. M. A. Schwartz and W. L. Hayton, Relative Stability of Hetacillin and Ampicillin in Solution, *J. Pharm. Sci., 61*, 906 (1972).

151. R. Sutherland and O. P. W. Robinson, Laboratory and Pharmacological Studies in Man with Hetacillin and Ampicillin, *Brit. Med. J., 2*, 804 (1967).

152. Z. Modr and K. Dvoracek, Pharmacokinetics of Ampicillin and Hetacillin, *Rev. Czech. Med., 16*, 84 (1970).

153. L. Magni, B. Ortangren, B. Sjoberg, and S. Wahlquist, Stability, Absorption, and Excretion Studies with Hetacillin, *Scand. J. Clin. and Lab. Invest., 20*, 195 (1967).

154. W. J. Jusko and G. P. Lewis, Comparison of Ampicillin and Hetacillin Pharmacokinetics in Man, *J. Pharm. Sci., 62*, 69 (1973).

155. P. H. Tardrew, J. C. H. Mao, and D. Kenny, Antibacterial Activity of 2′-Esters of Erythromycin, *Appl. Microb., 18*, 159 (1969).

156. R. S. Griffith and H. R. Black, Comparison of the Blood Levels Obtained After Single and Multiple Doses of Erythromycin Estolate and Erythromycin Stearate, *Amer. J. Med. Sci., 247*, 69 (1964).

157. W. E. Wick and G. E. Mallitt, New Analysis for the Therapeutic Efficacy of Proprionyl Erythromycin and Erythromycin Base, *Antimicrob. Agent Chemotherap.*, p. 410 (1968).

158. V. C. Stephens, C. T. Pugh, and N. E. Davis, A Study of the Behavior of Propionyl Erythromycin in Blood by a New Chromatographic Method, *J. Antibiot. (Tokyo), 22*, 551 (1969).

159. A. A. Sinkula and C. Lewis, Chemical Modification of Lincomycin: Synthesis and Bioactivity of Selected 2,7-Dialkylcarbonate Esters, *J. Pharm. Sci.*, *62*, 1757 (1973).
160. R. M. Dettaan and D. Schellenberg, Clindamycin Palmitate Flavored Granules. Multidose Tolerance, Absorption and Urinary Excretion Study in Healthy Children, *J. Clin. Pharmacol.*, *12*, 74 (1972).
161. A. A. Sinkula, in *Molecular Modification: Derivative Formation and Pharmaceutical Properties*, 14th Annual National Industrial Pharmaceutical Research Conference, June 1972.
162. F. H. Dost, *Grundlugen der Pharmacokinetic*, Stuttgart: Georg Thiene Verlag, 1968.
163. R. E. Notari, J. L. DeYoung, and R. H. Reuning, Effect of Parallel First-order Drug Loss from Site of Administration on Calculated Values for Absorption Rate Constants, *J. Pharm. Sci.*, *61*, 135 (1972).
164. S. A. Kaplan, R. E. Weinfeld, C. W. Abruzzo, and M. Lewis, Pharmacokinetic Profile of Sulfisoxazole Following Intravenous, Intramuscular, and Oral Administration to Man, *J. Pharm. Sci.*, *61*, 773 (1972).
165. W. J. Jusko and G. P. Lewis, Comparison of Ampicillin and Hetacillin Pharmacokinetics in Man, *J. Pharm. Sci.*, *62*, 69 (1973).

Chapter 6

ADDITIONAL PRACTICE PROBLEMS FOR COMPREHENSIVE REVIEW

The problems included in the previous chapters have always been placed immediately following the section dealing with the principles needed for their solution. This group of problems is included to allow an overview of the various topics previously discussed and, hopefully, to provide a means for the reader to observe how the individual calculations are assimilated into an overall pharmacokinetic analysis for a drug and the therapeutic implications of such considerations. Some rather simplistic examples of compartmental analysis are also included here. The examples chosen are necessarily simple since they are to be solved by graphical methods or by calculation with paper and pencil rather than by use of a computer.

Practice Problem 1

An 800-mg dose of a one-compartment model drug given I.V. to a 70-kg male results in the data given in Table 1.

Table 1

Time After Adm. (hr)	Cumulative Amt. in Urine (mg)	Cumulative Amt. Metabolized (mg)
0	000	000
1	(approx. 20)	(approx. 10)
2	50	50
4	112	112
6	163	163
8	206	206
10	242	242
12	270	270

(a) The biological $t_{1/2}$ of this drug is known to be 6.9 hr. What is the value and units for β?
Answer: 0.1 hr^{-1}

(b) It is desired to maintain the therapeutic blood level of 5 mg%, which corresponds to the 2-hr time in Table 1. What is the value of Vd? What initial dose must be injected to achieve 5 mg% in the blood? At what rate must the infusion be given to maintain this level?
Answer: Vd = 14 liters; Loading dose = 700 mg; Infusion rate = 70 mg/hr

(c) Draw a compartmental scheme representing the fate of the drug following the 800-mg I.V. Fill in the amounts of drug in each of the four compartments at 2 hr.
Answer: Assuming blood volume is 3.5 liters: B = 175 mg, T = 525 mg, Urine = 50 mg, Metab. = 50 mg.

Practice Problem 2

Assume the therapeutic blood level of sulfaethylthiadiazole (SETD) is 12 mg% as total sulfa. The drug is eliminated by urinary excretion and metabolism. The biological half-life ($t_{1/2}$) is 6 hr. A single 2.0-g dose is required to reach the therapeutic blood level in a 70-kg man. The amount excreted in the urine is 180 mg when the blood has reached 12 mg%. The drug is 100% absorbed, an 90% remains in the body when the desired level is achieved.

(a) What is the first-order rate constant for total elimination (β_{elim})?
Answer: 0.116 hr^{-1}

(b) What is the rate constant for excretion (β_e) and for metabolism (β_m)?
Answer: $\beta_e = 0.104\ hr^{-1}$; $\beta_m = 0.012\ hr^{-1}$

(c) What is the "apparent volume of distribution" if equilibrium has been achieved when the 2-g dose is used to achieve the desired blood level?
Answer: Vd = 15 liters

(d) Draw a compartmental scheme showing the *amount* in each compartment when the blood level is 12 mg%. Label each specific rate constant with the value.
Answer: Assuming that V_p = 3.5 liters: B = 420 mg; T = 1.38 g; Urine = 180 mg; Metab. = 20 mg; $\beta_e = 0.104\ hr^{-1}$; $\beta_m = 0.012\ hr^{-1}$

Practice Problem 3 (courtesy of Dr. Harold Boxenbaum)

(a) A patient has been maintained adequately on p.o. digoxin having a serum concentration of 1 ng/ml. A change in disease state necessitates raising the serum concentration to 1.5 ng/ml.

If the maintenance dose has been 0.25 mg/day, recommend a new maintenance dose.
Answer: 0.375 mg

(b) A patient on maintenance therapy (0.25 mg of digoxin p.o. per day) had a plasma level of 0.5 ng/ml. Upon being hospitalized, I.M. injections were begun (0.25 mg of digoxin I.M. per day) and after 10 days the plasma level was 0.75 ng/ml. On discharge it was decided to maintain a level of 0.75 mg but by p.o. therapy. Recommend an appropriate p.o. dose.
Answer: 0.375 mg

(c) A dose of 300 mg of aminophylline p.o. q 6h is generally considered to be an appropriate dose for an average patient with a half-life of 5 hr. Recommend a dose for a patient having a half-life of 9 hr.
Answer: 167 mg every 6 hr.

Practice Problem 4

A drug was administered to a 70-kg patient by an I.V. injection of 150 mg. All of the patient's urine was collected by catheterization over a period of 30 hr. The urine samples were assayed for drug content. The resulting data are found in Table 2.

Table 2

Intact Drug Appearing in the Urine as a Function of Time Following I.V. Injection of 150 mg

T (hr)	Cumulative Amt. of Drug in Urine (mg)	(continued) t	mg
0	0	12	91
1	18	14	94
2	33	16	96
3	45	18	97
4	55	20	98
5	64	24	100
6	70	30	100
8	80	36	100
10	87		

(a) What is the value of the elimination rate constant?
Answer: $\beta = 0.202\ \text{hr}^{-1}$

(b) What is the value of the rate constant for metabolism?
Answer: $\beta_m = 0.067\ \text{hr}^{-1}$

(c) What is the apparent volume of distribution of the drug if the plasma level at 8 hr is 0.06 mg% and equilibrium has already been achieved?
Answer: Vd = 50 liters

(d) It is desired to construct a sustained-release tablet of the drug in question of the type which has an immediately available dose in the outer shell and a sustained-release erosion core in the center. The *minimum effective concentration* of the drug is 0.06 mg%. How much drug must be placed into the core to make the tablet last for 8 hr?
Answer: 48.5 mg.

(e) Suppose that this patient had liver dysfunction and was unable to metabolize the drug. What would be the resultant blood level pattern following administration of the *whole* tablet and *why*?
Answer: 0.09 mg%, since β would now equal β_e

(f) It is desired to prepare a venous infusion of 1 pint (480 ml) of this drug to be infused over a 12-hr period. How much drug must be dissolved in a pint of "water for injection" to maintain a 0.06 mg% blood level, and what volume must be injected per hour?
Answer: For the normal patient: 72.7 mg/pint, 40 ml/hr

(g) Calculate the rate constants and the *amounts* (in mg, *not* mg%) which would be in each compartment following 10 hr of infusion.
Answer:

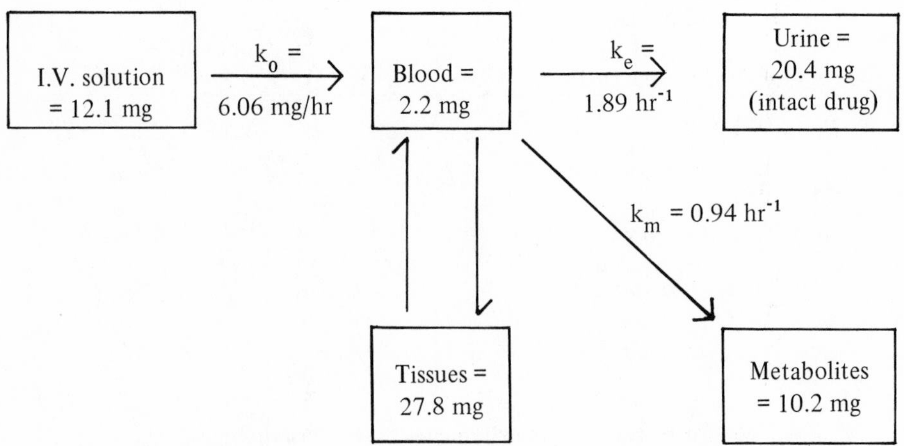

Practice Problem 5

B. M. Orme and R. E. Cutler reported (*Clin. Pharmacol. and Therap.*, *10*, 543, 1969) that kanamycin is not protein-bound to any significant extent and that it is primarily excreted unaltered by the kidney. Shortly after intramuscular injection, the blood concentration of kanamycin was said to achieve equilibrium with the concentration in other fluids. It was stated that kanamycin lost prior to equilibrium was not clinically significant and probably less than 10% of that injected. The data in Table 3 have been taken from Fig. 4 in that reference.

Table 3

Decrease in Serum Kanamycin Concentration After a Single Intramuscular Injection (7 mg/kg) in Patient B.M. (Body Wt. 50.0 g)

Time (hr)	Serum Kanamycin (mg%)
1.0	0.96
2.0	0.62
3.0	0.40
4.0	0.26
5.0	0.17

(a) Calculate the apparent volume of distribution (in % body wt.) for kanamycin in patient B.M.
Answer: 47% v/wt.

(b) What is the value of β and $t_{1/2}$ for kanamycin in B.M.?
Answer: Estimate from a first-order plot is $\beta = 0.44\ hr^{-1}$, $t_{1/2}$ = 1.6 hr.

(c) Orme and Cutler determined the Vd in 18 patients by infusing for 3 hr and measuring the serum levels obtained. Then the infusion was stopped and all urine collected for 48 hr (or until serum levels were no longer measurable). The volume of distribution was then calculated from

$$Vd = \frac{\text{Amount excreted}}{\text{Serum concentration}}$$

Using this method, the Vd averaged 20% of the body weight and the range for all patients was 9-35%. It was also found that $t_{1/2}$ varied with kidney function and had a range of 1.5-43 hr.

In part (a) you calculated the Vd following a single shot of kanamycin. You should have obtained a value of 47% v/wt. State two possible reasons why this value is larger than the range reported by Orme and Cutler.

(d) Which value would be appropriate to calculate an intramuscular dose and why? Which would you use for an intravenous dose?

Practice Problem 6

For each entry in the following table choose the most likely model: (a) one-compartment, (b) two-compartment, or (c) insufficient data.

	k_1	k_{12}	k_{21}	k_2	β	Vd[a]	T′/P′[b]
1	–	10	5	8	–	–	–
2	–	20	10	1	–	–	–
3	–	20	5	–	–	25%	–
4	3	5	2	5	–	–	–
5	–	10	5	–	–	–	3.0
6	–	10	5	–	–	–	2.0
7	–	4	1	1	–	–	–
8	–	6	4	4	1.0	–	–
9	–	6	4	1	0.4	–	–

[a] Vd = % v/wt.
[b] T′/P′ ratio of amounts postdistribution.

Answer: These are to be answered assuming a one-compartment model will achieve equilibrium where $K = k_{12}/k_{21} = T'/P'$.

Practice Problem 7 (Courtesy of Dr. Harold Boxenbaum)

(a) For a given patient, digitoxin has a half-life of 5.75 days and a Vd of 57,000 ml. What fraction of digitoxin body stores are eliminated each day?
Answer: $(1-f) = 0.113$

(b) If a physician initially digitalized this patient I.V. with 1.2 mg of digitoxin and wished to maintain similar body glycoside stores, what should the daily oral maintenance dose be? Assume that F = 1 for this estimate.
Answer: $(1.2)(0.113) = 0.136$ mg

(c) What is P_{max}, P_{min}, and $\overline{P}$ of digitoxin for this patient receiving 0.1 mg of oral digitoxin daily. Assume that F = 1..
Answer: P_{max} = 15.5 ng/ml, P_{min} = 13.7 ng/ml, and $\overline{P}$ = 14.5 ng/ml

(d) A physician wishes to digitalize a patient rapidly with I.V. digitoxin so as to achieve a plasma level corresponding to 70% of P_{max} when the daily oral dose is 0.1 mg. What should be the loading dose?
Answer: 0.615 mg

(e) What is the average equilibrium plasma level of digoxin when 0.5 mg is administered p.o. each day? Assume that 55% of the

dose is absorbed and use the pharmacokinetic parameters: Vd = 175 liters, $t_{1/2}$ = 1.6 days.
Answer: 1.33 ng/ml

(f) What would be the appropriate loading dose of digitoxin compatible with a maintenance dose of 0.1 mg/day p.o.?
Answer: 0.885 mg

(g) A patient had been stabilized on 0.1 mg of digitoxin p.o. per day but developed toxicity caused by a change in disease state. The patient was taken off digitoxin and demonstrated a desirable response 3 days later. Recommend a new maintenance dose to be started on the fourth day. Assume that F = 1.
Answer: After the first day 0.885 mg decreases to 0.785 mg. After the second day 0.785 mg decreases to 0.696 mg. After the third day 0.696 mg decreases to 0.617 mg. We want to replace digitoxin lost from the body during the third day.

0.696 - 0.617 = 0.08 mg (New maintenance dose)

Practice Problem 8

The data in Table 4 have been taken from J. G. Wagner, *Can. J. Pharm. Sci., 1*, 55 (1966).

Table 4

Blood Level Data Following Lincomycin Oral Administration of a 0.5-g Capsule in Eight Normal Adults. Treatment Over a 4-week Period Using a Latin Square Design

	Average Serum Concentration (mg%)	
Time (hr)	Lincomycin Given Alone	Lincomycin Given with Kaopectate
0.0	0.000	0.000
1.5	0.200	0.034
3.0	0.310	0.033
4.5	0.346	0.026
6.0	0.272	0.024
8.0	0.205	0.010
10.0	0.150	0.002
12.0	0.110	0.010

(a) What estimate of the $t_{1/2}$ for lincomycin is obtained from this data?
Answer: $t_{1/2}$ = 4.7 hr (oral estimates are unreliable)

(b) What is the relative percent absorption of lincomycin in the

presence of kaopectate during the first 12 hr.
Answer: Relative area under curves indicates only 9% absorption with kaopectate relative to without it. However, lincomycin alone still shows high levels in 12 hr. The actual percent based on the total areas would be less.

Appendix A

FICK'S LAW

I. PASSIVE TRANSPORT ENERGETICS: FICK'S LAW

In the discussion of reversible first-order rate processes, we have considered a system where the rate of drug transfer is governed by Fick's first law, which states that the flux (the quantity of substance diffusing per unit time through a unit area) through a plane perpendicular to the direction of diffusion is directly proportional to the concentration gradient.

In the case of a biological barrier, such as that illustrated in Fig. 1 (p. 7), the concentration gradient between the compartments is assumed to be due to the barrier itself. That is, we are defining the system such that the diffusion within a compartment is not rate-determining but that passage through the membrane itself is the slowest diffusion process. For the case represented by Figs. 1 and 2, the mass transport from compartment A to B through the rate-controlling barrier is described by

$$\frac{-da}{dt} = D'A\,\frac{dC}{dX} \tag{1a}$$

where $-da/dt$ equals the decrease in mass in the A compartment as a function of time, D' is the diffusion constant of the drug in the barrier, A is the area of the membrane, and dC/dX is the change in concentration as a function of distance. For a given drug and membrane the following may be stated: The diffusion constant, D', will be a constant; the area will remain constant; the thickness of the barrier (dX is sometimes referred to as h in the barrier case) is constant, and dC is the concentration gradient $(A_t - B_t)$ or the difference in concentration between the two compartments. The membrane-drug parameters, $D'A/h$, may be set equal to a constant, k, and Eq. (1a) may then be written as a rate process

$$\frac{-da}{dt} = k(A_t - B_t) \tag{2a}$$

In the case of equivalent compartments, the volume of A (V_A) equals the volume of B (V_B), so that $V_A = V_B = V$. The right side of Eq. (2a) may now be expressed in terms of mass:

$$\frac{-da}{dt} = k\left(\frac{a_t}{V} - \frac{b_t}{V}\right) \tag{3a}$$

where a_t and b_t represent the mass of drug in compartments A and B, respectively. Letting $k/V = k'$,

$$\frac{-da}{dt} = k'(a_t - b_t) \tag{4a}$$

Since $b_t = a_0 - a_t$, substitution gives

$$\frac{da_t}{2a_t - a_0} = -k'\,dt \tag{5a}$$

which integrates directly to

$$\ln(2a_t - a_0) = -2k't + \ln a_0 \tag{6a}$$

between the limits of a_0 and a_t and t = 0 and t. Now, $a_\infty = b_\infty = (\frac{1}{2})a_0$, so Eq. (6a) may be expressed as

$$\ln(a_t - a_\infty) = -2k't + \ln a_\infty \tag{7a}$$

Equation (7a) has been derived from Fick's law, while Eq. (15) (p. 14) has been used to demonstrate the fact that a first-order plot will allow the calculation of the pseudo-first-order rate constants, k_1, which is the sum of k_f and k_r. Since both equations refer to the same system, the relationship between k' and $(k_f + k_r)$ will now be examined.

II. RELATIONSHIP OF FICK'S LAW TO A ⇌ B REVERSIBLE FIRST-ORDER KINETICS

Equation (15) (p. 14) may be written in terms of mass as:

$$\ln\left(\frac{a_t}{V} - \frac{a_\infty}{V}\right) = -(k_f + k_r)t + \ln \frac{a_\infty}{V}$$

This reduces to

$$\ln(a_t - a_\infty) = -(k_f + k_r)t + \ln a_\infty \tag{8a}$$

which has the same form as Eq. (7a). We may therefore conclude that $2k' = k_f + k_r$. Since, in the present case where $A_\infty = B_\infty$ and $a_\infty = b_\infty$, $k_f = k_r$, then $k' = k_f = k_r$ and $k = k'V$ so that the rate constant, k, associated with the mass transport Eq. (3a) is related to the first-order constants by the expression

$$k = k_f V = k_r V = \frac{k_1 V}{2} \tag{9a}$$

This applies only to the simplest case where the compartments are identical and, therefore, the microconstants are equal. When, for example, V_A is not equal to V_B, the Fick's law equation may be written

$$\frac{-da_t}{dt} = k\left(\frac{a_t}{V_A} - \frac{b_t}{V_B}\right) \tag{10a}$$

$$\frac{-da_t}{dt} = k_1 a_t - k_2 b_t$$

This may be integrated to yield

$$\ln(a_t - a_\infty) = -(k_1 + k_2)t + \ln(a_0 - a_\infty) \tag{11a}$$

Equation (14) (p. 13) written in terms of mass is

$$\ln(a_t - a_\infty) = -(k_f + k_r)t + \ln(a_0 - a_\infty) \tag{12a}$$

which is comparable to Equation (11a), allowing us to conclude that in this case $k_1 + k_2 = k_f + k_r$.

It is important to realize that only the concentration gradient between transferable species is described by Fick's law. The derivatives to compare the Fick's law expressions to the kinetic equations when $A_\infty \neq B_\infty$ are considerably more complex and will not be covered.

Appendix B

Vd

1. Volume of Distribution in the One-compartment Open Model

a. Vd_1 Independent of Elimination. Equation (10) in Chap. 3 states that

$$Vd = \frac{D_t}{P_t} \tag{13a}$$

where D_t may be written as the sum of drug in the central compartment, P′, and drug in other tissues, T′, so that

$$Vd = \frac{P' + T'}{P_t} \tag{14a}$$

This can be written

$$Vd = \frac{P'(1 + T'/P')}{P_t} \tag{15a}$$

For a one-compartment model, $T'/P' \rightarrow k_{12}/k_{21}$, so Vd becomes

$$Vd = \frac{P'(1 + k_{12}/k_{21})}{P_t} \tag{16a}$$

Since

$$V_p = \frac{P'}{P} \tag{17a}$$

where V_p is the volume of the central compartment,

$$Vd_1 = V_p\left(1 + \frac{k_{12}}{k_{21}}\right) \tag{18a}$$

which corresponds to Eq. (13) in Chap. 3.

The analogous expression for a two-compartment model is given by Eq. (40a), which, in contrast to (18a), is dependent upon elimination.

b. Volume of Distribution by Extrapolation. We know that Eq. (29). Chap. 2, $P = Be^{-\beta t}$, describes the concentration of drug in blood over virtually the entire time the drug is in the body if a one-compartment model applies. At time zero,

$$P = B \tag{19a}$$

so Eq. (10) in Chap. 3 becomes

$$Vd_1 = \frac{D_0}{B} \tag{20a}$$

which is Eq. (11), Chap. 3.

c. Volume of Distribution by Area. The area under the plasma concentration curve is found by integrating Eq. 29 (Chap. 2), from t = 0 to t = ∞.

$$\text{Area} = \int_0^\infty P\,dt = \int_0^\infty Be^{-\beta t}\,dt \tag{21a}$$

$$\text{Area} = \frac{B}{\beta} e^{-\beta t} \Big|_0^\infty \tag{22a}$$

$$\text{Area} = \frac{B}{\beta} \tag{23a}$$

Substituting into Eq. (20a),

$$Vd_1 = \frac{D_0}{(\text{Area})\beta} \tag{24a}$$

which is Eq. 12, Chap. 3.

2. Volume of Distribution in the Two-compartment Open Model

a. Volume of Distribution by Extrapolation. The plasma concentration of drug in a two-compartment model is given by

$$P = \frac{D_0(k_{21} - \alpha)e^{-\alpha t}}{Vp(\beta - \alpha)} + \frac{D_0(k_{21} - \beta)e^{-\beta t}}{Vp(\alpha - \beta)} \tag{25a}$$

After the distribution phase is complete, the first term approaches zero, and extrapolation of the second phase back to zero time yields

$$P = B = \frac{D_0(k_{21} - \beta)}{Vp(\alpha - \beta)} \tag{26a}$$

Substituting into Eq. (20a),

$$Vd_2 = \frac{Vp(\alpha - \beta)}{(k_{21} - \beta)} \tag{27a}$$

By means of Eqs. (21) and (22) (p. 22) we can show that

$$\alpha - \beta = \sqrt{C_1^2 - 4C_2} \tag{28a}$$

and

$$k_{21} - \beta = \tfrac{1}{2}(k_{21} - k_{12} - k_2 + \sqrt{C_1^2 - 4C_2}) \tag{29a}$$

Therefore

$$Vd_2 = \frac{Vp\sqrt{C_1^2 - 4C_2}}{\tfrac{1}{2}(k_{21} - k_{12} - k_2 + \sqrt{C_1^2 - 4C_2})} \tag{30a}$$

b. Volume of Distribution by Area. It can be shown that the area under the plasma concentration-vs-time curve for a two-compartment model following intravenous injection is given by

$$\text{Area} = \frac{P_0}{k_2} \tag{31a}$$

Substituting into Eq. (24a),

$$Vd_2 = \frac{D_0 k_2}{P_0 \beta} \tag{32a}$$

$$Vd_2 = \frac{Vpk_2}{\beta} \tag{33a}$$

Nagashima, Levy, and O'Reilly (Chap. 3, Ref. 27) have shown that k_2 is related to β by the fraction of the total drug which is in the central compartment, or

$$\beta = \frac{k_2(P')}{T' + P'} \tag{34a}$$

Substituting into Eq. (33a),

$$Vd_2 = \frac{Vp(T' + P')}{(P')} \tag{35a}$$

or

$$Vd_2 = Vp(1 + \frac{T'}{P'}) \tag{36a}$$

The ratio T'/P' can be obtained using the following equations

$$P' = \frac{D_0}{(\alpha - \beta)} [(k_{21} - \beta)e^{-\beta t} - (k_{21} - \alpha)e^{-\alpha t}] \tag{37a}$$

and

$$T' = \frac{k_{12} D_0}{(\alpha - \beta)} (e^{-\beta t} - e^{-\alpha t}) \tag{38a}$$

As $t \to \infty$, $e^{-\alpha t} \to 0$, and T'/P' in the β phase approaches the ratio

$$\frac{T'}{P'} = \frac{k_{12}}{k_{21} - \beta} \tag{39a}$$

Substituting this into Eq. (36a), we obtain

$$Vd_2 = Vp[1 + \left(\frac{k_{12}}{k_{21} - \beta}\right)] \tag{40a}$$

This equation may also be derived by the method used for Eq. (18a).

c. *Volume of Distribution by Infusion.* When the concentration of drug in the plasma has reached a constant value during a zero-order infusion,

$$\frac{dP'}{dt} = 0 = k_0 + k_{21}T' - k_{12}P' - k_2P' \tag{41a}$$

At any time during an infusion, the plasma concentration given by (Chap. 3, Ref. 8)

$$P = \frac{k_0}{Vpk_2}\left[1 + \frac{(k_2 - \beta)e^{-\alpha t}}{(\beta - \alpha)} - \frac{(k_2 - \alpha)e^{-\beta t}}{(\beta - \alpha)}\right] \tag{42a}$$

When a constant plasma concentration has been established; that is, at infinite time, this reduces to

$$P = \frac{k_0}{Vp\,k_2} \tag{43a}$$

or

$$k_0 = k_2P' \tag{44a}$$

Substituting Eq. (44a) into Eq. (41a),

$$\frac{T'}{P'} = \frac{k_{12}}{k_{21}} \tag{45a}$$

Equation (10) in Chap. 3 can be rewritten as

$$Vd = \frac{P' + T'}{P} \tag{46a}$$

Substituting from Eq. (45a),

$$Vd_{inf} = \frac{P'(k_{21} + k_{12})}{k_{21}P} \tag{47a}$$

or

$$Vd_{inf} = Vp \frac{(k_{21} + k_{12})}{k_{21}} \quad V_p \left[1 + \frac{k_{12}}{k_{21}}\right] \tag{48a}$$

This is the same as Eq. (13) in Chap. 3, and also identical to Vd_{ss} as defined by Riggs (Chap. 3, Ref. 8). Notice that even in a two-compartment model, T′/P′ equals the equilibrium ratio k_{12}/k_{21} after infusion has continued long enough for the plasma level to become constant.

Appendix C

AREA UNDER I.V. CURVES

1. One-compartment Open Model

According to Eq. (29) in Chap. 2,

$$P = Be^{-\beta t} \qquad (49a)$$

describes the plasma time course following a rapid I.V. injection of a drug distributed according to a one-compartment model. The area under a plot of P as a function of t would be

$$\int_0^\infty P = B \int_0^\infty e^{-\beta t} \qquad (50a)$$

which, upon integration yields

$$\text{Area} = B \left(\frac{e^{-\beta \infty}}{-\beta} - \frac{e^{-\beta 0}}{-\beta} \right)$$

Thus the area under a blood level curve following a rapid I.V. injection of a one-compartment drug can be calculated from the simple expression

$$\text{Area} = \frac{B}{\beta} \qquad (51a)$$

The area of such a curve from any time t to time ∞ may be calculated from

$$\text{Area} = \frac{P_t}{\beta} \qquad (52a)$$

where P_t is the blood concentration at time t.

2. Two-compartment Open Model

Equation (20) in Chap. 2 describes the time course for a rapid I.V. injection of a two-compartment model drug.

$$P = Ae^{-\alpha t} + Be^{-\beta t} \qquad (53a)$$

Since it is the sum of two exponentials, thy area equation may be derived as shown above with the results

$$\text{Area} = \frac{A}{\alpha} + \frac{B}{\beta} \qquad (54a)$$

Appendix D

MULTIPLE-DOSE EQUATIONS FOR THE ONE-COMPARTMENT MODEL

In Chap. 4, Sec. A on dosage regimens, several equations were presented without a formal derivation or explanation of how they were obtained. The following will give the interested student more insight into the nature of the equations and the system they describe.

The first-order equation for loss of drug from the body following a single rapid I.V. injection for a drug described by a one-compartment model is

$$D = D_0 e^{-\beta t} \tag{55a}$$

where D is the total amount of drug remaining in the body, D_0 is the dose, and t is the time elapsed after the administration of a dose. For the first dosage interval the maximum amount of drug in the body will be equal to the dose, D_0. The minimum amount will be equal to the amount remaining in the body when t = τ. Thus from Eq. (55a),

$$D^1_{min} = D_0 e^{-\beta\tau} \tag{56a}$$

where τ is the dosing interval. The value of D^1_{min} is the amount of drug which has accumulated in the body before the administration of the second dose. When the second I.V. injection is given, the time course of the drug in the body is described by

$$D^2 = (D_0 + D^1_{min})e^{-\beta t} \tag{57a}$$

or

$$D^2 = (D_0 + D_0 e^{-\beta\tau})e^{-\beta t} \tag{58a}$$

The maximum amount of drug in the body during the second dosage interval will be that amount present when t = 0 and thus

$$D^2_{max} = D_0 + D_0 e^{-\beta\tau} = D_0 + D^1_{min} \tag{59a}$$

The minimum during the second interval will occur when t = τ as before, yielding

$$D^2_{min} = D_0 e^{-\beta\tau} + D_0 e^{-2\beta\tau} \tag{60a}$$

When a third dose is administered, the amount of drug in the body as a function of time will be given by

$$D^3 = (D_0 + D_0 e^{-\beta\tau} + D_0 e^{-2\beta\tau})e^{-\beta t} \tag{61a}$$

or

$$D^3 = (D_0 + D^2_{min})e^{-\beta t} \tag{62a}$$

Using the same reasoning as was used previously, it can be shown that

$$D^3_{max} = (D_0 + D_0 e^{-\beta\tau} + D_0 e^{-2\beta\tau}) = D_0 + D^2_{min} \tag{63a}$$

and

$$D^3_{min} = (D_0 e^{-\beta\tau} + D_0 e^{-2\beta\tau} + D_0 e^{-3\beta\tau}) \tag{64a}$$

It should be apparent by now that the amount of drug in the body after n doses will be described by the equations

$$D^n = (D_0 + D^{n-1}_{min})e^{-\beta t} \tag{65a}$$

$$D^n_{max} = D_0 + D^{n-1}_{min} \tag{66a}$$

$$D^n_{min} = D_0 e^{-\beta\tau} + D_0 e^{-2\beta\tau} + \cdots + D_0 e^{-n\beta\tau} \tag{67a}$$

Expanding Eq. (65a) gives

$$D^n = D_0(1 + e^{-\beta\tau} + e^{-2\beta\tau} + \cdots + e^{-(n-1)\beta\tau})e^{-\beta t} \tag{68a}$$

If we let the sum inside the parentheses equal a, then

$$ae^{-\beta\tau} = e^{-\beta\tau} + e^{-2\beta\tau} + \cdots + e^{-n\beta\tau} \tag{69a}$$

Subtracting Eq. (69a) from the equation for "a" gives

$$a - ae^{-\beta\tau} = a(1 - e^{-\beta\tau}) = 1 - e^{-n\beta\tau} \tag{70a}$$

Thus

$$a = \frac{1 - e^{-n\beta\tau}}{1 - e^{-\beta\tau}} \tag{71a}$$

Therefore

$$D^n = D_0\left(\frac{1 - e^{-n\beta\tau}}{1 - e^{-\beta\tau}}\right)e^{-\beta t} \tag{72a}$$

Using similar arguments, Eqs. (65a) and (67a) may be rewritten

$$D^n_{max} = D_0\left(\frac{1 - e^{-n\beta\tau}}{1 - e^{-\beta\tau}}\right) \tag{73a}$$

$$D^n_{min} = D_0\left(\frac{1 - e^{-n\beta\tau}}{1 - e^{-\beta\tau}}\right)e^{-\beta\tau} \tag{74a}$$

Now the steady state will be reached when a sufficiently large number of doses have been given (i.e. as $n \rightarrow \infty$). Thus at the *steady state*,

$$D = \left(\frac{D_0}{1 - e^{-\beta\tau}} \right) e^{-\beta t} \qquad (75a)$$

$$D_{max} = \frac{D_0}{1 - e^{-\beta\tau}} \qquad (76a)$$

$$D_{min} = \frac{D_0 e^{-\beta\tau}}{1 - e^{-\beta\tau}} \qquad (77a)$$

Recalling that we defined τ in terms of f as follows,

$$\tau = \frac{\ln(f)}{-\beta} \qquad (78a)$$

Then

$$f = e^{-\beta\tau} \qquad (79a)$$

Thus Eqs. (76a) and (77a) may be written

$$D_{max} = \frac{D_0}{1 - f} \qquad (80a)$$

$$D_{min} = \frac{fD_0}{1 - f} = D_{max} - D_0 \qquad (81a)$$

Author Index

Numbers in brackets are reference numbers and indicate that an author's work is referred to although his name is not cited in the text. Underlined numbers give the page on which the complete reference is listed.

A

B

C

D

Y

Z

Subject Index

B

C

D

E

P

R

T

U

V

W

NATURAL LOG TABLES

Natural Logarithms* 0.000—0.999

x	0.000	0.001	0.002	0.003	0.004	0.005	0.006	0.007	0.008	0.009
0.000	−∞	−6.90776	−6.21461	−5.80914	−5.52146	−5.29832	−5.11600	−4.96185	−4.82831	−4.71053
010	−4.60517	−4.50986	−4.42285	−4.34281	−4.26870	−4.19971	−4.13517	−4.07454	−4.01738	−3.96332
020	−3.91202	−3.86323	−3.81671	−3.77226	−3.72970	−3.68888	−3.64966	−3.61192	−3.57555	54046
030	50656	47377	44202	41125	38139	35241	32424	29684	27017	24419
040	21888	19418	17009	14656	12357	10109	07911	05761	03655	01593
0.050	−2.99573	−2.97593	−2.95651	−2.93746	−2.91877	−2.90042	−2.88240	−2.86470	−2.84731	−2.83022
060	81341	79688	78062	76462	74887	73337	71810	70306	68825	67365
070	65926	64508	63109	61730	60369	59027	57702	56395	55105	53831
080	52573	51331	50104	48891	47694	46510	45341	44185	43042	41912
090	40795	39690	38597	37516	36446	35388	34341	33304	32279	31264
0.100	−2.30259	−2.29263	−2.28278	−2.27303	−2.26336	−2.25379	−2.24432	−2.23493	−2.22562	−2.21641
110	20727	19823	18926	18037	17156	16282	15417	14558	13707	12863
120	12026	11196	10373	09557	08747	07944	07147	06357	05573	04794
130	04022	03256	02495	01741	00992	00248	−1.99510	−1.98777	−1.98050	−1.97328
140	−1.96611	−1.95900	−1.95193	−1.94491	−1.93794	−1.93102	92415	91732	91054	90381
0.150	−1.89712	−1.89048	−1.88387	−1.87732	−1.87080	−1.86433	−1.85790	−1.85151	−1.84516	−1.83885
160	83258	82635	82016	81401	80789	80181	79577	78976	78379	77786
170	77196	76609	76026	75446	74870	74297	73727	73161	72597	72037
180	71480	70926	70375	69827	69282	68740	68201	67665	67131	66601
190	66073	65548	65026	64507	63990	63476	62964	62455	61949	61445
0.200	−1.60944	−1.60445	−1.59949	−1.59455	−1.58964	−1.58475	−1.57988	−1.57504	−1.57022	−1.56542
210	56065	55590	55117	54646	54178	53712	53248	52786	52326	51868
220	51413	50959	50508	50058	49611	49165	48722	48281	47841	47403
230	46968	46534	46102	45672	45243	44817	44392	43970	43548	43129
240	42712	42296	41882	41469	41059	40650	40242	39837	39433	39030
0.250	−1.38629	−1.38230	−1.37833	−1.37437	−1.37042	−1.36649	−1.36258	−1.35868	−1.35480	−1.35093
260	34707	34323	33941	33560	33181	32803	32426	32051	31677	31304
270	30933	30564	30195	29828	29463	29098	28735	28374	28013	27654
280	27297	26940	26585	26231	25878	25527	25176	24827	24479	24133
290	23787	23443	23100	22758	22418	22078	21740	21402	21066	20731
0.300	−1.20397	−1.20065	−1.19733	−1.19402	−1.19073	−1.18744	−1.18417	−1.18091	−1.17766	−1.17441
310	17118	16796	16475	16155	15836	15518	15201	14885	14570	14256
320	13943	13631	13320	13010	12701	12393	12086	11780	11474	11170
330	10866	10564	10262	09961	09661	09362	09064	08767	08471	08176
340	07881	07587	07294	07002	06711	06421	06132	05843	05555	05268
0.350	−1.04982	−1.04697	−1.04412	−1.04129	−1.03846	−1.03564	−1.03282	−1.03002	−1.02722	−1.02443
360	02165	01888	01611	01335	01060	00786	00512	00239	−0.99967	−0.99696
370	−0.99425	−0.99155	−0.98886	−0.98618	−0.98350	−0.98083	−0.97817	−0.97551	97286	97022
380	96758	96496	96233	95972	95711	95451	95192	94933	94675	94418
390	94161	93905	93649	93395	93140	92887	92634	92382	92130	91879
0.400	−0.91629	−0.91379	−0.91130	−0.90882	−0.90634	−0.90387	−0.90140	−0.89894	−0.89649	−0.89404
410	89160	88916	88673	88431	88189	87948	87707	87467	87227	86988
420	86750	86512	86275	86038	85802	85567	85332	85097	84863	84630
430	84397	84165	83933	83702	83471	83241	83011	82782	82554	82326
440	82098	81871	81645	81419	81193	80968	80744	80520	80296	80073
0.450	−0.79851	−0.79629	−0.79407	−0.79186	−0.78966	−0.78746	−0.78526	−0.78307	−0.78089	−0.77871
460	77653	77436	77219	77003	76787	76572	76357	76143	75929	75715
470	75502	75290	75078	74866	74655	74444	74234	74024	73814	73605
480	73397	73189	72981	72774	72567	72361	72155	71949	71744	71539
490	71335	71131	70928	70725	70522	70320	70118	69917	69716	69515

0.500	−0.69315	−0.69115	−0.68916	−0.68717	−0.68518	−0.68320	−0.68122	−0.67924	−0.67727	−0.67531
510	67334	67139	66943	66748	66553	66359	66165	65971	65778	65585
520	65393	65201	65009	64817	64626	64436	64245	64055	63866	63677
530	63488	63299	63111	62923	62736	62549	62362	62176	61990	61804
540	61619	61434	61249	61065	60881	60697	60514	60331	60148	59966
0.550	−0.59784	−0.59602	−0.59421	−0.59240	−0.59059	−0.58879	−0.58699	−0.58519	−0.58340	−0.58161
560	57982	57803	57625	57448	57270	57093	56916	56740	56563	56387
570	56212	56037	55862	55687	55513	55339	55165	54991	54818	54645
580	54473	54300	54128	53957	53785	53614	53444	53273	53103	52933
590	52763	52594	52425	52256	52088	51919	51751	51584	51416	51249
0.600	−0.51083	−0.50916	−0.50750	−0.50584	−0.50418	−0.50253	−0.50088	−0.49923	−0.49758	−0.49594
610	49430	49266	49102	48939	48776	48613	48451	48289	48127	47965
620	47804	47642	47482	47321	47160	47000	46840	46681	46522	46362
630	46204	46045	45887	45728	45571	45413	45256	45099	44942	44785
640	44629	44473	44317	44161	44006	43850	43696	43541	43386	43232
0.650	−0.43078	−0.42925	−0.42771	−0.42618	−0.42465	−0.42312	−0.42159	−0.42007	−0.41855	−0.41703
660	41552	41400	41249	41098	40947	40797	40647	40497	40347	40197
670	40048	39899	39750	39601	39453	39304	39156	39008	38861	38713
680	38566	38419	38273	38126	37980	37834	37688	37542	37397	37251
690	37106	36962	36817	36673	36528	36384	36241	36097	35954	35810
0.700	−0.35667	−0.35525	−0.35382	−0.35240	−0.35098	−0.34956	−0.34814	−0.34672	−0.34531	−0.34390
710	34249	34108	33968	33827	33687	33547	33408	33268	33129	32989
720	32850	32712	32573	32435	32296	32158	32021	31883	31745	31608
730	31471	31334	31197	31061	30925	30788	30653	30517	30381	30246
740	30111	29975	29841	29706	29571	29437	29303	29169	29035	28902
0.750	−0.28768	−0.28635	−0.28502	−0.28369	−0.28236	−0.28104	−0.27971	−0.27839	−0.27707	−0.27575
760	27444	27312	27181	27050	26919	26788	26657	26527	26397	26266
770	26136	26007	25877	25748	25618	25489	25360	25231	25103	24974
780	24846	24718	24590	24462	24335	24207	24080	23953	23826	23699
790	23572	23446	23319	23193	23067	22941	22816	22690	22565	22439
0.800	−0.22314	−0.22189	−0.22065	−0.21940	−0.21816	−0.21691	−0.21567	−0.21443	−0.21319	−0.21196
810	21072	20949	20825	20702	20579	20457	20334	20212	20089	19967
820	19845	19723	19601	19480	19358	19237	19116	18995	18874	18754
830	18633	18513	18392	18272	18152	18032	17913	17793	17674	17554
840	17435	17316	17198	17079	16960	16842	16724	16605	16487	16370
0.850	−0.16252	−0.16134	−0.16017	−0.15900	−0.15782	−0.15665	−0.15548	−0.15432	−0.15315	−0.15199
860	15032	14966	14850	14734	14618	14503	14387	14272	14156	14041
870	13926	13811	13697	13582	13467	13353	13239	13125	13011	12897
880	12783	12670	12556	12443	12330	12217	12104	11991	11878	11766
890	11653	11541	11429	11317	11205	11093	10981	10870	10759	10647
0.900	−0.10536	−0.10425	−0.10314	−0.10203	−0.10093	−0.09982	−0.09872	−0.09761	−0.09651	−0.09541
910	09431	09321	09212	09102	08992	08883	08774	08665	08556	08447
920	08338	08230	08121	08013	07904	07796	07688	07580	07472	07365
930	07257	07150	07042	06935	06828	06721	06614	06507	06401	06294
940	06188	06081	05975	05869	05763	05657	05551	05446	05340	05235
0.950	−0.05129	−0.05024	−0.04919	−0.04814	−0.04709	−0.04604	−0.04500	−0.04395	−0.04291	−0.04186
960	04082	03978	03874	03770	03666	03563	03459	03356	03252	03149
970	03046	02943	02840	02737	02634	02532	02429	02327	02225	02122
980	02020	01918	01816	01715	01613	01511	01410	01309	01207	01106
990	01005	00904	00803	00702	00602	00501	00401	00300	00200	00100

* To find the natural logarithm ($\log_e$) of a number which is a power of ten less or greater than a number given in the table: if the number concerned is *less*, e.g., $^1/_{10}$ (10^{-1}), $^1/_{100}$ (10^{-2}), $^1/_{1000}$ (10^{-3}), etc., *subtract* from the given logarithm $\log_e 10$, $2 \log_e 10$, $3 \log_e 10$, etc.; if the number concerned is *greater*, e.g., 10 times (10^1), 100 times (10^2), 1000 times (10^3), etc., *add* to the given logarithm $\log_e 10$, $2 \log_e 10$, $3 \log_e 10$, etc. Examples: $\log_e 0.02 = \log_e 0.2 - \log_e 10$; $\log_e 2000 = \log_e 200 + \log_e 10$.

Natural Logarithms* 1.00—9.99

x	0.00	0.01	0.02	0.03	0.04	0.05	0.06	0.07	0.08	0.09
1.00	0.00000	0.00995	0.01980	0.02956	0.03922	0.04879	0.05827	0.06766	0.07696	0.08618
10	09531	10436	11333	12222	13103	13976	14842	15700	16551	17395
20	18232	19062	19885	20701	21511	22314	23111	23902	24686	25464
30	26236	27003	27763	28518	29267	30010	30748	31481	32208	32930
40	33647	34359	35066	35767	36464	37156	37844	38526	39204	39878
1.50	0.40547	0.41211	0.41871	0.42527	0.43178	0.43825	0.44469	0.45108	0.45742	0.46373
60	47000	47623	48243	48858	49470	50078	50682	51282	51879	52473
70	53063	53649	54232	54812	55389	55962	56531	57098	57661	58222
80	58779	59333	59884	60432	60977	61519	62058	62594	63127	63658
90	64185	64710	65233	65752	66269	66783	67294	67803	68310	68813
2.00	0.69315	0.69813	0.70310	0.70804	0.71295	0.71784	0.72271	0.72755	0.73237	0.73716
10	74194	74669	75142	75612	76081	76547	77011	77473	77932	78390
20	78846	79299	79751	80200	80648	81093	81536	81978	82418	82855
30	83291	83725	84157	84587	85015	85442	85866	86289	86710	87129
40	87547	87963	88377	88789	89200	89609	90016	90422	90826	91228
2.50	0.91629	0.92028	0.92426	0.92822	0.93216	0.93609	0.94001	0.94391	0.94779	0.95166
60	95551	95935	96317	96698	97078	97456	97833	98208	98582	98954
70	99325	99695	1.00063	1.00430	1.00796	1.01160	1.01523	1.01885	1.02245	1.02604
80	1.02962	1.03318	03674	04028	04380	04732	05082	05431	05779	06126
90	06471	06815	07158	07500	07841	08181	08519	08856	09192	09527
3.00	1.09861	1.10194	1.10526	1.10856	1.11186	1.11514	1.11841	1.12168	1.12493	1.12817
10	13140	13462	13783	14103	14422	14740	15057	15373	15688	16002
20	16315	16627	16938	17248	17557	17865	18173	18479	18784	19089
30	19392	19695	19996	20297	20597	20896	21194	21491	21788	22083
40	22378	22671	22964	23256	23547	23837	24127	24415	24703	24990
3.50	1.25276	1.25562	1.25846	1.26130	1.26413	1.26695	1.26976	1.27257	1.27536	1.27815
60	28093	28371	28647	28923	29198	29473	29746	30019	30291	30563
70	30833	31103	31372	31641	31909	32176	32442	32708	32972	33237
80	33500	33763	34025	34286	34547	34807	35067	35325	35584	35841
90	36098	36354	36609	36864	37118	37372	37624	37877	38128	38379
4.00	1.38629	1.38879	1.39128	1.39377	1.39624	1.39872	1.40118	1.40364	1.40610	1.40854
10	41099	41342	41585	41828	42070	42311	42552	42792	43031	43270
20	43508	43746	43984	44220	44456	44692	44927	45161	45395	45629
30	45862	46094	46326	46557	46787	47018	47247	47476	47705	47933
40	48160	48387	48614	48840	49065	49290	49515	49739	49962	50185
4.50	1.50408	1.50630	1.50851	1.51072	1.51293	1.51513	1.51732	1.51951	1.52170	1.52388
60	52606	52823	53039	53256	53471	53687	53902	54116	54330	54543
70	54756	54969	55181	55393	55604	55814	56025	56235	56444	56653
80	56862	57070	57277	57485	57691	57898	58104	58309	58515	58719
90	58924	59127	59331	59534	59737	59939	60141	60342	60543	60744
5.00	1.60944	1.61144	1.61343	1.61542	1.61741	1.61939	1.62137	1.62334	1.62531	1.62728
10	62924	63120	63315	63511	63705	63900	64094	64287	64481	64673
20	64866	65058	65250	65441	65632	65823	66013	66203	66393	66582
30	66771	66959	67147	67335	67523	67710	67896	68083	68269	68455
40	68640	68825	69010	69194	69378	69562	69745	69928	70111	70293

5.50	1.70475	1.70656	1.70838	1.71019	1.71199	1.71380	1.71560	1.71740	1.71919	1.72098
60	72277	72455	72633	72811	72988	73166	73342	73519	73695	73871
70	74047	74222	74397	74572	74746	74920	75094	75267	75440	75613
80	75786	75958	76130	76302	76473	76644	76815	76985	77156	77326
90	77495	77665	77834	78002	78171	78339	78507	78675	78842	79009
6.00	1.79176	1.79342	1.79509	1.79675	1.79840	1.80006	1.80171	1.80336	1.80500	1.80665
10	80829	80993	81156	81319	81482	81645	81808	81970	82132	82294
20	82455	82616	82777	82938	83098	83258	83418	83578	83737	83896
30	84055	84214	84372	84530	84688	84845	85003	85160	85317	85473
40	85630	85786	85942	86097	86253	86408	86563	86718	86872	87026
6.50	1.87180	1.87334	1.87487	1.87641	1.87794	1.87947	1.88099	1.88251	1.88403	1.88555
60	88707	88858	89010	89160	89311	89462	89612	89762	89912	90061
70	90211	90360	90509	90658	90806	90954	91102	91250	91398	91545
80	91692	91839	91986	92132	92279	92425	92571	92716	92862	93007
90	93152	93297	93442	93586	93730	93874	94018	94162	94305	94448
7.00	1.94591	1.94734	1.94876	1.95019	1.95161	1.95303	1.95445	1.95586	1.95727	1.95869
10	96009	96150	96291	96431	96571	96711	96851	96991	97130	97269
20	97408	97547	97685	97824	97962	98100	98238	98376	98513	98650
30	98787	98924	99061	99198	99334	99470	99606	99742	99877	2.00013
40	2.00148	2.00283	2.00418	2.00553	2.00687	2.00821	2.00956	2.01089	2.01223	01357
7.50	2.01490	2.01624	2.01757	2.01890	2.02022	2.02155	2.02287	2.02419	2.02551	2.02683
60	02815	02946	03078	03209	03340	03471	03601	03732	03862	03992
70	04122	04252	04381	04511	04640	04769	04898	05027	05156	05284
80	05412	05540	05668	05796	05924	06051	06179	06306	06433	06560
90	06686	06813	06939	07065	07191	07317	07443	07568	07694	07819
8.00	2.07944	2.08069	2.08194	2.08318	2.08443	2.08567	2.08691	2.08815	2.08939	2.09063
10	09186	09310	09433	09556	09679	09802	09924	10047	10169	10291
20	10413	10535	10657	10779	10900	11021	11142	11263	11384	11505
30	11626	11746	11866	11986	12106	12226	12346	12465	12585	12704
40	12823	12942	13061	13180	13298	13417	13535	13653	13771	13889
8.50	2.14007	2.14124	2.14242	2.14359	2.14476	2.14593	2.14710	2.14827	2.14943	2.15060
60	15176	15292	15409	15524	15640	15756	15871	15987	16102	16217
70	16332	16447	16562	16677	16791	16905	17020	17134	17248	17361
80	17475	17589	17702	17816	17929	18042	18155	18267	18380	18493
90	18605	18717	18830	18942	19054	19165	19277	19389	19500	19611
9.00	2.19722	2.19834	2.19944	2.20055	2.20166	2.20276	2.20387	2.20497	2.20607	2.20717
10	20827	20937	21047	21157	21266	21375	21485	21594	21703	21812
20	21920	22029	22138	22246	22354	22462	22570	22678	22786	22894
30	23001	23109	23216	23324	23431	23538	23645	23751	23858	23965
40	24071	24177	24284	24390	24496	24601	24707	24813	24918	25024
9.50	2.25129	2.25234	2.25339	2.25444	2.25549	2.25654	2.25759	2.25863	2.25968	2.26072
60	26176	26280	26384	26488	26592	26696	26799	26903	27006	27109
70	27213	27316	27419	27521	27624	27727	27829	27932	28034	28136
80	28238	28340	28442	28544	28646	28747	28849	28950	29051	29152
90	29253	29354	29455	29556	29657	29757	29858	29958	30058	30158

* To find the natural logarithm ($\log_e$) of a number which is a power of ten less or greater than a number given in the table: if the number concerned is *less*, e.g., $^1/_{10}$ (10^{-1}), $^1/_{100}$ (10^{-2}), $^1/_{1000}$ (10^{-3}), etc., *subtract* from the given logarithm $\log_e 10$, $2 \log_e 10$, $3 \log_e 10$, etc.; if the number concerned is *greater*, e.g., 10 times (10^1), 100 times (10^2), 1000 times (10^3), etc., *add* to the given logarithm $\log_e 10$, $2 \log_e 10$, $3 \log_e 10$, etc. Examples: $\log_e 0.02 = \log_e 0.2 - \log_e 10$; $\log_e 2000 = \log_e 200 + \log_e 10$.

Natural Logarithms* 10.0—99.9

x	0.0	0.1	0.2	0.3	0.4	0.5	0.6	0.7	0.8	0.9
10.0	2.30259	2.31254	2.32239	2.33214	2.34181	2.35138	2.36085	2.37024	2.37955	2.38876
11.0	39790	40695	41591	42480	43361	44235	45101	45959	46810	47654
12.0	48491	49321	50144	50960	51770	52573	53370	54160	54945	55723
13.0	56495	57261	58022	58776	59525	60269	61007	61740	62467	63189
14.0	63906	64617	65324	66026	66723	67415	68102	68785	69463	70136
15.0	2.70805	2.71469	2.72130	2.72785	2.73437	2.74084	2.74727	2.75366	2.76001	2.76632
16.0	77259	77882	78501	79117	79728	80336	80940	81541	82138	82731
17.0	83321	83908	84491	85071	85647	86220	86790	87356	87920	88480
18.0	89037	89591	90142	90690	91235	91777	92316	92852	93386	93916
19.0	94444	94969	95491	96011	96527	97041	97553	98062	98568	99072
20.0	2.99573	3.00072	3.00568	3.01062	3.01553	3.02042	3.02529	3.03013	3.03495	3.03975
21.0	3.04452	04927	05400	05871	06339	06805	07269	07731	08191	08649
22.0	09104	09558	10009	10459	10906	11352	11795	12236	12676	13114
23.0	13549	13983	14415	14845	15274	15700	16125	16548	16969	17388
24.0	17805	18221	18635	19048	19458	19867	20275	20680	21084	21487
25.0	3.21888	3.22287	3.22684	3.23080	3.23475	3.23868	3.24259	3.24649	3.25037	3.25424
26.0	25810	26194	26576	26957	27336	27714	28091	28466	28840	29213
27.0	29584	29953	30322	30689	31054	31419	31782	32143	32504	32863
28.0	33220	33577	33932	34286	34639	34990	35341	35690	36038	36384
29.0	36730	37074	37417	37759	38099	38439	38777	39115	39451	39786
30.0	3.40120	3.40453	3.40784	3.41115	3.41444	3.41773	3.42100	3.42426	3.42751	3.43076
31.0	43399	43721	44042	44362	44681	44999	45316	45632	45947	46261
32.0	46574	46886	47197	47507	47816	48124	48431	48738	49043	49347
33.0	49651	49953	50255	50556	50856	51155	51453	51750	52046	52342
34.0	52636	52930	53223	53515	53806	54096	54385	54674	54962	55249
35.0	3.55535	3.55820	3.56105	3.56388	3.56671	3.56953	3.57235	3.57515	3.57795	3.58074
36.0	58352	58629	58906	59182	59457	59731	60005	60278	60550	60821
37.0	61092	61362	61631	61899	62167	62434	62700	62966	63231	63495
38.0	63759	64021	64284	64545	64806	65066	65325	65584	65842	66099
39.0	66356	66612	66868	67122	67377	67630	67883	68135	68387	68638
40.0	3.68888	3.69138	3.69387	3.69635	3.69883	3.70130	3.70377	3.70623	3.70868	3.71113
41.0	71357	71601	71844	72086	72328	72569	72810	73050	73290	73529
42.0	73767	74005	74242	74479	74715	74950	75185	75420	75654	75887
43.0	76120	76352	76584	76815	77046	77276	77506	77735	77963	78191
44.0	78419	78646	78872	79098	79324	79549	79773	79997	80221	80444
45.0	3.80666	3.80888	3.81110	3.81331	3.81551	3.81771	3.81991	3.82210	3.82428	3.82647
46.0	82864	83081	83298	83514	83730	83945	84160	84374	84588	84802
47.0	85015	85227	85439	85651	85862	86073	86283	86493	86703	86912
48.0	87120	87328	87536	87743	87950	88156	88362	88568	88773	88978
49.0	89182	89386	89589	89792	89995	90197	90399	90600	90801	91002
50.0	3.91202	3.91402	3.91602	3.91801	3.91999	3.92197	3.92395	3.92593	3.92790	3.92986
51.0	93183	93378	93574	93769	93964	94158	94352	94546	94739	94932
52.0	95124	95316	95508	95700	95891	96081	96272	96462	96651	96840
53.0	97029	97218	97406	97594	97781	97968	98155	98341	98527	98713
54.0	98898	99083	99268	99452	99636	99820	4.00003	4.00186	4.00369	4.00551

55.0	4.00733	4.00915	4.01096	4.01277	4.01458	4.01638	4.01818	4.01998	4.02177	4.02356
56.0	02535	02714	02892	03069	03247	03424	03601	03777	03954	04130
57.0	04305	04480	04655	04830	05004	05178	05352	05526	05699	05872
58.0	06044	06217	06389	06560	06732	06903	07073	07244	07414	07584
59.0	07754	07923	08092	08261	08429	08598	08766	08933	09101	09268
60.0	4.09434	4.09601	4.09767	4.09933	4.10099	4.10264	4.10429	4.10594	4.10759	4.10923
61.0	11087	11251	11415	11578	11741	11904	12066	12228	12390	12552
62.0	12713	12875	13036	13196	13357	13517	13677	13836	13996	14155
63.0	14313	14472	14630	14789	14946	15104	15261	15418	15575	15732
64.0	15888	16044	16200	16356	16511	16667	16821	16976	17131	17285
65.0	4.17439	4.17592	4.17746	4.17899	4.18052	4.18205	4.18358	4.18510	4.18662	4.18814
66.0	18965	19117	19268	19419	19570	19720	19870	20020	20170	20320
67.0	20469	20618	20767	20916	21065	21213	21361	21509	21656	21804
68.0	21951	22098	22244	22391	22537	22683	22829	22975	23120	23266
69.0	23411	23555	23700	23844	23989	24133	24276	24420	24563	24707
70.0	4.24850	4.24992	4.25135	4.25277	4.25419	4.25561	4.25703	4.25845	4.25986	4.26127
71.0	26268	26409	26549	26690	26830	26970	27110	27249	27388	27528
72.0	27667	27805	27944	28082	28221	28359	28496	28634	28772	28909
73.0	29046	29183	29320	29456	29592	29729	29865	30000	30136	30271
74.0	30407	30542	30676	30811	30946	31080	31214	31348	31482	31615
75.0	4.31749	4.31882	4.32015	4.32149	4.32281	4.32413	4.32546	4.32678	4.32810	4.32942
76.0	33073	33205	33336	33467	33598	33729	33860	33990	34120	34251
77.0	34381	34510	34640	34769	34899	35028	35157	35286	35414	35543
78.0	35671	35800	35927	36055	36182	36310	36437	36564	36691	36818
79.0	36945	37071	37198	37324	37450	37576	37701	37827	37952	38078
80.0	4.38203	4.38328	4.38452	4.38577	4.38701	4.38826	4.38950	4.39074	4.39198	4.39321
81.0	39445	39568	39692	39815	39938	40060	40183	40305	40428	40550
82.0	40672	40794	40916	41037	41159	41280	41401	41522	41643	41764
83.0	41884	42004	42125	42245	42365	42485	42604	42724	42843	42963
84.0	43082	43201	43319	43438	43557	43675	43793	43912	44030	44147
85.0	4.44265	4.44383	4.44500	4.44617	4.44735	4.44852	4.44969	4.45085	4.45202	4.45318
86.0	45435	45551	45667	45783	45899	46014	46130	46245	46361	46476
87.0	46591	46706	46820	46935	47050	47164	47278	47392	47506	47620
88.0	47734	47847	47961	48074	48187	48300	48413	48526	48639	48751
89.0	48864	48976	49088	49200	49312	49424	49536	49647	49758	49870
90.0	4.49981	4.50092	4.50203	4.50314	4.50424	4.50535	4.50645	4.50756	4.50866	4.50976
91.0	51086	51196	51305	51415	51525	51634	51743	51852	51961	52070
92.0	52179	52287	52396	52504	52613	52721	52829	52937	53045	53152
93.0	53260	53367	53475	53582	53689	53796	53903	54010	54116	54223
94.0	54329	54436	54542	54648	54754	54860	54966	55071	55177	55282
95.0	4.55388	4.55493	4.55598	4.55703	4.55808	4.55913	4.56017	4.56122	4.56226	4.56331
96.0	56435	56539	56643	56747	56851	56954	57058	57161	57265	57368
97.0	57471	57574	57677	57780	57883	57985	58088	58190	58292	58395
98.0	58497	58599	58701	58802	58904	59006	59107	59208	59310	59411
99.0	59512	59613	59714	59815	59915	60016	60116	60217	60317	60417

* To find the natural logarithm ($\log_e$) of a number which is a power of ten less or greater than a number given in the table: if the number concerned is *less*, e.g., $^1/_{10}$ (10^{-1}), $^1/_{100}$ (10^{-2}), $^1/_{1000}$ (10^{-3}), etc., *subtract* from the given logarithm $\log_e 10$, $2 \log_e 10$, $3 \log_e 10$, etc.; if the number concerned is *greater*, e.g., 10 times (10^1), 100 times (10^2), 1000 times (10^3), etc., *add* to the given logarithm $\log_e 10$, $2 \log_e 10$, $3 \log_e 10$, etc. Examples: $\log_e 0.02 = \log_e 0.2 - \log_e 10$; $\log_e 2000 = \log_e 200 + \log_e 10$.

Natural Logarithms* 0—999

x	0	1	2	3	4	5	6	7	8	9
00	∞	0.00000	0.69315	1.09861	1.38629	1.60944	1.79176	1.94591	2.07944	2.19722
10	2.30259	2.39790	2.48491	2.56495	2.63906	2.70805	2.77259	2.83321	89037	94444
20	99573	3.04452	3.09104	3.13549	3.17805	3.21888	3.25810	3.29584	3.33220	3.36730
30	3.40120	43399	46574	49651	52636	55535	58352	61092	63759	66356
40	68888	71357	73767	76120	78419	80666	82864	85015	87120	89182
50	3.91202	3.93183	3.95124	3.97029	3.98898	4.00733	4.02535	4.04305	4.06044	4.07754
60	4.09434	4.11087	4.12713	4.14313	4.15888	17439	18965	20469	21951	23411
70	24850	26268	27667	29046	30407	31749	33073	34381	35671	36945
80	38203	39445	40672	41884	43082	44265	45435	46591	47734	48864
90	49981	51086	52179	53260	54329	55388	56435	57471	58497	59512
100	4.60517	4.61512	4.62497	4.63473	4.64439	4.65396	4.66344	4.67283	4.68213	4.69135
110	70048	70953	71850	72739	73620	74493	75359	76217	77068	77912
120	78749	79579	80402	81218	82028	82831	83628	84419	85203	85981
130	86753	87520	88280	89035	89784	90527	91265	91998	92725	93447
140	94164	94876	95583	96284	96981	97673	98361	99043	99721	5.00395
150	5.01064	5.01728	5.02388	5.03044	5.03695	5.04343	5.04986	5.05625	5.06260	5.06890
160	07517	08140	08760	09375	09987	10595	11199	11799	12396	12990
170	13580	14166	14749	15329	15906	16479	17048	17615	18178	18739
180	19296	19850	20401	20949	21494	22036	22575	23111	23644	24175
190	24702	25227	25750	26269	26786	27300	27811	28320	28827	29330
200	5.29832	5.30330	5.30827	5.31321	5.31812	5.32301	5.32788	5.33272	5.33754	5.34233
210	34711	35186	35659	36129	36598	37064	37528	37990	38450	38907
220	39363	39816	40268	40717	41165	41610	42053	42495	42935	43372
230	43808	44242	44674	45104	45532	45959	46383	46806	47227	47646
240	48064	48480	48894	49306	49717	50126	50533	50939	51343	51745
250	5.52146	5.52545	5.52943	5.53339	5.53733	5.54126	5.54518	5.54908	5.55296	5.55683
260	56068	56452	56834	57215	57595	57973	58350	58725	59099	59471
270	59842	60212	60580	60947	61313	61677	62040	62402	62762	63121
280	63479	63835	64191	64545	64897	65249	65599	65948	66296	66643
290	66988	67332	67675	68017	68358	68698	69036	69373	69709	70044
300	5.70378	5.70711	5.71043	5.71373	5.71703	5.72031	5.72359	5.72685	5.73010	5.73334
310	73657	73979	74300	74620	74939	75257	75574	75890	76205	76519
320	76832	77144	77455	77765	78074	78383	78690	78996	79301	79606
330	79909	80212	80513	80814	81114	81413	81711	82008	82305	82600
340	82895	83188	83481	83773	84064	84354	84644	84932	85220	85507
350	5.85793	5.86079	5.86363	5.86647	5.86930	5.87212	5.87493	5.87774	5.88053	5.88332
360	88610	88888	89164	89440	89715	89990	90263	90536	90808	91080
370	91350	91620	91889	92158	92426	92693	92959	93225	93489	93754
380	94017	94280	94542	94803	95064	95324	95584	95842	96101	96358
390	96615	96871	97126	97381	97635	97889	98141	98394	98645	98896
400	5.99146	5.99396	5.99645	5.99894	6.00141	6.00389	6.00635	6.00881	6.01127	6.01372
410	6.01616	6.01859	6.02102	6.02345	02587	02828	03069	03309	03548	03787
420	04025	04263	04501	04737	04973	05209	05444	05678	05912	06146
430	06379	06611	06843	07074	07304	07535	07764	07993	08222	08450
440	08677	08904	09131	09357	09582	09807	10032	10256	10479	10702
450	6.10925	6.11147	6.11368	6.11589	6.11810	6.12030	6.12249	6.12468	6.12687	6.12905
460	13123	13340	13556	13773	13988	14204	14419	14633	14847	15060
470	15273	15486	15698	15910	16121	16331	16542	16752	16961	17170
480	17379	17587	17794	18002	18208	18415	18621	18826	19032	19236
490	19441	19644	19848	20051	20254	20456	20658	20859	21060	21261

N	0	1	2	3	4	5	6	7	8	9
500	6.21461	6.21661	6.21860	6.22059	6.22258	6.22456	6.22654	6.22851	6.23048	6.23245
510	23441	23637	23832	24028	24222	24417	24611	24804	24998	25190
520	25383	25575	25767	25958	26149	26340	26530	26720	26910	27099
530	27288	27476	27664	27852	28040	28227	28413	28600	28786	28972
540	29157	29342	29527	29711	29895	30079	30262	30445	30628	30810
550	6.30992	6.31173	6.31355	6.31536	6.31716	6.31897	6.32077	6.32257	6.32436	6.32615
560	32794	32972	33150	33328	33505	33683	33859	34036	34212	34388
570	34564	34739	34914	35089	35263	35437	35611	35784	35957	36130
580	36303	36475	36647	36819	36990	37161	37332	37502	37673	37843
590	38012	38182	38351	38519	38688	38856	39024	39192	39359	39526
600	6.39693	6.39859	6.40026	6.40192	6.40357	6.40523	6.40688	6.40853	6.41017	6.41182
610	41346	41510	41673	41836	41999	42162	42325	42487	42649	42811
620	42972	43133	43294	43455	43615	43775	43935	44095	44254	44413
630	44572	44731	44889	45047	45205	45362	45520	45677	45834	45990
640	46147	46303	46459	46614	46770	46925	47080	47235	47389	47543
650	6.47697	6.47851	6.48004	6.48158	6.48311	6.48464	6.48616	6.48768	6.48920	6.49072
660	49224	49375	49527	49677	49828	49979	50129	50279	50429	50578
670	50728	50877	51026	51175	51323	51471	51619	51767	51915	52062
680	52209	52356	52503	52649	52796	52942	53088	53233	53379	53524
690	53669	53814	53959	54103	54247	54391	54535	54679	54822	54965
700	6.55108	6.55251	6.55393	6.55536	6.55678	6.55820	6.55962	6.56103	6.56244	6.56386
710	56526	56667	56808	56948	57088	57228	57368	57508	57647	57786
720	57925	58064	58203	58341	58479	58617	58755	58893	59030	59167
730	59304	59441	59578	59715	59851	59987	60123	60259	60394	60530
740	60665	60800	60935	61070	61204	61338	61473	61607	61740	61874
750	6.62007	6.62141	6.62274	6.62407	6.62539	6.62672	6.62804	6.62936	6.63068	6.63200
760	63332	63463	63595	63726	63857	63988	64118	64249	64379	64509
770	64639	64769	64898	65028	65157	65286	65415	65544	65673	65801
780	65929	66058	66185	66313	66441	66568	66696	66823	66950	67077
790	67203	67330	67456	67582	67708	67834	67960	68085	68211	68336
800	6.68461	6.68586	6.68711	6.68835	6.68960	6.69084	6.69208	6.69332	6.69456	6.69580
810	69703	69827	69950	70073	70196	70319	70441	70564	70686	70808
820	70930	71052	71174	71296	71417	71538	71659	71780	71901	72022
830	72143	72263	72383	72503	72623	72743	72863	72982	73102	73221
840	73340	73459	73578	73697	73815	73934	74052	74170	74288	74406
850	6.74524	6.74641	6.74759	6.74876	6.74993	6.75110	6.75227	6.75344	6.75460	6.75577
860	75693	75809	75926	76041	76157	76273	76388	76504	76619	76734
870	76849	76964	77079	77194	77308	77422	77537	77651	77765	77878
880	77992	78106	78219	78333	78446	78559	78672	78784	78897	79010
890	79122	79234	79347	79459	79571	79682	79794	79906	80017	80128
900	6.80239	6.80351	6.80461	6.80572	6.80683	6.80793	6.80904	6.81014	6.81124	6.81235
910	81344	81454	81564	81674	81783	81892	82002	82111	82220	82329
920	82437	82546	82655	82763	82871	82979	83087	83195	83303	83411
930	83518	83626	83733	83841	83948	84055	84162	84268	84375	84482
940	84588	84694	84801	84907	85013	85118	85224	85330	85435	85541
950	6.85646	6.85751	6.85857	6.85961	6.86066	6.86171	6.86276	6.86380	6.86485	6.86589
960	86693	86797	86901	87005	87109	87213	87316	87420	87523	87626
970	87730	87833	87936	88038	88141	88244	88346	88449	88551	88653
980	88755	88857	88959	89061	89163	89264	89366	89467	89568	89669
990	89770	89871	89972	90073	90174	90274	90375	90475	90575	90675

* To find the natural logarithm ($\log_e$) of a number which is a power of ten less or greater than a number given in the table: if the number concerned is *less*, e.g., $^1/_{10}$ (10^{-1}), $^1/_{100}$ (10^{-2}), $^1/_{1000}$ (10^{-3}), etc., *subtract* from the given logarithm $\log_e 10$, $2 \log_e 10$, $3 \log_e 10$, etc.; if the number concerned is *greater*, e.g., 10 times (10^1), 100 times (10^2), 1000 times (10^3), etc., *add* to the given logarithm $\log_e 10$, $2 \log_e 10$, $3 \log_e 10$, etc. Examples: $\log_e 0.02 = \log_e 0.2 - \log_e 10$; $\log_e 2000 = \log_e 200 + \log_e 10$.